CHRONIC EPILEPSY, ITS PROGNOSIS AND MANAGEMENT

Publication of this book has been made possible through an educational grant from Hoechst.

CHRONIC EPILEPSY, ITS PROGNOSIS AND MANAGEMENT

Edited by

Michael R. Trimble FRCP FRCPsych

*Institute of Neurology
Queen Square
London*

JOHN WILEY & SONS
Chichester · New York · Brisbane · Toronto · Singapore

Copyright © 1989 by John Wiley & Sons Ltd.
Baffins Lane, Chichester,
West Sussex PO19 1UD, England

All rights reserved.

Distributed in the United States of America,
Canada and Japan by Alan R. Liss Inc.,
41 East 11th Street, New York, NY 10003, USA

No part of this book may be reproduced by any means,
or transmitted, or translated into a machine language
without the written permission of the publisher.

Other Wiley Editorial Offices

John Wiley & Sons, Inc., 605 Third Avenue,
New York, NY 10158-0012, USA

Jacaranda Wiley Ltd, G.P.O. Box 859, Brisbane,
Queensland 4001, Australia

John Wiley & Sons (Canada) Ltd, 22 Worcester Road,
Rexdale, Ontario M9W 1L1, Canada

John Wiley & Sons (SEA) Plc Ltd, 37 Jalan Pemimpin #05-04,
Block B, Union Industrial Building, Singapore 2057

Library of Congress Cataloging-in-Publication Data:

Chronic epilepsy: its prognosis and management / edited by
  Michael R. Trimble
    p. cm.
  Includes bibliographies and index.
  ISBN 0 471 92464 4
  1. Epilepsy. I. Trimble, Michael R.
  [DNLM: 1. Epilepsy—therapy. WL 385 C557]
RC372.C47 1989
616.8′53—dc20
DNLM/DLC
for Library of Congress   89-14826
                                                                                    CIP

British Library Cataloguing in Publication Data:

Chronic epilepsy, its prognosis and
  management.
  1. Man. Epilepsy
  I. Title II. Trimble, Michael R.
  616.3′53

  ISBN 0 471 92464 4

Typest by Inforum Typesetting, Portsmouth
Printed in Great Britain by Courier International Ltd,
Tiptree, Essex

Contents

Contributors		vii
Preface		ix
1	Pathophysiology of Chronic Epilepsy B.S. Meldrum	1
2	The Prognosis of Epilepsy: Is Chronic Epilepsy Preventable? E.H. Reynolds	13
3	How Does One Assess the Severity of Epilepsy? D. Janz	21
4	The Monitoring of Chronic Epilepsy C.D. Binnie	37
5	CT and PET in Drug-resistant Epilepsy D. Fish	59
6	Syndromes of Chronic Epilepsy in Children J.M. Pellock	73
7	Prognosis and Prophylaxis of Traumatic Epilepsy D. Janz	87
8	Cognitive Hazards of Seizure Disorders M.R. Trimble	103
9	Social Difficulties and Severe Epilepsy: Survey Results and Recommendations P.J. Thompson and J. Oxley	113
10	Some Behavioural Consequences of Epileptic Seizures M.R. Trimble	133
11	Strategies of Antiepileptic Drug Treatment in Patients with Chronic Epilepsy J.S. Duncan	143
12	Management of Chronic Epilepsy in Children K. Farrell	151

13	Adjunctive Therapy in Resistant Epilepsy *N. Callaghan* and *T. Goggin*	165
14	Clobazam for Chronic Epilepsy: Factors Relating to a Dramatic Response *A.J. Heller, H.A. Ring* and *E.H. Reynolds*	177
15	Strategies to Avoid the Development of Tolerance to Antiepileptic Benzodiazapine Effects *D. Schmidt, S. Ried* and *E. Rohrer*	183
16	Surgical Treatment of Chronic Epilepsy *C. E. Polkey*	189
17	Epilepsy in Developing Countries: A Review of Epidemiological, Sociocultural and Treatment Aspects *S.D. Shorvon* and *P.J. Farmer*	209
18	Advances in Genetics and Their Application to Epilepsy *H. Meierkord*	243
Index		255

Contributors

C.D. BINNIE
The Maudsley Hospital, Denmark Hill, London SE5 8AZ, UK

N. CALLAGHAN
Department of Neurology, Cork Regional Hospital, Cork, Ireland, and Department of Medicine, University College, Cork, Ireland

J.S. DUNCAN
National Hospital for Nervous Diseases, Queen Square, London WC1N 3GB, UK

P.J. FARMER
Institute of Neurology, Queen Square, London, UK, and National Society for Epilepsy Research Group, London, UK

K. FARRELL
Department of Paediatrics, University of British Columbia, Vancouver, Canada, and Seizure Clinic, British Columbia's Childrens Hospital, 4480 Oak Street, Vancouver, British Columbia V6H 3V4, Canada

D. FISH
Montreal Neurological Institute, Montreal, Canada

T. GOGGIN
Department of Neurology, Cork Regional Hospital, Cork, Ireland, and Department of Medicine, University College, Cork, Ireland

A.J. HELLER
Department of Neurology, King's College Hospital, London SE5, UK

D. JANZ
Department of Neurology, Klinikum Rudolph Virchow, Free University of Berlin, Berlin, West Germany

H. MEIERKORD
Institute of Neurology, Queen Square, London WC1N 3GB, UK

B.S. MELDRUM
Institute of Psychiatry, De Crespigny Park, London SE5, UK

J. OXLEY
National Society for Epilepsy, Chalfont St Peter, Bucks SL9 ORJ, UK

J.M. PELLOCK
Medical College of Virginia, Richmond, Virginia, USA

C.E. POLKEY
The Maudsley Hospital, De Crespigny Park, London SE5, UK

E.H. REYNOLDS
Department of Neurology, King's College Hospital, London SE5, UK

S. RIED
Klinikum Grosshadern, Ludwig-Maximilians Universitat, Munich, West Germany

H.A. RING
Department of Neurology, King's College Hospital, London SE5, UK

E. ROHRER
Klinikum Grosshadern, Ludwig-Maximilians Universitat, Munich, West Germany

D. SCHMIDT
Universitätsklinikum Rudolf Virchow, Charlottenburg, Spandauerdamn 130, Berlin

S.D. SHORVON
Institute of Neurology, Queen Square, London WC1N 3BG, UK, and the National Society for Epilepsy Research Group, London, UK

P.J. THOMPSON
National Society for Epilepsy, Chalfont St Peter, Bucks SL9 ORJ, UK

M.R. TRIMBLE
Institute of Neurology, Queen Square, London WC1N 3BG, UK

Preface

It is known that some 60–80% of patients with epilepsy will achieve a good result from treatment, becoming seizure-free. These figures, derived from more recent studies of remission rates, contrast with earlier, more gloomy, views of prognosis from more selective hospital referral clinics and institutionalized patients. Nonetheless, these data also reveal that there are 20–40% of patients who will not be so lucky, and who, in spite of the advantages that modern-day assessment and management of seizures brings, will continue to have recurrent seizures. These patients form the majority of those who attend hospital outpatient clinics, often on a regular recurring basis, with little hope, eventually, that their seizures will abate. The continuing seizures, the persistent disappointment with each returning bout, the ever-present need to take, often, large doses of anticonvulsant medications, and the failure to achieve so many of life's, often relatively modest, goals, inevitably lead to further handicaps, additional disappointments and secondary medical problems. As such these issues specifically relate to chronic epilepsy—the theme of this book.

The first chapter (Meldrum) considers the pathology of chronic epilepsy, especially some of the more recent speculations regarding neurotransmitter and neuromodular mechanisms that may lead to chronicity. Reynolds (Chapter 2) considers the prognosis of epilepsy, and looks at how chronicity may be prevented: at how the process may be contained. Janz (Chapter 3) emphasizes that there is more to patient evaluation than simply counting seizures, while the chapters on EEG (4—Binnie) and neuroimaging (5—Fish) reveal the importance of bringing modern technologies to these difficult patients, especially to clarify diagnosis, to plan treatment and to explore the possibility of surgery, the details of which are discussed in Chapter 16 (Polkey).

Since epilepsy often begins in childhood, and, by the time the patient is adult, chronicity is already established, two chapters describe the seizures and syndromes of epilepsy in children (6—Pellock) and their management (12—Farrell).

The social (9—Thompson and Oxley), cognitive (8—Trimble) and behavioural (10—Trimble) consequences of chronic epilepsy are then considered, as is the role of head trauma in causation (7—Janz). There follows several chapters on management, including strategies for anticonvulsant drug manipulations (11—Duncan), adjunctive therapy (13—Callaghan and Goggin), and the role of clobazam (14—Reynolds and colleagues). The problem of trying to overcome tolerance to the effects of benzodiazepines is discussed by Schmidt and colleagues (Chapter 15). Other authors, in their various chapters, also tackle differing aspects of management, especially some of the social issues.

The final two chapters are included to emphasize the broad scope of the problem of chronic epilepsy outlining the situation in developing countries (17—Shorvon and Farmer), and the possibility of new methods of preventing and treating epilepsy by genetic engineering (18—Meierkord).

It is hoped that this book will be of interest to all those who deal with the problems of patients with intractable seizure disorders, and, as a consequence, help some patients who suffer so much.

MICHAEL TRIMBLE, 1989

1
Pathophysiology of Chronic Epilepsy

B.S. Meldrum
Institute of Psychiatry, London, UK

Introduction

What is the pathophysiological basis of chronic intractable epilepsy? The answer to this question must contain anatomical information detailing the areas in the brain showing primary abnormalities, cytological information detailing the specific types of cells affected and biochemical information detailing the molecular changes. Additionally, electrophysiological information may help relate the biochemical and cytological abnormalities to the development of epileptic attacks and their clinical expression. Although we have substantial information on all these topics, we are not yet in a position to explain what is the factor determining intractability.

Three broad hypotheses compete as explanations. These are:

(1) a defect of the neuronal membrane and its ionic conductance properties,
(2) a defect in the GABAergic inhibitory systems or in other endogenous anticonvulsant agents, and
(3) a defect in excitatory mechanisms, especially the excitatory amino acid systems.

We shall here review recent evidence that is relevant to these issues.

Classical Pathological Observations

A particular pattern of cerebral pathology has long been associated with severe chronic epilepsy (Bouchet and Cazauvieilh, 1825; Sommer, 1880; Meldrum and Corsellis, 1984). It is seen in the majority of patients whose lives end in institutions providing chronic care. The most characteristic element is a unilateral hippocampal sclerosis. Within the hippocampus there is a severe loss of pyramidal neurons in the Sommer sector (zone CA1 and part of the subiculum), loss of neurons in the endfolium (CA3–4) with prominent gliosis, and commonly also some loss of dentate granule cells. The cerebellum shows a loss of Purkinje cells, particularly in the posterior superior quadrant. There is sometimes a diffuse cortical atrophy, often involving loss of small neurons in the third lamina. Other regions (e.g. thalamus, amygdala) may show cell loss. Cerebellar and cortical degenerative changes tend to be symmetrical, in contrast to the hippocampal Sommer sector lesions.

This pattern of cell loss can readily be interpreted as a consequence of repeated, prolonged seizures. Similar patterns of damage can be induced in experimental animals by prolonged seizures induced by convulsant drugs. The lesions could, however, also facilitate seizures. In particular, the pattern of hippocampal cell loss could be a cause of temporal lobe epilepsy, manifest as complex partial seizures. The therapeutic effect of removing a temporal pole containing Ammon's horn sclerosis is presumptive evidence that a focus responsible for the seizures was contained in that temporal pole. In functional terms, several different possibilities exist. A selective loss of inhibitory GABAergic neurons has been presumed to play a key role by numerous authors (Lloyd et al., 1985). Evidence for this will be examined below.

The development of supersensitivity (denervation supersensitivity) is also a possibility, and some evidence for this affecting excitatory amino acid receptors has been accumulated. Disorders of neuronal or glial membrane function may also develop.

A wide variety of other pathological changes is found in the brains of patients with epilepsy. They are often interpreted as being the primary cause of the epilepsy. Traumatic lesions (following blunt or penetrating head injury) are a major cause of epilepsy. Commonly, there is a significant interval (often of several years) between the injury and the onset of recurrent seizures. The processes occurring during this period are not known but may include selective degeneration, denervation supersensitivity and sprouting of axonal processes, primarily involving excitatory systems. Developmental abnormalities, neoplastic disease and infections (viral, bacterial, parasitic) provide other 'causal' pathologies.

Dysplasias and Epilepsy

Developmental abnormalities associated with epilepsy are of two main types, vascular and neuronal. Vascular abnormalities may be gross (focal or diffuse) or seen only at the microlevel (microaneurysms on capillaries). The link between a vascular abnormality and the pathogenesis of epilepsy may involve the leakage of red blood cells and the epileptogenic effect of haemoglobin or iron.

Neuronal dysgenesis can take several forms: one class is referred to as microdysgenesis, and the more gross abnormalities may be described as hamartomas. Microdysgenesis was first described in epilepsy by Veith and Wicke (1968). This takes two forms, abnormal neuronal clustering associated with bare areas within cortical layers, and small groups of ectopic neurons within the the subcortical white matter. Such changes were described in post mortem studies of primary generalized epilepsies and in post-traumatic epilepsy (Meenke, 1983, 1985; Meenke and Janz, 1984). Similar abnormalities have been described in surgical specimens from patients with intractable temporal lobe epilepsy, neuronal ectopia affecting 42% and neuronal clustering 28% (Hardiman et al., 1988). These abnormalities are found in some other neuropsychiatric disorders such as dyslexia and mental retardation but are rare in normal subjects. Thus the simplest interpretation is that they are a developmental abnormality that predisposes patients to febrile convulsions, traumatic epilepsy, primary generalized epilepsy and complex partial seizures.

Hamartomas are a more severe form of focal dysplasia, often with abnormal neurons and glia. Somewhat similar focal lesions may be found in tuberous sclerosis, which may be associated with many different forms of epilepsy. The link to epileptogenesis is uncertain in all these developmental abnormalities. A recent finding that may be relevant comes from a study employing in situ hybridization to identify specific chromosomes (Borden and Manuelidis, 1988). This shows that the X chromosome is normally located next to the nuclear membrane in males, but in the focus (and not in non-focal cortical tissue) it moves centrally. This may be a consequence of sustained abnormal electrical activity, or of local pathology, and may subsequently contribute to abnormal activity (by an unknown mechanism).

Recent Studies with Operative/Post Mortem Material

Recently many research groups have begun to exploit the possibilities of studying neurotransmitter function in tissue obtained through operative procedures on patients with intractable epilepsy. Such data concern immunocytochemistry and biochemistry. Some results are currently controversial but much new information has been gained about inhibitory and excitatory mechanisms.

Membrane Defects

Two sorts of abnormality in membrane function have been postulated to explain epileptogenicity. One assumes that the primary defect is in the ionophores (most probably either K^+ or Ca^{2+} channels) giving rise to oscillatory instability (see Adams and Galvan, 1986; Prince and Connors, 1986). The other assumes that ionic transport mechanisms, particularly those linked to membrane ATPases, are primarily at fault. Many studies have reported abnormalities in either Na^+/K^+-ATPases or Ca^{2+}-ATPases. In the audiogenic seizure-prone mouse strain, DBA/2, a reduction in brain Ca^{2+}-ATPase activity is inherited together with the seizure susceptibility (Palayoor, Seyfried and Bernard, 1986).

It is also possible that the primary defect is in a phosphorylation mechanism. An enhancement in the brain content of a cAMP-dependent protein kinase has been observed in a seizure-prone strain of rats (Wistar, GEPR) (Ribak and Ludvig, unpublished). Enhanced protein kinase activity could produce secondary changes in monoaminergic, GABAergic and glutamatergic transmission.

Abnormalities of GABAergic Systems

A failure of inhibitory mechanisms has long seemed a plausible mechanism to account for the onset of epilepsy (Meldrum, 1975). GABA, 4-aminobutyric acid, is the principal inhibitory neurotransmitter in the brain. GABAergic neurons have a wide diversity of structures but they provide a high proportion of interneurons in cortex and hippocampus and also provide output systems from some deep brain nuclei (Houser et al., 1983; Somogyi et al., 1985; Hendry et al., 1987). Pharmacological impairment of GABA-mediated inhibition readily induces epileptic activity. Thus neuronal damage that selectively involved the GABAergic interneurons might be responsible for the development of epilepsy. Two lines of evidence have offered support for such a mechanism occurring, for example, after perinatal cerebral hypoxia and after cerebral trauma.

In infant monkey cortex 2 weeks after a 30 min episode of hypoxia, Sloper, Johnson and Powell (1980) detected a selective loss of symmetric (inhibitory) synapses. In the rat hippocampus, however, somatostatin-containing interneurons rather than GABAergic inhibitory interneurons appear to be selectively vulnerable to ischaemic damage (Johansen, Zimmer and Diemer, 1987). Using immunocytochemistry of glutamic acid decarboxylase (GAD), Ribak et al. (1979) found a marked decrease in GAD-positive terminals in the region of an alumina focus compared with distant unaffected areas in the monkey cortex. With electron microscopy, symmetric synapses showed a relatively greater reduction than asymmetric (excitatory) synapses around the alumina gel lesion (Ribak, Bradburne and Harris, 1982).

Studies utilizing human surgical material have, however, not given definitive support to this. Lloyd et al. (1985), in a biochemical study, found a decrease in GAD content in some foci relative to control, but no change or an increase in others. In 24 anterior temporal lobes resected for temporal lobe epilepsy, Babb

(1986), however, found no excess loss of GABAergic terminals (GAD-positive puncta).

Changes in GAD activity or immunoreactivity have been reported in association with kindling in the rat. Babb et al. (1989), studying GAD-containing terminals in the fascia dentata, found GAD staining to be reduced 24 h after a kindled seizure but not 3–7 days later. Thus the reduction in GAD staining appeared to be a consequence of the seizure and not a factor contributing to the kindled state. Such observations may be relevant to the studies of human temporal lobe epilepsy.

Sustained electrical stimulation of the afferent hippocampal system in rodents provides a model for epileptic brain damage following status epilepticus. Using immunocytochemical methods in this model, Sloviter (1987) found that the GABAergic interneurons in the hilus remained intact but that the somatostatin-containing interneurons were lesioned. These interneurons are thought to be excitatory to the GABAergic interneurons in a feedback loop acting on dentate granule cells. Thus such a lesion could be disinhibitory even though the GABAergic neurons remain intact.

Studies of GABA content in CSF in patients with epilepsy have tended to show a reduced GABA concentration, but similar observations have been made in other classes of neurological patient not showing epilepsy (Wood et al., 1979; Manyam et al., 1980; Löscher and Siemes, 1985). The role of an acquired deficit in GABAergic inhibitory mechanisms in cortex and hippocampus requires further investigation.

Abnormalities of Excitatory Amino Acid Systems

Glutamate and aspartate provide fast excitatory neurotransmission at sites throughout the central nervous system. The postsynaptic receptors fall into two major categories, N-methyl-D-aspartate-preferring receptors (NMDA receptors) and non-NMDA receptors (possibly comprising two subtypes referred to as quisqualate and kainate receptors). Activation of NMDA receptors on normal neurons leads to paroxysmal depolarizing shifts and burst firing similar to that seen in a cortical epileptic focus (Meldrum, 1986). Focal injections of agonists acting on either NMDA or non-NMDA receptors can induce focal epileptic activity. Inherited or acquired supersensitivity of the excitatory amino acid neurotransmitter systems could thus provide the basis for focal cortical epilepsy.

Evidence relating to such possibilities has been obtained in a variety of animal models of epilepsy and from neurosurgical material.

Kindling and Changes in Sensitivity of NMDA Systems

An enormous variety of changes in neurotransmitter metabolism or receptor density have been reported to occur in association with kindling in the rodent brain. However, the change which is best documented and appears to be capable of explaining the phenomenon of kindling is an increase in physiological responsiveness of the NMDA-mediated excitatory amino acid receptor. Evidence for this is seen in the hippocampal slices prepared from kindled rats.

Studies of changes in the extracellular concentration of Ca^{2+} induced by the local iontophoresis of NMDA show a marked increase in the effect of NMDA in the dendritic fields of CA1 pyramidal neurons in the kindled hippocampus (Wadman and Heinemann, 1985). In the dentate molecular layer in non-kindled rats, NMDA-mediated responses contribute minimally to synaptically evoked activation. However, following kindling they make a major contribution to excitatory postsynaptic potentials (Mody and Heinemann, 1987; Mody, Stanton and Heinemann, 1988).

In Vitro Studies and Excitatory Amino Acids

Seizure-like activity can be induced in CA3 or CA1 neurons in hippocampal slices from normal rats by various manipulations of the extracellular environment, including raising $[K^+]$ or lowering $[Mg^{2+}]$ or $[Ca^{2+}]$. A major reduction in $[Mg^{2+}]$ can produce repeated paroxysmal depolarizing shifts with burst discharges. These are almost certainly due to facilitation of NMDA-induced responses (which are normally suppressed in a membrane-voltage-dependent manner by Mg^{2+}). Such bursts are resistant to the action of phenytoin, ethosuximide or barbiturates, but they are suppressed by NMDA receptor antagonists such as 2APV (2-amino-5-phosphonovalerate) (Heinemann et al., 1989). Data of this kind suggest that in so far as temporal lobe epilepsy in man depends on enhanced sensitivity or activity in the NMDA receptor systems, it will be resistant to conventional drug treatments but susceptible to NMDA antagonists.

Abnormal NMDA Sensitivity in Human Epilepsy

Cortical slices obtained from focal epileptic tissue resected surgically have been used to study the role of excitatory amino acid systems in epileptic activity. Measuring changes in extracellular $[Ca^{2+}]$ with ion-selective electrodes induced by the iontophoresis of NMDA indicates an enhanced sensitivity and an altered laminar pattern of NMDA responsiveness. Burst activity induced in slices by altered ionic circumstances can be suppressed by an NMDA-receptor antagonist (Avoli and Olivier, 1987).

Aspartate Transaminase in Cortex

In addition to the various studies indicating abnormalities of excitatory receptor sensitivity, there are some biochemical studies suggesting that the metabolism of glutamate and aspartate may be abnormal in epilepsy. Firstly, the activity of two enzymes involved in the metabolism of the dicarboxylic amino acids, namely glutamate dehydrogenase and aspartate aminotransferase, is increased (Kish, Dixon and Sherwin, 1988). Secondly, there is an increase in the content of glutamate (+25%) and aspartate (+25%) in focal cortical tissue (Sherwin et al., 1988).

Quinolinic Acid Abnormalities

Quinolinic acid is a metabolite formed from tryptophan when it is metabolized via the tryptophan pyrrolase pathway. The main site for such metabolism is the liver, but it has recently been established that quinolinic acid and the enzymes directly involved in its synthesis and further metabolism are found in the brain. The enzymes concerned are 3-hydroxyanthranilic acid oxygenase and quinolinic phosphoribosyltransferase (QPRT). Immunocytochemical studies show these to be primarily located in glial cells (Köhler et al., 1988). Measurements made on cortical tissue identified from operative EEG recordings as being a focal site of seizure origin show both an increase in quinolinic acid content and a decrease in the activity of the enzyme responsible for its further metabolism (QPRT) (Feldblum et al., 1988). It is thus possible that a primary or secondary defect in the metabolism of quinolinate leads to an accumulation of quinolinate in the extracellular space, which might facilitate burst firing.

Kainate Receptors

Kainic acid is a toxin derived from a seaweed that was used in Japan as an ascaricide. When injected focally into the brain it induces focal seizures; injected systemically or intracerebroventricularly it induces limbic seizures which probably originate in the hippocampus. It is also excitotoxic. Autoradiography with [^{3}H]kainate *in vivo* or *in vitro* reveals a high density of high-affinity kainate receptors in the mossy fibre system of the hippocampus (Patel, Meldrum and Collins, 1986). Represa, Le Gall La Salle and Ben-Ari (1989) and Represa et al. (1989) found that changes in these receptors can be detected both in the hippocampus of kindled rats and in the hippocampus of infants with epilepsy. Aberrant kainate-binding sites appear in the supragranular region and in the inferior region of CA3 in kindled rats, suggesting sprouting of the mossy fibre system (Represa, Le Gall La Salle and Ben-Ari, 1989). In five infant epileptics having suffered from various forms of generalized epilepsy (including two with myoclonic syndromes) the kainate binding was increased more than two-fold (relative to non-neurological controls) in the terminal field of the mossy fibre system. In a comparison of temporal lobectomy material with post mortem controls, Geddes et al. (1990) have found that the density of kainate receptors in the mossy fibre system is reduced (presumably as a consequence of cell loss), but that their density is markedly increased in the entorhinal cortex. There is a similar fall in NMDA receptor density in the CA1 zone of the hippocampus and an increase in the entorhinal cortex.

Antiepileptic Activity of Excitatory Amino Acid Antagonists

A powerful antiepileptic effect of NMDA antagonists or of non-selective excitatory amino acid antagonists has been found in animal models of epilepsy, including primates (Meldrum et al., 1983; Meldrum, 1984; Chapman, 1988). This provides strong evidence for the involvement of NMDA receptors in the initiation and spread of seizure activity. It is possible that such antagonists may prove effective in 'drug-resistant' epilepsies. The possibility of organizing appropriate clinical trials has been greatly enhanced by the recent discovery of orally active analogues of 2APV and 3-(2-carboxypiperazin-4-yl) propyl-1-phosphonate (Schmutz et al., 1988).

Summary

Intractable epilepsy is associated with various cortical and hippocampal lesions. These comprise developmental abnormalities (such as microdysgenesis), which may facilitate different types of epilepsy and degenerative changes, such as pyramidal cell loss in the Sommer sector. Possible secondary changes include instability of neuronal membranes, impaired GABAergic inhibition and enhanced or supersensitive excitatory neurotransmission. These mechanisms suggest that pharmacological manipulation of inhibitory or excitatory transmission may provide appropriate therapeutic approaches.

References

Adams PR, Galvan M. Voltage-dependent currents of vertebrate neurons and their role in membrane excitability. Adv Neurol 1986; 44: 137–70.
Avoli M, Olivier A. Bursting in human epileptogenic neocortex is depressed by an N-methyl-D-aspartate antagonist. Neurosci Lett 1987; 76: 249–54.
Babb TL. GABA-Mediated inhibition in the Ammon's horn and pre-subiculum in human temporal lobe epilepsy: GAD immunocytochemistry. In: Nistico G, Morselli PL, Lloyd KG, Fariello RG, Engel J (eds) Neurotransmitters, seizures, and epilepsy III. New York: Raven Press, 1986: 293–302.
Babb TL, Pretorius JK, Kupfer WR, Feldblum S. Recovery of decreased glutamate decarboxylase immunoreactivity after rat hippocampal kindling. Epilepsy Res 1989; 3: 18–30.
Borden, J, Manuelidis L. Movement of the X chromosome in epilepsy. Science 1988; 242: 1687–91.
Bouchet C, Cozauvieilh. De l'épilepsie considerée dans ses rapports avec l'aliénation mentale. Arch Gen Med 1825; 9: 510–42.
Chapman AG. Anticonvulsant activity of excitatory amino acid antagonists. In: Cavalheiro EA, Lehman S, Turshi L (eds) Frontiers in excitatory amino acid research. New York: Alan R Liss, 1988: 203–10.
Faingold CL, Millan MH, Boersma CA, Meldrum BS. Excitant amino acid and audiogenic seizures in the genetically epilepsy-prone rat: I. Afferent seizure initiation pathway. Exp Neurol 1988; 99: 678–86.
Feldblum S, Rougier A, Loiseau H, Loiseau P, Cohadon F, Morselli PL, Lloyd KG.

Quinolinic-phosphoribosyl transferase activity is decreased in epileptic human brain tissue. Epilepsia 1988; 29: 523–29.
Geddes JW, Cooper SM, Cotman CW, Patel S, Meldrum BS. N-methyl-D-aspartate receptors in the cortex and hippocampus of baboon (*Papio anubis* and *Papio papio*). Neuroscience 1989 (in press).
Geddes JW, Cahan LD, Cooper SM, Kim RC, Choi BH, Cotman CW. Altered density and distribution of excitatory amino acid receptors in temporal lobe epilepsy. Exp Neurol 1990 (in press).
Godfrey PP, Wilkins CJ, Tyler W, Watson SP. Stimulatory and inhibitory actions of excitatory amino acids on inositol phospholipid metabolism in rat cerebral cortex. Br J Pharmacol 1988; 95: 131–8.
Hardiman O, Burke T, Phillips J, Murphy S, O'Moore B, Staunton H, Farrell MA. Microdysgenesis in resected temporal neocortex: incidence and clinical significance in focal epilepsy. Neurology 1988; 38: 1041–7.
Hendry SHC, Schwark HD, Jones EG, Yan J. Numbers and proportions of GABA-immunoreactive neurons in different areas of monkey cerebral cortex. J Neurosci 1987; 7:1503–19.
Horton RW, Prestwich SA, Meldrum BS. γ-Aminobutyric acid and benzodiazepine binding sites in audiogenic seizure-susceptible mice. J Neurochem 1982; 39: 864–70.
Houser CR, Hendry SHC, Jones EG, Vaughn JE. Morphological diversity of immunocytochemically identified GABA neurones in the monkey sensory-motor cortex. J Neurocytol 1983; 12: 617–38.
Johansen FF, Zimmer J, Diemer NH. Early loss of somatostatin neurons in dentate hilus after cerebral ischemia in the rat precedes CA-1 pyramidal cell loss. Acta Neuropathol 1987; 73: 110–14.
Kish SJ, Dixon LM, Sherwin AL. Aspartic acid aminotransferase activity is increased in actively spiking vs non-spiking human epileptic cortex. J Neurol Neurosurg Psychiatry 1988; 51: 552–56.
Köhler C, Eriksson LG, Flood PR, Hardie JA, Okuno E, Schwartz R. Quinolinic acid metabolism in the rat brain. Immunohistochemical identification of 3-hydroxyanthranilic acid oxygenase and quinolinic acid phosphoribosyltransferase in the hippocampal region. J Neurosci 1988; 8: 975–87.
Lloyd KG, Bossi L, Morselli PL, Rougier M, Loiseau P, Munari C. Biochemical evidence for dysfunction of GABA neurons in human epilepsy. In: Bartholini G, Bossi L, Lloyd KG, Morselli PL (eds) Epilepsy and GABA receptor agonists: basic and therapeutic research. New York: Raven Press, 1985: 43–51.
Löscher W, Siemes H. Cerebrospinal fluid γ-aminobutyric acid levels in children with different types of epilepsy: effect of anticonvulsant treatment. Epilepsia 1985; 26: 314–19.
Manyam NVB, Katz L, Hare TA, Gerber JC, Grossman MH. Levels of γ-aminobutyric acid in cerebrospinal fluid in various neurologic disorders. Arch Neurol 1980; 37: 352–5.
Meenke HJ. The density of dystopic neurons in the white matter of the gyrus frontalis inferior in epilepsy. J Neurol 1983; 230: 171–81.
Meenke HJ. Neuron density in the molecular layer of the frontal cortex in primary generalised epilepsy. Epilepsia 1985; 26: 450–4.
Meenke HJ, Janz D. Neuropathological findings in primary generalized epilepsy: a study of eight cases. Epilepsia 1984; 25: 8–21.
Meldrum BS. Epilepsy and GABA-mediated inhibition. Int Rev Neurobiol 1975; 17: 1–36.
Meldrum BS. Amino acid neurotransmitters and new approaches to anticonvulsant drug action. Epilepsia 1984; 25: S140–9.
Meldrum B. Is epilepsy a disorder of excitatory transmission? In: Trimble MR, Reynolds EH (eds) What is Epilepsy? Edinburgh: Churchill Livingstone, 1986: 293–302.

Meldrum BS, Corsellis JAN. Epilepsy. In: Blackwood W, Corsellis JAN (eds) Greenfield's neuropathology. 4th ed. London: Arnold, 1984: 921–50.
Meldrum BS, Croucher MJ, Badman G, Collins JF. Antiepileptic action of excitatory amino acid antagonists in the photosensitive baboon. Neurosci Lett 1983; 39: 101–4.
Mody I, Stanton PK, Heinemann U. Activation of N-methyl-D-aspartate receptors parallels changes in cellular and synaptic properties of dentate gyrus granule cells after kindling. J Neurophysiol 1988; 59: 1033–54.
Mody I, Heinemann U. NMDA receptors of dentate gyrus granule cells participate in synaptic transmission following kindling. Nature 1987; 326: 701–4.
Nicoletti F, Meek JL, Iadarola MJ, Chuang DM, Roth BL, Costa E. Coupling of inositol phospholipid metabolism with excitatory amino acid recognition sites in rat hippocampus. J Neurochem 1986; 46: 40–6.
Olsen RW, Wamsley JK, McCabe RT, Lee RJ, Lomax P. Benzodiazepine/γ-aminobutyric acid receptor deficit in the midbrain of the seizure-susceptible gerbil. Proc Natl Acad Sci USA 1985; 82: 6701–5.
Palayoor ST, Seyfried TN, Bernard DJ. Calcium ATPase activities in synaptic plasma membranes of seizure-prone mice. J Neurochem 1986; 46: 1370–5.
Patel S, Meldrum BS, Collins JF. Distribution of [^{3}H]kainic acid binding sites in the rat brain: in vivo and in vitro receptor autoradiography. Neurosci Lett 1986; 70: 301–7.
Prince DA, Connors BW. Mechanisms of interictal epileptogenesis. Adv Neurol 1986; 44: 275–99.
Pumain R, Menini C, Heinemann U, Louvel J, Silva-Barrat C. Chemical synaptic transmission is not necessary for epileptic seizures to persist in the baboon, *Papio papio*. Exp Neurol 1985; 89: 250–8.
Represa A, Le Gall La Salle G, Ben-Ari Y. Hippocampal plasticity in the kindling model of epilepsy in rats. Neurosci Lett 1989; 99: 345–50.
Represa A, Robain O, Tremblay E, Ben-Ari Y. Hippocampal plasticity in childhood epilepsy. Neurosci Lett 1989; 99: 351–55.
Ribak CE, Bradburne RM, Harris AB. A preferential loss of GABAergic, inhibitory synapses in epileptic foci: A quantitative ultrastructural analysis of monkey neocortex. J Neurosci 1982; 2: 1725–35.
Ribak CE, Harris AB, Vaughn JE, Roberts E. Inhibitory, GABAergic nerve terminals decrease at sites of focal epilepsy. Science 1979; 205: 211–14.
Schmutz M, Klebs K, Olpe HR, Fagg GE, Allgeier H, Heckendorn R, Angst C, Brundish D, Dingwall JG. CGP 37849/CGP 39551: Competitive NMDA receptor antagonists with potent oral anticonvulsant activity. Soc Neurosci Abstracts 1988: 864.
Sherwin A, Robitaille Y, Quesney F, Olivier A, Villemure J, Leblanc R, Feindel W, Andermann E, Gotman J, Andermann F, Ethier R, Kish S. Excitatory amino acids are elevated in human epileptic cerebral cortex. Neurology 1988; 38: 920–3.
Silva-Barrat C, Brailowsky S, Levesque G, Menini C. Epileptic discharges induced by intermittent light stimulation in photosensitive baboons: a current source density study. Epilepsy Res 1987; 2: 1–8.
Sircar R, Ludvig N, Zukin SR, Moshe SL. Down-regulation of hippocampal phencyclidine (PCP) receptors following amygdala kindling. Eur J Pharmacol 1987; 141: 167–8.
Sloper JJ, Johnson P, Powell TPS. Selective degeneration of interneurons in the motor cortex of infant monkeys following controlled hypoxia: a possible cause of epilepsy. Brain Res 1980; 198: 204–9.
Sloviter RS. Decreased hippocampal inhibition and a selective loss of interneurons in experimental epilepsy. Science 1987; 235: 73–6.

Sommer W. Erkrankung des Ammonshornes als aetiologisches Moment der Epilepsie. Arch Psychiat Nervenkrankheit 1880; 10: 631–75.

Somogyi P, Freund TF, Hodgson AJ, Somogyi J, Beroukas D, Chubb IW. Identified axo-axonic cells are immunoreactive for GABA in the hippocampus and visual cortex of the cat. Brain Res. 1985; 332: 143–9.

Veith G, Wicke R. Cerebrale Differenzierungsstörungen bei Epilepsie. Jahrbuch 1968. Köln-Opladen: Westdeutscher Verlag, 1968: 515–34.

Wadman WJ, Heinemann U. Laminar profiles of $[K^+]_0$ and $[Ca^{2+}]_0$ in region CA1 of the hippocampus of kindled rats. In: Kessler M et al. (eds) Physiology and medicine. Berlin: Springer-Verlag, 1985: 221–8.

Wood JH, Hare TA, Glaeser BS, Ballenger JC, Post RM. Low cerebrospinal fluid γ-aminobutyric acid content in seizure patients. Neurology 1979; 29: 1203–8.

2
The Prognosis of Epilepsy: Is Chronic Epilepsy Preventable?

E.H. Reynolds
King's College Hospital, London, UK

Introduction

It is well known that the treatment of chronic epilepsy is very difficult. Such patients are often characterized as 'drug resistant', justifying in suitably selected cases more drastic approaches, such as neurosurgery. The hunt is on for new and more powerful or less toxic drugs than those currently available (Meldrum and Porter, 1986).

In this chapter I would like to consider the following question: is chronic epilepsy preventable? I should make it absolutely clear that I am not here discussing the prevention of *epilepsy*, but rather the prevention of *chronic* epilepsy. In other words, after the occurrence of the first seizure or few seizures, which herald the onset of epilepsy, is it possible to prevent the development of chronic epilepsy by prompt effective action at this early stage? This question requires consideration of two subsidiary questions: (1) how common is chronic epilepsy; and (2) how does epilepsy become chronic (Reynolds, Elwes and Shorvon, 1983; Reynolds, 1987, 1988)?

The Prognosis of Epilepsy: How Common is Chronic Epilepsy?

The traditional and rather gloomy view of prognosis was summarized in the detailed, authoritative, and classic review by Rodin (1968), which spans the period from Gowers, who first applied a statistical approach to prognosis in the late nineteenth century, to Rodin's own valuable studies. Table 1 summarizes

Table 1. Prognostic studies of predominantly chronic epileptic patients. Modified from Rodin (1968)

Author	Number	Duration of remission (years)	Percentage in remission
Habermass (1901)	937	2	10
Turner (1907)	87	2	32
Grosz (1930)	125	10	11
Kirstein (1942)	174	3	22
Alstroem (1950)	897	5	22
Strobos (1959)	228	1	38
Kiorboe, Lund and Poulsen (1960)	130	4	32
Probst (1960)	83	2	31
Trolle (1960)	799	2	37
Juul-Jensen (1963)	969	2	32
Lorgé (1964)	177	2	34

For references, see Rodin (1968).

many of the larger studies of prognosis prior to Rodin's review. On the basis of these and his own studies, Rodin concluded that only approximately one-third of epileptic patients are likely to achieve a terminal remission of at least 2 years; that the longer patients are followed up, the more likely relapse will occur; and that 80% of all patients with epilepsy are likely to have a chronic seizure disorder. Although the latter does not rule out short-term remission, it emphasizes that epilepsy should be regarded as a chronic condition with remissions and exacerbations. Rodin recognized that his review was based almost wholly on studies of chronic patients in institutions or attending special outpatient clinics. He noted that the longer the history of epilepsy prior to hospital consultation, the worse the prognosis, and he rightly drew attention to the good prognosis reported by Gowers (1881) in patients with a short history of epilepsy treated with bromides. At the time of his review, there had been no systematic study of epilepsy at its onset.

In the last decade, new studies (Table 2) have focused attention on epilepsy as viewed and followed from the onset of the disorder, both in the community and the hospital clinic. This has given some new insights into the temporal evolution of epilepsy, dispelled some of the gloomier views of prognosis based on studies of chronic patients, and raised some fundamental questions about the nature and treatment of epilepsy.

Community-based studies (Annegers, Hauser and Elveback, 1979; Goodridge and Shorvon, 1983), a retrospective multi-institutional study from Japan (Okuma and Kumashiro, 1981) and the prospective hospital-based study of Elwes et al. (1984), all present a much more optimistic picture of prognosis, with 58–82% of patients in 2–5 year remission (Table 2). The key difference

Table 2. Prognostic studies of newly diagnosed patients

	Number	Duration of remission (years)	Percentage of remission
Community (retrospective)			
Annegers, Hauser and Elveback (1979)	457	5	70
Goodridge and Shorvon (1983)	122	4	69
Hospital (retrospective)			
Okuma and Kumashiro (1981)	1868	3	58.3
Hospital (prospective)			
Elwes et al. (1984)	106	2	82

between these and earlier studies reviewed by Rodin (1968) (Table 1) is that the former are based on epileptic populations followed from the *onset* of their disorder. As the lifetime prevalence of epilepsy is of the order of 2% (Goodridge and Shorvon, 1983), then if only 20–30% go on to develop chronic 'active' epilepsy, giving a prevalence of approximately 0.5% (Zielinski, 1982; Goodridge and Shorvon, 1983), this still represents an enormous number of patients needing at times sophisticated and expensive health services.

How Does Epilepsy Become Chronic?

Whether or not chronic epilepsy is preventable will depend upon how epilepsy becomes chronic. Here there are two conflicting, but not necessarily mutually exclusive, views. The traditional view is that some patients are endowed with or acquire more 'severe' epilepsy from the start, the chronicity being the inevitable outcome of the inadequacy of the presently available treatment for such 'severe' epilepsy. However, the concept of 'severe' epilepsy is a difficult one that has never been very clearly defined, perhaps because it would require the prolonged observation of untreated patients, which for obvious reasons has never been undertaken; besides which it seems that some patients can at different times have either 'severe' or 'mild' epilepsy.

An alternative view, to which I am inclined, is that epilepsy should be viewed as a *process* (Reynolds, Elwes and Shorvon, 1983; Shorvon and Reynolds, 1986; Reynolds, 1987, 1989). According to this view, epilepsy may escalate out of control and become chronic unless effectively treated at the onset, i.e. 'arrested', to use Gowers' (1881) much neglected word. It should be emphasized that according to this more dynamic view of epilepsy, it is possible for the disorder to *remit* spontaneously, as is well known to occur, for example, in petit mal or benign rolandic epilepsy of childhood. The brain is the seat of competing excitatory and inhibitory processes.

Such limited evidence as is available does lend some support to the view of a process that may lead to chronic epilepsy, although the concept is far from confirmed. It was Gowers (1881), in fact, who first suggested the concept of such a process when he proposed that seizures may beget further seizures: 'When one attack has occurred, whether in apparent consequence of an excitant or not, others usually follow without any immediate traceable cause. The effect of a convulsion on the nerve centres is such as to render the occurrence of another more easy, to intensify the predisposition that already exists. Thus every fit may be said to be, in part, the result of those that have preceded it, the cause of those which follow it.'

Gowers presented evidence from his own careful observations that the prognosis for seizure control was inversely proportional to the duration of the disorder. He emphasized the very favourable prognosis in patients with a seizure disorder of less than 1 year (83% 'arrested') and the relatively high probability that seizures would not be controlled if the disorder had been present for more than 5 years. Gowers' views and their implications were overlooked for most of this century, as the history of drug trials and treatment until quite recently testifies. Rodin (1968) also noted from his own and other studies that the longer the history of epilepsy prior to hospital consultation, the worse the prognosis. This could, however, be an artefact due to the selection of chronic patients into the studies.

My colleagues and I have followed up prospectively 106 newly diagnosed adult epileptic patients whom we treated with carefully monitored single drug therapy, either phenytoin or carbamazepine (Elwes et al., 1984). Overall, the patients did very well, with 82% in 2-year remission by 8 years of follow-up. However, it was noticeable that the longer seizures continued after the onset of treatment, the worse the subsequent prognosis. Thus, if seizures were continuing 2 years after the start of treatment, the subsequent 1-year remission rate was halved. Although this might be in keeping with a process of escalation along the lines proposed by Gowers, it would not exclude the possibility that the patients doing badly and becoming chronic had more 'severe' epilepsy.

A number of factors were related to a more adverse prognosis, including partial seizures as compared to tonic–clonic seizures, and the presence of additional neurological, psychological and social handicaps, i.e. factors well known from the study of chronic patients (Rodin, 1968). Nevertheless, even in the presence of such factors most epileptic patients did well, and it was noteworthy that among our patients failing to respond to single-drug therapy, the most significant association was poor compliance (Chesterman, Elwes and Reynolds, 1987). It seems probable that with better compliance at the onset of treatment the overall outcome would be even more favourable.

It was clear from our study that the first 2 years of treatment were crucial in determining the future course and progress. Nineteen of 21 patients who failed

Table 3. Median interseizure intervals (weeks) in 183 newly diagnosed untreated patients with between two and five tonic–clonic seizures. From Elwes et al. (1988)

	\multicolumn{5}{c}{Pretreatment seizure number}
	All (N = 183)	2 (N = 101)	3 (N = 53)	4 (N = 18)	5 (N = 11)
From first to second seizure	12 (4–28)	12 (4–25)	12 (4–44)	22 (4–36)	24 (4–42)
From second to third seizure	8 (4–16)	—	8 (4–16)	16 (4–40)	4 (4–12)
From third to fourth seizure	4 (2–23)	—	—	6 (2–24)	4 (2–20)
From fourth to fifth seizure	3 (2–4)	—	—	—	3 (2–4)

Median interval is for 25th to 75th centiles.

to respond to single-drug therapy did so within the first 2 years and *all* went on to develop chronic epilepsy (Elwes et al., 1984). In a retrospective study based on patients referred to a special centre (Chalfont), Shorvon and Sander (1985) showed that chronic epilepsy had usually been persistent from the onset of the disorder, and that remission periods in such patients were uncommon.

Ideally, the question of 'severe' or evolving epilepsy should be studied prospectively in untreated patients but, as already noted, for ethical reasons the natural history of untreated epilepsy is unknown. My colleagues and I have attempted a limited retrospective study in patients presenting to the neurology department at King's College Hospital with between two and five untreated tonic–clonic seizures (Elwes, Johnson and Reynolds, 1988). We have examined the time intervals between each seizure in 183 patients in whom we could accurately date the attacks. This is possible in many patients presenting with the more dramatic tonic–clonic seizures but rarely possible in patients presenting with partial seizures, many of which are uncountable or even unknown to the patient. Overall, we found a steadily declining time interval between attacks, whether patients presented with three, four or five seizures (Table 3). In only 20% of patients did we find examples of lengthening between two successive time intervals. Such a study has several methodological weaknesses related to its retrospective, hospital-based nature, dictated by ethical considerations. Nevertheless, the findings are in keeping with the concept of an escalating process of epilepsy, at least in its early stages, and again emphasize the need to find some way of examining the issues prospectively. Perhaps this could be done by studying patients with single seizures.

The Single Seizure

The literature on the prognosis of a single seizure is controversial, as illustrated by Hauser (1986), who compared two studies of his own in the USA with one undertaken by my colleagues and me (Elwes, Chesterman and Reynolds, 1985) in England. At 3 years of follow-up, the relapse rate following a single first attack was 27% at Minneapolis, 55% at Rochester, and 71% at London. Other studies have produced equally variable results (see Elwes, Chesterman and Reynolds, 1985). It is worth considering the reasons for such variation (Elwes and Reynolds, 1988). There are probably several that relate to the patient populations in the different studies. However, two factors seem particularly important. First, in both the Rochester and Minneapolis studies, approximately two-thirds of the patients were actually treated with anticonvulsants, whereas none of our own patients were so treated. This is likely to have reduced the overall recurrence rate in the American studies. Probably a more important factor is the time interval between the first seizure and the time of entry into the single-seizure study. In our retrospective study of the natural history of untreated epilepsy described above (Elwes, Johnson and Reynolds, 1988), we have confirmed Gowers' (1881) observation that in one-third of epileptic patients with tonic–clonic attacks, the second attack follows the first *within 1 month*. In the American studies and other reports, the time interval between the first attack and the point of entry to the study is usually several weeks or else unstated. If 4 weeks have already elapsed, at least one-third of the potential candidates for a single-seizure study will have been excluded by virtue of the fact that they have already developed a second attack. It is for this very reason that in our own single-seizure study (Elwes, Chesterman and Reynolds, 1985) we identified our 133 patients within a median of *1 day* after their tonic–clonic attack. In keeping with Gowers' views and the epidemiological findings of Goodridge and Shorvon (1983), we therefore suspect that, following a single tonic–clonic attack, the risk of further attacks is high. The question therefore arises whether such patients should be treated with anticonvulsant therapy (Reynolds, 1984). There has been no adequate investigation of the value of such a policy, and practice is very variable. In view of the issues raised in this chapter and elsewhere (Reynolds, 1987) about prognosis and the preventive possibilities of early effective treatment for epilepsy, such studies are indicated even though they pose difficult practical and ethical problems. Perhaps within the context of such studies it will be possible to learn more about the early natural history of untreated epilepsy and the implications of treatment or no treatment for longer-term prognosis.

Conclusions

In this chapter I have focused attention on the possible preventive implications of early effective treatment for epilepsy. This seems to be an objective worthy of consideration because even if it is only partially attainable, then it would relieve an enormous amount of individual suffering as well as a considerable burden on health services for what may be a relatively small price in terms of individual effort or discipline, or financial cost (Reynolds, Elwes and Shorvon, 1983; Reynolds, 1987, 1989). I have reviewed our own and other studies that lend some support to the concept that epilepsy is a *process* that may escalate into a chronic state and that at least in some patients chronicity is preventable. Epilepsy may also remit spontaneously, and an intriguing but unanswered question is whether early effective treatment may increase the prospects for natural remission. The issue of inherently more 'severe' as opposed to an escalating process of epilepsy is, however, far from clarified and will require prospective studies in patients with single seizures or newly diagnosed epilepsy to try to learn more about the natural history of untreated epilepsy and the effect of early treatment on longer-term prognosis.

Finally, the model of kindling (Goddard, 1967) may be relevant to the issues discussed here, even though there are clear differences between kindling and the process of epilepsy envisaged. In the kindling model, each successive subthreshold electrical or chemical stimulus is necessary and plays its part in the eventual precipitation of a seizure. Is it conceivable that, whereas a subthreshold stimulus may leave its unknown mark on the nervous system, a seizure itself does not (Reynolds, 1989)?

Summary

Recent epidemiological and hospital-based studies of newly diagnosed epileptic patients suggest that the prognosis for epilepsy is much more favourable than had previously been reported and believed. Approximately three-quarters of such patients may expect to go into prolonged remission with currently available drugs, utilized as monotherapy. For chronic epileptic patients, however, the outlook for seizure control is poor. Factors that contribute to the development of chronic epilepsy are partial or multiple seizure types, brain pathology, neuropsychiatric or social handicaps, poor compliance, and the early response to treatment. Evidence is presented that epilepsy should be viewed as a process in which early effective treatment may be important to prevent the evolution of chronic epilepsy, which is so difficult to control.

References

Annegers JF, Hauser WA, Elveback LR. Remission of seizures and relapse in patients with epilepsy. Epilepsia 1979; 20: 729–37.

Chesterman P, Elwes RDC, Reynolds EH. Failure of monotherapy in newly diagnosed epilepsy. In: Wolf P, Dam M, Janz D, Dreifuss FE (eds) The XVIth Epilepsy International Symposium. Advances in Epileptology. vol. 16. New York: Raven Press, 1987: 461–4.

Elwes RDC, Chesterman P, Reynolds EH. Prognosis after a first untreated tonic–clonic seizure. Lancet 1985; 2: 752–3.
Elwes RDC, Johnson AL, Reynolds EH. The course of untreated epilepsy. Br Med J 1988; 297: 948–50.
Elwes RDC, Reynolds EH. Should people be treated after a first seizure? Arch Neurol 1988; 45: 490–1.
Elwes RDC, Johnson AL, Shorvon SD, Reynolds EH. The prognosis for seizure control in newly diagnosed epilepsy. N Engl J Med 1984; 311: 944–7.
Goddard GV. Development of epileptic seizures through brain stimulation at low intensity. Nature 1967; 214: 1020–1.
Goodridge DMG, Shorvon SD. Epilepsy in a population of 6000. 1. Demography, diagnosis and classification, and the role of the hospital services. 2. Treatment and prognosis. Br Med J 1983; 287: 641–7.
Gowers WR. Epilepsy and other chronic convulsive diseases. London: Churchill, 1881.
Hauser WA. Should people be treated after a first seizure? Arch Neurol 1986; 43: 1287–8.
Meldrum BS, Porter RJ (eds). New anticonvulsant drugs. London: J. Libby, 1986.
Okuma T, Kumashiro H. Natural history and prognosis of epilepsy: report of a multi-institutional study in Japan. Epilepsia 1981; 22: 35–53.
Reynolds EH. The initiation of anticonvulsant drug therapy. In: Pedley TA, Meldrum BS (eds) Recent advances in epilepsy. vol. 2. Edinburgh: Churchill Livingstone, 1984: 101–10.
Reynolds EH. Early treatment and prognosis of epilepsy. Epilepsia 1987; 28: 97–106.
Reynolds EH. The prevention of chronic epilepsy. Epilepsia 1988; 29 (suppl. 1): S25–S28.
Reynolds EH. The process of epilepsy: Is kindling relevant? In: Bolwig T, Trimble MR (eds) The clinical relevance of kindling. Wiley: Chichester, 1989: 149–160.
Reynolds EH, Elwes RDC, Shorvon SD. Why does epilepsy become intractable? Prevention of chronic epilepsy. Lancet 1983; 2: 952–4.
Rodin EA. The prognosis of patients with epilepsy. Springfield, IL: Charles C Thomas, 1968.
Shorvon SD. The temporal aspects of prognosis in epilepsy. J Neurol Neurosurg Psychiatry 1984; 47: 1157–65.
Shorvon SD, Reynolds EH. The nature of epilepsy: evidence from studies of epidemiology, temporal patterns of seizures, prognosis and treatment. In: Trimble MR, Reynolds EH (eds) What is epilepsy? Edinburgh: Churchill Livingstone, 1986: 36–45.
Shorvon SD, Sander JWAS. Temporal pattern of remission and relapse of seizures in patients with epilepsy. In: Schmidt D, Morselli P (eds) A workshop on intractable epilepsy. New York: Raven Press, 1985: 13–23.
Zielinski JJ. Epidemiology. In: Laidlaw J, Richens A (eds) A textbook of epilepsy, 2nd ed. Edinburgh: Churchill Livingstone, 1982: 16–33.

3
How Does One Assess the Severity of Epilepsy?

Dieter Janz
Free University of Berlin, Berlin, West Germany

As fashions change with time, so do the opinions of doctors. In the 1950s and 1960s views regarding epilepsy were fairly optimistic. One would hear and read about the success of pharmacotherapy. This changed in the 1970s and 1980s: people now talk about limitations, unsuccessful treatments and the reasons for them. Concepts of more or less severe epilepsy on the one hand, and of benign epilepsy on the other, are used without making detailed definitions. It therefore might be helpful to consider the criteria by which the severity of epilepsy is assessed.

The 'severity of a disease' is a relative term, and its definition will differ depending on whether one is describing its responsiveness to medical treatment, its ramifications on the patient's social situation, or the patient's subjective experience of the disease. The proposal by the WHO to classify impaired health due to chronic diseases on the basis of 'impairments, disabilities and handicaps' (WHO, 1980) follows the same line of reasoning.

It is important with regard to epilepsy to specify in each instance to which of the three aspects one is referring when one speaks of 'benign' or 'severe', and this is very often done (e.g. as in the new classification of epileptic syndromes). To give an example: in a book on intractable epilepsy, Porter (1986) says 'a biweekly complex partial seizure in a retarded institutionalized patient is far less disabling than a single such seizure occurring annually in the family breadwinner.' In this case he is setting the social aspect of disability against the personal aspect of a handicap. Let me give another example: the claim I made at one time that the less patients are aware of their attacks, the more violent those attacks are (Janz, 1963), relates to the astonishing paradox which exists between the minimal 'handicap' and the maximum 'impairment' in the case of a severe, generalized, tonic–clonic seizure. The different ways of considering the disease are obviously not parallel. That is why the doctor's perspective, that of society, and that of the patient, frequently diverge.

Subjective Handicap

With regard to the patient's perception of the disease or subjective handicap, the criteria which apply differ from those which concern the patient's role as a citizen or his social disability, and they differ again from those applied in the medical sphere, e.g. in the case of drug resistance. Patients may experience isolated auras as a serious nuisance or with fear, while the same phenomena are rated by neurosurgeons as being of minor importance in assessing the results of surgical treatment. On the other hand, patients with juvenile myoclonic epilepsy consider their occasional morning jerks as trivial, provided they are not followed by major attacks, whereas medical assessors have to refuse patients a driving licence simply because of those jerks. Due to the increasing appreciation of the psychological aspects of epilepsy, and thanks to the growing activities of the self-help movement, reports in recent years of self-awareness and coping with epilepsy have been gaining in importance (Schneider and Conrad, 1983). However, to my knowledge no systematic grading of subjective handicap has yet emerged from this.

Social Disability

From the social aspect, in order to determine the degree of social disability caused by epilepsy alone, one traditionally uses data concerning the frequency and type of seizures as quantitative and qualitative criteria (Goodglass et al., 1963; Janz, 1972; Pond et al., 1960; Zielinski, 1972). Sometimes attention is paid to the timing of attacks (i.e. whether they occur during sleep or only after waking). However, the medical classification of seizures is completely inappropriate for assessing social capabilities, especially the patient's suitability for certain occupations. For many activities or occupations, for example, it is completely unimportant whether the patient suffers complex focal or secondary generalized seizures, but it is important whether the seizures occur exclusively during sleep or primarily in the waking state. It is also unimportant in assessing a patient's suitability for an occupation whether his attacks are simple or complex absences, myoclonic jerks, or atonic fits, but it is relevant whether the person affected falls down during these attacks or remains standing. We have therefore drawn up a scale in relation to occupational hazards, on which we classify occupational abilities and disabilities as a consequence of attacks

Assessment of Severity

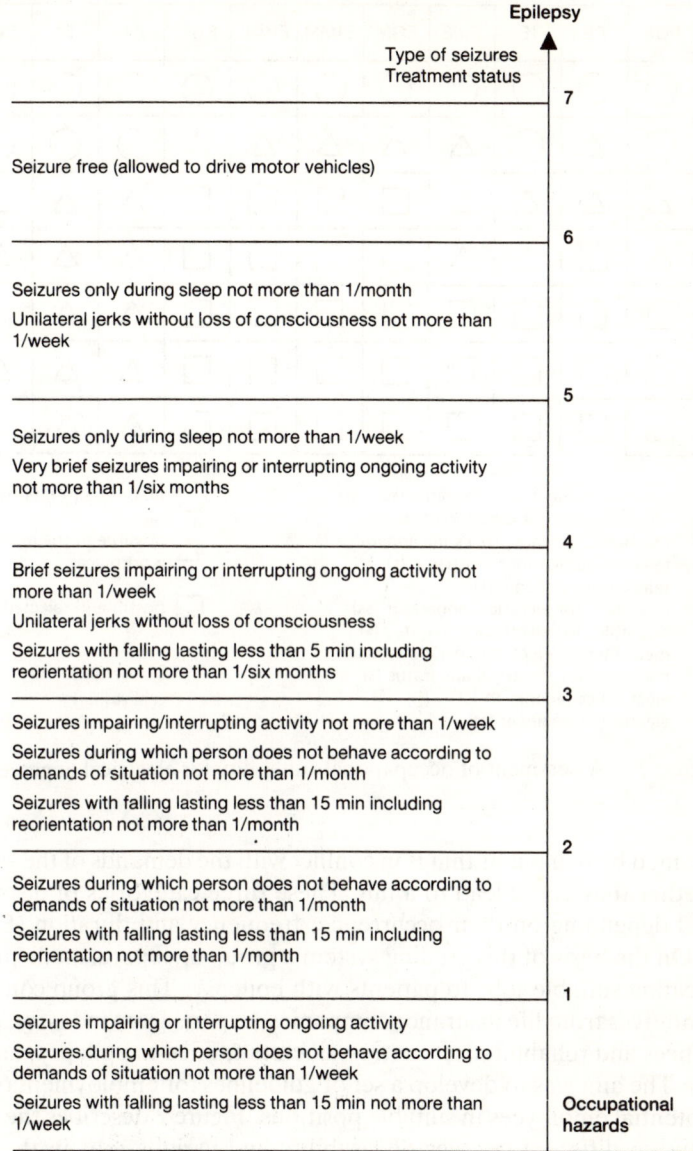

Figure 1.

into seven grades (Thorbecke and Janz, 1984). We based this grading system not on the criteria of neurological diagnosis, but on the criteria of the risk of accidents (Figure 1). It is crucial when assessing a patient's suitability for a job whether the attacks impair or interrupt job-related activities, whether they are

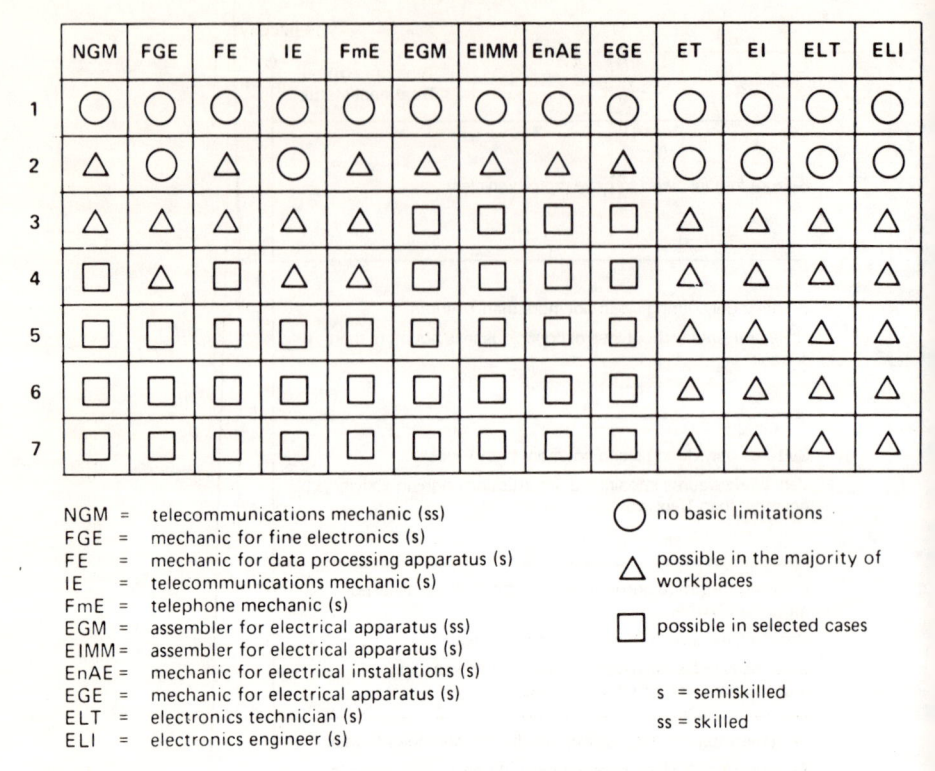

	NGM	FGE	FE	IE	FmE	EGM	EIMM	EnAE	EGE	ET	EI	ELT	ELI
1	○	○	○	○	○	○	○	○	○	○	○	○	○
2	△	○	△	○	△	△	△	△	△	○	○	○	○
3	△	△	△	△	△	□	□	□	□	△	△	△	△
4	□	△	□	△	△	□	□	□	□	△	△	△	△
5	□	□	□	□	□	□	□	□	□	△	△	△	△
6	□	□	□	□	□	□	□	□	□	△	△	△	△
7	□	□	□	□	□	□	□	□	□	△	△	△	△

NGM = telecommunications mechanic (ss)
FGE = mechanic for fine electronics (s)
FE = mechanic for data processing apparatus (s)
IE = telecommunications mechanic (s)
FmE = telephone mechanic (s)
EGM = assembler for electrical apparatus (ss)
EIMM = assembler for electrical apparatus (s)
EnAE = mechanic for electrical installations (s)
EGE = mechanic for electrical apparatus (s)
ELT = electronics technician (s)
ELI = electronics engineer (s)

○ no basic limitations

△ possible in the majority of workplaces

□ possible in selected cases

s = semiskilled
ss = skilled

Figure 2. Assessment of occupational suitability for electrical engineering

accompanied by behaviour that is in conflict with the demands of the situation, and whether they could lead to a fall. These three categories of disorder are weighted depending on their occurrence, frequency and duration (Figures 2 and 3). On the basis of this grading system a group of experts made proposals for allocating suitable jobs to patients with epilepsy. This group consisted of representatives from life insurance companies, experts from industry, employment offices and rehabilitation centres, doctors trained in epilepsy, and social workers. The aim was to develop a set of guidelines for employment offices to place potential employees in suitable positions. Figure 2 describes the correlation between different degrees of disability and various jobs in the field of electronics: Figure 3 shows a similar correlation in the field of tool-making. The grading system illustrated in Table 1 could be extended to cover more professions on the one hand and/or more severe forms of epilepsy on the other, and it could also be supplemented by enumerating neurological and psychological deficits. However, the essential point, as far as the severity of epilepsy is concerned, is that the yardsticks that are appropriate when characterizing social ability and disability are different from those used when characterizing

Assessment of Severity

	I	II	III	IV	V	VI	VII
1	○	○	○	○	○	○	○
2	○	○	○	○	○	○	○
3	□	△	△	△	○	○	○
4	□	□	□	□	△	△	△
5	□	□	□	□	△	△	△
6	□	□	□	□	△	△	△
7	□	□	□	□	△	△	△

I = driller, drilling machine lathe-hand, lathe-hand, revolver lathe-hand, automaton fitter, milling operative, universal milling operative, planer, universal planer, universal polisher

II = surgical mechanic, mechanic, precision tool-maker, office machinery mechanic, electromechanical engineer, tool-maker

III = aircraft fitter, agricultural machinery fitter, fitter, industrial fitter, plastics mechanic

IV = welder

V = quality controller

VI = draughtsman, component part designer, mechanical engineering technician in the construction department, quality control, preparation of production, numerical control technology

VII = mechanical engineering

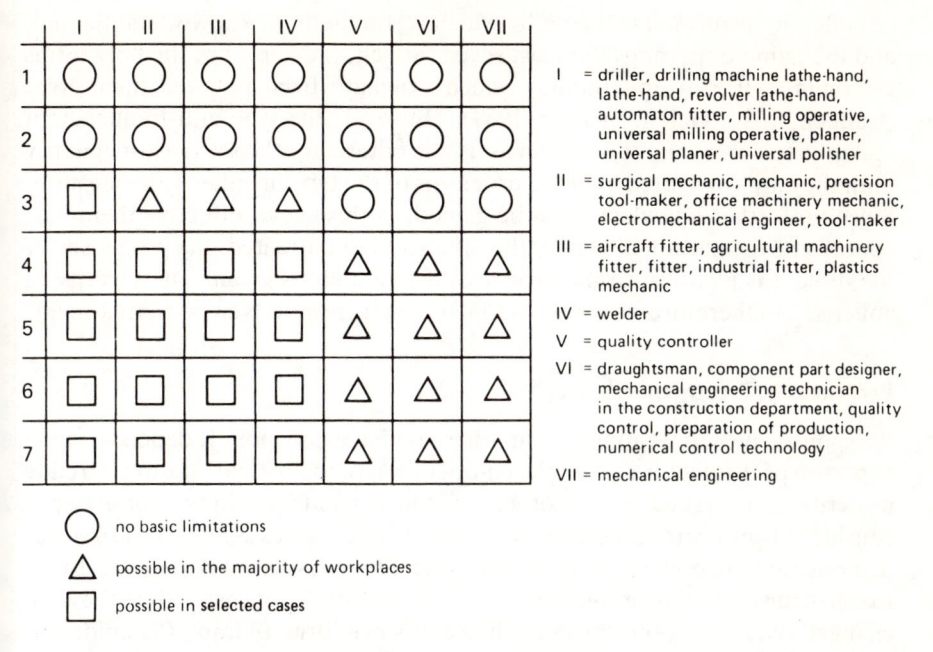

○ no basic limitations
△ possible in the majority of workplaces
□ possible in selected cases

Figure 3. Assessment of occupational suitability for machine construction

the subjective handicap as perceived by the patient, or the objective impairment as recorded by the doctor.

Medical Impairment

What yardstick should be used by the doctor to measure the severity of epilepsy? The most commonly used method is to characterize attacks on the basis of their severity as perceived by an observer. Following this principle, doctors have distinguished between epilepsia major and minor since the Middle Ages (Temkin, 1971), or between grand mal and petit mal since the middle of the last century (Esquirol, 1838). Opinions may differ concerning the dividing line between the different types of minor attack, and even the terminology may be questioned, as Gastaut (1985) does, when he states in a discussion about astatic seizures: 'In my opinion, seizures which make children fall and have injuries should not be named minor!' However, nobody doubts that an attack with generalized tonic–clonic jerks, apnea, and profound unconsciousness is objectively the most severe type of epileptic attack, and is therefore rightly called grand mal.

A further criterion of severity is the frequency of individual seizures, and their tendency to combine into series or status. Once again, nobody can doubt that convulsive status epilepticus constitutes the most severe manifestation of epileptic seizures. The name by which it is sometimes known, état de mal, and the name of perhaps the least severe attack, the aura, are the only terms in common use in epileptology which originate from patients themselves (Calmeil, 1824; Galen, in Janz, 1969). However, the type and frequency of epileptic seizures cannot be taken as usable criteria for the severity of epilepsy until they are correlated with the prognosis of the type of epilepsy in question. Since no further knowledge can be gained, in this age of effective therapies, concerning the natural history of the disease if left untreated, the prognosis for the disease is identical to the prognosis if treatment is given. The severity of epilepsy can therefore be seen as a function of its responsiveness to treatment.

Prognosis if Treatment is Given

'Responsiveness to treatment' is another relative expression. It depends on the expertise of the doctor and on the co-operation of the patient. If drugs already prescribed are issued as monotherapy, the percentage of cases of epilepsy considered uncontrollable can be reduced by 23%, as Schmidt (1984) has demonstrated in epilepsy with complex focal seizures. Even patients resistant to one drug can achieve freedom from attacks in 13% of cases when they are changed over to another drug of choice in single-drug therapy (Schmidt and Richter, 1986). Simply by improving compliance, one-third of the patients hitherto treated without success can become free of attacks (Lund, 1972), as in cases where medication is controlled by putting the daily doses in individual containers, and making the intervals between consultations shorter.

However, it can also be demonstrated that the prognosis for epilepsy if treated has become better in general during the course of this century. Table 1 lists the cases involving adult patients who were terminally free of attacks for at least 1 year follow up in the course of treatment over many years. It can be seen that there has been a marked increase in the chance of remission in recent years. The number of remissions reported by all authors did not exceed one-third of the cases in the first half of the century, but it has risen to two-thirds and even three-quarters since the 1970s. However, results in recent times diverge considerably. One explanation for this may be that the most favourable results were obtained in patients not previously treated (Elwes et al., 1983), and the least favourable results come from patients with many years of chronic epilepsy (Broeker and Müller, 1986). This finding, that a treatment administered at a later time in the course of the disease is less beneficial than that given earlier, is seen by Reynolds, Elwes and Shorvon (1983) as justifying their call for their prevention of chronic epilepsy by means of optimal treatment in the first 2 years of the illness, preferably in the form of single-drug therapy. Elwes et al. (1984) recently found that if seizures continued for up to 2 years after the commencement of treatment, the probability of controlling seizures subsequently fell by half. Thus, they claim this early treatment phase to be critical in determining

Table 1. Terminal remission for adults, cross-sectional surveys

Author	Year	Number of patients	Minimal duration of remission (years)	Patients remitted (%)
Habermass	1901	937	2	10
Turner	1907	87	2	32
Grosz	1930	91	10	11
Kirstein	1942	174	3	22
Alstroem	1950	897	5	22
Kiorboe, Lund and Poulson	1958	130	4	32
Strobos	1959	86	1	38
Probst	1960	83	2	31
Trolle	1961	799	2	37
Lorgé	1964	177	2	34
Rodin	1968	90	2	32
Schilling	1968	243	5	32
Janz	1983	574	2	62
Elwes et al.	1984	106	2	82
Oller-Daurella and Oller Ferrer-Vidal	1985	2048	1	73
Broeker and Müller	1986	495	5	40

the outcome of the disease. Moreover, the probability of control appears to be lower if one applies a stricter measure to the duration of terminal remission. In the two cross-sectional surveys based on a 5-year terminal remission period, it is reported that only 40% of patients achieved this objective. One must therefore accept even today that about 40–50% of adult patients in a neurological clinic, predominantly affected with chronic epilepsy, will not achieve freedom from attacks or will not remain free of attacks in the long term. With a paediatric clientele (Groh, 1975; Sofijanow, 1982) or in a population of patients previously untreated or recently affected for the first time (Elwes et al., 1984), who are identified in community surveys, the long-term prospects are understandably more encouraging.

Resistance to Therapy

In Different Kinds of Symptomatic Epilepsy

What are the neurological reasons for resistance to therapy? It is said that symptomatic epilepsy is more difficult to treat than cryptogenic epilepsy.

However, this distinction has not been the focus of any thorough investigation, and perhaps the subject is too vague to allow one to expect a worthwhile answer. In epilepsy with psychomotor seizures, our experience is that aetiology plays no role in the long-term prognosis with therapy (Tsai, 1984). We have heard, and we know from our own case experience, that postencephalitic epilepsy, especially that following herpes simplex encephalitis (Jacobi, 1984), is often very difficult to control with drugs, but to my knowledge there have been no systematic studies of this.

We know rather more about the natural history of post-traumatic epilepsy, in particular the condition and the prognosis for early attacks and late attacks following trauma (see Janz, Chapter 7). Just as with early seizures, which tend to cease spontaneously, the prognosis for late seizures is not necessarily unfavourable. Epilepsy does not develop in all cases. Out of 51 cases in the Mayo Clinic study (Annegers et al., 1980), whose course has been followed for at least 6 years, 19 suffered only one seizure. Of the 28 cases reported by Jennett and Lewin (1960) with late seizures, 7 cases had only one seizure, and only 9 cases had more than three seizures after a 7-year follow-up investigation. Evans (1962) also showed a tendency to natural remission on the basis of a 7–11-year follow-up study. More than one major seizure occurred per year in only 18 out of 75 cases; 32 were free of seizures, 19 of whom were no longer taking antiepileptic drugs. Traumatic late epilepsy fails to become chronic in approximately one-quarter of cases, with a variability of between 13% for closed and 54% for open injuries. Follow-up investigations give the impression of a 'generally favorable course' (Wessely, 1981). According to Walker (1962), 60% of the patients no longer had attacks 10 years after the injury.

In Cases with Structural Lesions

We still hear and read claims that seizures in patients with organic brain damage are less well controlled than in patients without (Loiseau, 1986; Reynolds and Shorvon, 1981; Strobos, 1959; Rodin, 1968; Annegers, Hauser and Elveback, 1979; Rowal et al., 1980). Chesterman, Elwes and Reynolds (1987) found three times more patients with structural lesions failing to achieve remission with single-drug therapy. In a comparison of patients resistant to drug therapy and patients not resistant to drug therapy with complex focal seizures, we saw no difference in the frequency of structural lesions which could be identified by computerized tomography (CT) or magnetic resonance imaging (MRI) (Meencke, Schörner and Janz, 1987) (Table 2). Every neurologist is alert to the possibility of a slowly growing tumour in cases of refractory epilepsy. However, even more than that, one must always bear in mind that a positive response to therapy does not rule out the possibility of a tumour, as Schmidt so memorably describes on the basis of a case (Schmidt, 1984). In the age of neuroimaging techniques, it seems even more appropriate to remind

Table 2. Frequency of localized atrophies and focal lesions seen by CT and MRI in 62 patients with complex focal seizures. From Meencke, Schörner and Janz (1987)

	No. of patients	Localized atrophies CT	Localized atrophies MRI	Focal lesions CT	Focal lesions MRI
Drug therapy					
Resistant	24	1	13	6	10
Non-resistant	38	0	14	8	13

ourselves that focal epilepsy with visible lesions should not be considered a priori as resistant to drug therapy, and that visible lesions should not be removed surgically until one has evidence that they coincide with the epileptogenic focus.

In Cases with Convulsive Status Epilepticus

Convulsive status epilepticus, the most severe manifestation of epileptic seizures, is about five to six times more frequent in patients with seizures of defined cause. In our experience, grand mal status occurred in only 1.6% of the cases of cryptogenic epilepsy; however, it occurred in 15.8% of patients with tumour-related epilepsy and in 10.7% of those with traumatic epilepsy, as compared with its occurrence in 5.4% of patients with epilepsy of other known causes (Janz, 1983).

In Different Types of Seizure

We are on firmer ground when we come to consider the prognosis with therapy of different types of seizure and epileptic syndromes. As far as the type of seizure is concerned, a comparison of terminal remissions in different types of generalized seizures (Table 3) shows that, as expected, the risk of suffering absences continuously is lowest in epilepsy with simple absences, known as pyknolepsy. The risk becomes markedly higher when absences are combined with tonic–clonic seizures. The risk of further attacks in the long term is also relatively low in cases of epilepsy involving only generalized tonic–clonic seizures (i.e. in pure grand mal epilepsy).

As is well known, the greatest resistance to therapy occurs in epilepsy with infantile spasms (West's syndrome) and in epilepsy with myoclonic astatic seizures (Lennox–Gastaut syndrome), in which 50–89% of all patients still fail to achieve freedom from attacks in the long term. The prognosis with therapy for epilepsy with focal seizures is neither especially good nor especially poor (Table 4). There appear to be no significant differences between epilepsies with

Table 3. Terminal remission in generalized seizures, by per cent

	Groh (1975)	Okuma and Kumashiro (1981)	Sofijanow (1982)	Janz (1983)	Oller-Daurella and Oller Ferrer-Vidal (1985)
Infantile spasms	52	51	40	31	34
Myoclonic astatic	55	37	36	16	21
Absences	99	67	61	84	87
Absences and GTC seizures	44	67		60	42
Myoclonic and GTC seizures	—	—	—	75	80
Tonic–clonic seizures	77	69	72	84	88

GTC = generalized tonic–clonic.

Table 4. Terminal remission in focal seizures, by per cent

	Groh (1975)	Okuma and Kumashiro (1981)	Sofijanow (1982)	Janz (1983)	Oller-Daurella and Oller Ferrer-Vidal (1985)
Simple	68	60	66	50	67
Simple and GTC	57	42		40	68
Complex	71	61	36	42	64
Complex and GTC	50	30		48	63
Secondary GTC	—	39	50	74	97

GTC = generalized tonic–clonic.

simple and those with complex attacks, nor even between those which occur in isolation and those which occur in combination with major seizures. Experience of the prognosis with therapy of secondary generalized seizures of a major nature varies widely. There are reports of resistance to therapy in 3–61% of cases. These differences can only be associated with the application of different classification criteria. As far as the forms of grand mal are concerned, which differ in their timing, sleeping and waking seizures appear not to differ in their prognosis with therapy. On the other hand, epilepsy with random seizures tends to have a poor prognosis (Janz et al., 1983).

In Different Epileptic Syndromes

With regard to epileptic syndromes, one can identify special factors which determine the severity or the prognosis in the long term if treated. For

Table 5. Negative factors for treatment prognosis in absence seizures. After Wolf and Inoue (1984)

Pyknoleptic recurrence of absences
Absences with mild clonic components
More than 10 GTC seizures
GTC seizures in sleep or at random
History of absence status
History of GTC status
Developmental delay
Mental retardation
Slow EEG-background activity
Spike–waves unprovoked
Spike–wave bursts of more than 5 s
Asymmetry of spike–waves
Onset of epilepsy before age 11 years
Persistence of absences beyond age 25 years
Persistence of absences for more than 12 years

GTC = generalized tonic–clonic.

example, we know that in West's syndrome, which is generally rated as a severe form of epilepsy, an early commencement (before the third month), abnormal development before the onset of attacks, and neurological abnormalities, enable one to predict an unfavourable course (Aicardi, 1986; Jeavons, 1985). With regard to Lennox–Gastaut syndrome, which is considered equally difficult to treat, the situation is very similar, with an early commencement (before the age of 3 years) and retarded psychomotor development regarded as predictors of an unfavourable course (Aicardi and Chevrie, 1986; Beaumanoir, 1985). Although absences, as the most common type of attack, are usually associated with particularly benign syndromes, circumstances do arise which make the success of therapy less than optimal (Table 5). Thus, Wolf and Inoue (1984) state that pyknoleptic absences are not quite so easy to treat as non-pyknoleptic, juvenile absences; furthermore, absences with myoclonic features are not as straightforward as simple absences. Treatment is made more difficult if more than ten major attacks, major attacks during sleep or a random, petit mal status, or even convulsive status, have occurred, and if the absences have persisted for more than 12 years or beyond the patient's 25th year. There is no similar differentiation as yet in the factors which determine the prognosis in epilepsy with impulsive petit mal or in juvenile myoclonic epilepsy. However, we know that after drug withdrawal this form has such a high incidence of relapse, even after many years of freedom from attacks, despite its good response to treatment, that the patient will be unable to go without drugs at any time for the rest of his life (Janz, 1985). It is therefore not appropriate to label this form as benign (Asconape and Penry, 1984). Focal epilepsy with contratemporal spikes is genuinely benign because it always or almost always ceases whether treated with drugs or not (Lerman, 1985), as do

Table 6. Factors for long-term treatment prognosis in complex focal seizures. According to Tsai (1984)

Favourable	Unfavourable	No significance
No automatisms	Oral sensory, epigastric, vegetative aura with/without automatisms Automatisms	No aura Type of automatisms Tonic change during seizure
Seldom seizures	Frequent seizures Seizures in clusters Frequent GTC	Seizure during sleep GTC GTC status or series Age onset
Short duration of epilepsy, treatment before 14 years, seizure free period for at least 1 year	Long duration of epilepsy	
	Febrile seizures, neonatal seizures Delayed delivery, asphyxia More than one aetiological factor	No aetiological factor Genetic disposition
No psychopathological symptoms	Psychopathological symptoms EEG with: Combined focal slow wave and sharp/spike Focal slow wave on left side	Psychosis Normal EEG

GTC = generalized tonic–clonic.

the febrile convulsions referred to in passing by Lennox (1960) as the mildest form of epilepsy.

Tsai (1984) has given us a good summary of the factors that are of importance in the long-term prognosis with therapy of epilepsy with complex focal attacks (Table 6). The prognosis is unfavourable in the following circumstances: complex focal attacks which begin with auras, attacks with automatisms, diseases of long duration, a high frequency of seizures with attacks occurring in clusters, psychopathological changes, the occurrence of neonatal convulsions or infantile convulsions, delayed birth or asphyxia during birth, and a combination of several aetiological factors. It is hardly necessary to say that the prospects for treatment are favourable if the disease has been in existence for less than 3 years and the attacks have been relatively infrequent. It is astonishing to learn that the occurrence of secondarily generalized attacks or even convulsive status epilepticus has no effect on the prognosis if treatment is given. Contrary to the general view, accompanying neurological findings do not play a part, and it is irrelevant whether the aetiology is known or not, except when several aetiological factors occur simultaneously.

In conclusion, the data presented by Wolf and Inoue (1984) and by Tsai (1984) explain the fact that the severity of epilepsy cannot ultimately be defined on the basis of a single aspect, even from the medical point of view, but is a complex matter in which several aspects must be taken into account. When the complex term 'severity' is at last defined on the basis of several factors that have a predictive value, then the term will be of practical use in assessing the prognosis of different types of seizures and of the respective epilepsy.

Conclusions

The 'severity' of a disease is a relative expression and its definition will vary depending on the perspective of the observer. The patient's subjective perception of the disease, the way it is regarded socially by the community, and the doctor's objective assessment, rarely coincide. In fact, they are frequently diametrically opposed. As far as the patient's personal perception of epilepsy is concerned, there has apparently been no satisfactory attempt thus far at a systematic grading of the subjective handicap, despite the growth of interest in psychological matters and the self-help movement. Similarly, social ability or disability cannot be adequately assessed on the basis of medical criteria such as frequency and type of seizures. We present a grading system which will serve as an appropriate method of assessing social abilities, and which will permit the patient's occupational potential to be estimated in relation to the risk of accidents resulting from seizures. From the medical point of view, the impairment of a patient's abilities due to epilepsy is a function of the patient's responsiveness to treatment. We have presented a critical review of the factors which have an effect on the therapeutic prognosis: the causes of epilepsy, underlying structural lesions, the incidence of convulsive status epilepticus, various types of attack, and the different epileptic syndromes. Taking two examples—epilepsy presenting in the form of absence and epilepsy with complex focal seizures—we show that ultimately the 'severity of epilepsy' can only be defined from the medical standpoint on the basis of several factors whose value is of a predictive nature.

References

Aicardi J. Treatment of infantile spasms. In: Schmidt D, Morselli PL (eds). Intractable epilepsy: experimental and clinical aspects. New York: Raven Press, 1986: 147–56.
Aicardi J, Chevrie JJ. Lennox–Gastaut syndrome and myoclonic epilepsies of infancy and early childhood. In: Schmidt D, Morselli PL (eds) Intractable epilepsy: experimental and clinical aspects. New York: Raven Press, 1986: 157–66.

Alstroem CH. A study of epilepsy in its clinical, social and genetic aspects. Acta Psychiatr Neurol Scand 1950; suppl. 63.
Annegers JF, Hauser WA, Elveback LR. Remission of seizures and relapse in patients with epilepsy. Epilepsia 1979; 20: 729–37.
Annegers JF, Grabow JD, Groover RV, Laws ER, Elveback LR, Kurland LT. Seizures after head trauma: a population study. Neurology (Minneap) 1980; 30: 683–9.
Asconape J, Penry K. Some clinical and EEG aspects of benign juvenile myoclonic epilepsy. Epilepsia 1984; 25: 108–14.
Beaumanoir A. The Lennox–Gastaut syndrome. In: Roger J, Dravet C, Bureau M, Dreifuss FE, Wolf P (eds) Epileptic syndromes in infancy, childhood and adolescence. London, Paris: John Libbey, 1985: 42–50.
Broeker H, Müller D. Die Bedeuting des EEG für die Therapieprognose bei erwachsenen Epilepsiekranken. Psychiatr Neurol Med Psychol (Leipz) 1986; 38: 509–17.
Calmeil LF. De l'epilepsie, étudiée sous le rapport de son siège et de son influence sur la production de l'alienation mentale. Thèse de Paris, 1824.
Chesterman P, Elwes RDC, Reynolds EH. Failure of monotherapy in newly diagnosed epilepsy. In: Wolf P, Dam M, Janz D, Dreifuss FE (eds) Advances in epileptology: XVIth Epilepsy International Symposium. New York: Raven Press, 1987: 461–4.
Elwes RDC, Johnson AL, Shorvon SD, Reynolds EH. The early prognosis of epilepsy. In: Parsonage M, Grant RHE, Craig AG, Ward AA (eds) Advances in epileptology: XIVth Epilepsy International Symposium. New York: Raven Press, 1983: 133–41.
Elwes RDC, Johnson AL, Shorvon SD, Reynolds EH. The prognosis for seizure control in newly diagnosed epilepsy. N Engl J Med 1984; 311: 944–7.
Esquirol E. Des maladies mentales, medical, hygiénique et medico-legal. 2 vols. Paris: Baillière, 1838.
Evans, JH. Post-traumatic epilepsy. Neurology (Minneap) 1962; 12: 665–74.
Gastaut H. Discussion of myoclonic epilepsies and Lennox–Gastaut syndrome. In: Roger J, Dravet C, Bureau M, Dreifuss FE, Wolf P (eds) Epileptic syndromes in infancy, childhood and adolescence. London, Paris: John Libbey, 1985: 100.
Goodglass H, Morgan M, Folsom AT, Quadfasel FA. Epileptic seizures: Psychological factors and occupational adjustment. Epilepsia 1963; 4: 322–41.
Goodridge DGM, Shorvon SD. Epileptic seizures in a population of 6000: I. Demography, diagnosis and classification, and role of the hospital services. Br Med J 1983; 287: 641–4.
Groh Ch. Zur Frage der Heilbarkeit kindlicher Epilepsien. Wien Klin Wochenschr 1975; 87 (suppl. 49): 3–23.
Grosz W. Uber den Augang der genuinen Epilepsie. Arch Psychiatr Nervenkr 1930; 90: 765–76.
Habermass. Uber die Prognose der Epilepsie. Allg Z Psychiatr 1901; 58: 243–53.
Jacobi G. Therapeutisch schwer zu beeinflussende zerebrale Anfälle nach Herpessimplex. Enzephalitis bei Kindern. In: Meier, K (eds) Therapieresistenz bei Anfallsleiden. München, Bern, Wien: Zuckschwerdt, 1984: 53–64.
Janz D. Soziale Aspekte der Epilepsie. Psychiatr Neurol Neurochir 1963; 66: 240–8.
Janz D. Social prognosis in epilepsy especially in regard to social status and the necessity for institutionalisation. Epilepsia 1972; 13: 141–7.
Janz D. Etiology of convulsive status epilepticus. Adv Neurol 1983; 34: 47–54.
Janz D. Epilepsy with impulsive petit mal (juvenile myoclonic epilepsy). Acta Neurol Scand 1985; 72: 449–59.
Janz D. Neurological morbidity of severe epilepsy. Epilepsia 1988; 29 (suppl. 1): S1–S8.

Janz D, Mössinger HJ, Puhlmann U. Rückfall-Prognose nach Reduktion der Medikament bei Epilepsiebehandlung. Nervenarzt 1983; 54: 525–9.
Jeavons PM. West-syndrome infantile spasms. In: Roger J, Dravet C, Bureau M, Dreifuss FE, Wolf P (eds) Epileptic syndromes in infancy, childhood and adolescence. London, Paris: John Libbey, 1985: 42–50.
Jennett WB, Lewin WS. Traumatic epilepsy after closed head injuries. J Neurol Neurosurg Psychiatr 1960; 23: 295–301.
Juul-Jensen P. Epilepsy. A clinical and social analysis of 1020 adult patients with epileptic seizures. Acta Neurol Scand 1964; suppl. 5.
Kiorboe E, Lund M, Poulsen A. The prognosis of epilepsy of short duration in adults: with special regard to the risk in traffic and industry. Ugeskr Laeger 1958; 2: 10. Acta Psychiatr Scand 1961; 36 (suppl. 150): 166–78.
Kirstein L. A contribution to knowledge of the prognosis of epilepsy. Acta Med Scand 1942; 111: 515–23.
Lerman P. Benign partial epilepsy with centro-temporal spikes. In: Roger J, Dravet C, Bureau M, Dreifuss FE, Wolf P (eds) Epileptic syndromes in infancy, childhood and adolescence. London, Paris: John Libbey, 1985: 150–8.
Loiseau P. Intractable epilepsy. Prognostic evaluation. In: Schmidt D, Morselli PL (eds) Intractable epilepsy: experimental and clinical aspects. New York: Raven Press, 1986: 227–36.
Lorgé M. Epilepsie und Lebensschicksal: Ergebnisse katammestischer Untersuchungen. Psychiatr Neurol (Basel) 1964; 147: 360–81.
Lund M. Errors in medication with special regard to outpatient treatment of epileptic patients. Acta Neurol Scand 1972; 4: 461.
Meencke HJ, Schörner W, Janz D. Magnetic resonance tomography studies in patients with temporal lobe epilepsy. In: Wolf P, Dam M, Janz D, Dreifuss FE (eds) Advances in epileptology: XVIth Epilepsy International Symposium. New York: Raven Press, 1987: 279–82.
Okuma T, Kumashiro H. Natural history and prognosis of epilepsy: a report of a multiinstitutional study. Epilepsia 1981; 22: 35–53.
Oller-Daurella L, Oller Ferrer-Vidal L. Que se puede lograr en al tratamiento del epileptico? Barcelona: Geigy Division Farmaceutica, 1985.
Pond DA, Bidwell BH, Stein L. A survey of epilepsy in fourteen general practices. I. Demographic and medical data. Psychiatr Neurol Neurochir 1960; 63: 217–36.
Porter R. Concluding remarks. In: Schmidt D, Morselli PL (eds) Intractable epilepsy: experimental and clinical aspects. New York: Raven Press, 1986: 259–62.
Probst C. Uber den Verlauf von hirnelektrisch stummen Epilepsien. Schweiz Arch Neurol Neurochir Psychiatr 1960; 85: 385–94.
Reynolds EH, Elwes RDC, Shorvon SD. Why does epilepsy become intractable? Prevention of chronic epilepsy. Lancet 1983; ii: 952–4.
Rodin EA. The prognosis of patients with epilepsy. Springfield, IL: Thomas, 1968.
Schilling D. Langzeitresultate ambulanter Epilepsiebehandlung. Med. Diss. Universität Heidelberg, 1968.
Schmidt D. Die Behandlung der Epilepsien. 2nd Aufl. Stuttgart, New York: Thieme, 1984: 22.
Schmidt D. Prognosis of chronic epilepsy with complex partial seizures. J Neurol Neurosurg Psychiatry 1984; 47: 1274–8.
Schmidt D, Richter K. Alternative single anticonvulsant drug therapy for refractory epilepsy. Ann Neurol 1986; 19: 85–7.
Schneider JW, Conrad P. Having epilepsy. The experience and control of illness. Philadelphia: Temple University Press, 1983.

Sofijanow NG. Clinical evolution and prognosis of childhood epilepsies. Epilepsia 1982; 23: 61–9.
Strobos RRJ. Prognosis in convulsive disorders. Arch Neurol 1959; 1: 216–25.
Temkin O. The falling sickness. 2nd ed., revised. Baltimore, London: The Johns Hopkins Press, 1971.
Thorbecke R, Janz D. Guidelines for assessing the occupational possibilities of persons with epilepsy. In: Porter RJ et al. (eds) Advances in epileptology: XVth Epilepsy International Symposium. New York: Raven Press, 1984; 571–5.
Trolle E. Drug therapy in epilepsy. Acta Psychiatr Neurol Scand 1961; Suppl. 150: 187–99.
Tsai JJ. Langzeitresultate der medikamentösen Behandlung von Patienten mit psychomotorischen Anfällen. Eine Längsschnittuntersuchung an 155 Fällen. Med. Diss., Berlin, 1984.
Turner WA. Epilepsy, a study of idiopathic disease. London: Macmillan, 1907. Facsimile edition, New York: Raven Press, 1973: 272.
Walker AE. Post-traumatic epilepsy. World Neurol 1962; 3: 185–94.
Wessely P. Zur Bedeutung von Zeitfaktoren bei posttraumatischen Anfällen. In: Remschmidt H, Renz R, Jungmann J (eds) Epilepsi 1980. Thieme Stuttgart, New York, 1981: 138–43.
WHO. International classification of impairment, disabilities and handicaps. Geneva: World Health Organization, 1980.
Wolf P, Inoue Y. Therapeutic response of absence seizures in patients of an epilepsy clinic for adolescents and adults. J Neurol 1984; 231: 255–9.

4
The Monitoring of Chronic Epilepsy

C.D. Binnie
The Maudsley Hospital, London, UK

Introduction

Notwithstanding the sombre views traditionally held both by the layman and the physician, epilepsy has in general a favourable prognosis (Elwes et al., 1984). Chronicity should not, therefore, be regarded as the natural outcome, but rather as a therapeutic failure which demands radical reassessment of both diagnosis and treatment. Intensive monitoring of the EEG, of clinical ictal events, and possibly of serum antiepileptic blood levels, may play a crucial role in such reappraisal.

Differential Diagnosis of Epilepsy

Understandably, misdiagnosis frequently results in failed treatment of supposed epilepsy. In hospital-based studies using telemetric EEG and video monitoring, pseudoseizures apparently represent the major source of diagnostic error, whereas outpatient series using ambulatory monitoring with cassette recorders focus rather on the problems of differential diagnosis from cardiac dysrhythmias and syncope. Possibly this difference in clinical populations reflects the fact that, once the subject comes under inpatient observation, the clinical differential diagnosis between syncope and epilepsy rarely represents a major difficulty. For instance, the present author evaluating 370 consecutive referrals for intensive monitoring, of which 270 were for differential diagnosis, encountered none in which syncope or cardiac dysrhythmia was either suspected prior to the investigation, or established following monitoring. Over the

---

Chronic Epilepsy, Its Prognosis and Management
Edited by M.R. Trimble. © 1989 John Wiley & Sons

period of the study, six cases of cardiogenic attacks were proven in the same unit but without the need for monitoring, the diagnosis being suspected either on clinical grounds or because of abnormalities found in a half-hour single-channel ECG routinely recorded during EEG investigations. Evaluation studies suggest the yield of new information (as opposed to confirmation of a reasonably secure diagnosis) from prolonged ECG monitoring to be rather modest (Gibson and Heitzman, 1984). In any event where the differential diagnosis between cardiogenic and epileptic attacks is in doubt, it is important that both EEG and ECG should be monitored. Epileptic seizures may be accompanied by changes in cardiac rhythm ranging from tachy- or bradycardia to frank dysrhythmias or asystole (Blumhardt, Smith and Owen, 1986). Conversely, any change in cerebral function due to an acute cardiovascular disturbance will produce EEG changes. Excessive reliance on either EEG or ECG alone for the purpose of this particular differential diagnosis of seizures of uncertain origin invites misinterpretation (Blumhardt and Oozeer, 1982). In patients with epilepsy, interictal ECG abnormalities are no more common than in controls (Blumhardt, Smith and Owen, 1986), whereas patients with attacks of cardiac origin can usually be identified during monitoring by subclinical, or interictal, ECG arrhythmias (Schott, Mcleod and Jewett, 1977). The same is not true of the EEG, which often shows interictal abnormalities in patients with syncope (Graf et al., 1982).

Differential diagnosis of pseudoseizures represents the major single clinical application of intensive epilepsy monitoring, and is an issue which frequently arises when apparently epileptic attacks prove intractable to therapy. Again, the clinical picture appears to vary very much between different types of practice: while studies based on psychiatric referrals may suggest a combination of pseudoseizures and epilepsy to be exceedingly rare, in epileptological practice this is a common combination (Roy, 1979; Callaghan and McCarthy, 1982). The two are indeed sometimes causally linked. Successful treatment of previously intractable and disabling epilepsy is incomplete without appropriate psychosocial support to enable the patient to come to terms with a changed lifestyle. The response of a patient who has 'learned to live with epilepsy' to the abolition of his attacks may be to develop pseudoseizures. In patients without epilepsy, pseudoseizures are often dramatic and convulsive, and bear little resemblance to any ictal pattern commonly occurring in epilepsy (Desai, Porter and Penry, 1982). Those seen in patients with epilepsy are, however, often much more subtle, commonly representing a fragment, usually the initial events, of the patient's habitual epileptic seizure pattern. In a group of patients with pseudoseizures, often associated with epilepsy, and being investigated as inpatients of a specialized epilepsy unit, Binnie and Van der Wens (1986) found little difficulty in classifying the clinical manifestations according to the criteria of the International Classification of Epileptic Seizures. In this population few attacks occurred which, on clinical grounds alone, could confidently be classified as clearly not epileptic in origin.

The capture of seizures during monitoring frequently establishes whether or not they are epileptic in nature, but the dangers of extrapolating to assume that all of a patient's attacks are of the same nature will be appreciated. There is, moreover, a substantial group of patients in whom, even when technically adequate ictal recordings of the EEG and behaviour have been obtained, the issue remains in doubt. Changes in the scalp EEG during epileptic seizures do not necessarily involve the appearance of epileptiform activity, and may be extremely subtle or indeed apparently absent. The early literature on epilepsy monitoring (particularly studies using ambulatory cassette recorders) conceded this fact with apparent reluctance, and suggested that seizures without readily identifiable EEG changes were so very rare that a negative ictal EEG was prima facie evidence of a pseudoseizure. This is far from the case. An absence seizure is invariably accompanied by generalized spike–wave activity and a tonic–clonic seizure by generalized spikes and spike–wave discharges. However, other types even of generalized seizures may be accompanied by less obvious ictal changes: atonic seizures without other symptoms often produce only an electrodecremental change in the EEG (Egli et al., 1985), and this may, moreover, be confined to the region of the vertex where it will readily escape notice unless an appropriate recording montage is used. The presumed physiological mechanism underlying the concept of the complex partial seizure as defined in the 1981 classification (Dreifuss, 1981) involves extensive spread of the discharges, at least through the limbic system. Although ictal EEG change will usually be found, this does not necessarily produce spiky wave forms at surface contacts. The scalp EEG may show an electrodecremental change or the appearance of a rhythm remarkable only for its consistent association with the clinical seizure, or on account of an unusual topography.

Simple partial seizures with sensory or motor symptoms confined to a relatively small part of the body or with viscerosensory or psychic symptomatology may produce no change in the scalp EEG (Figure 1) (Wieser, 1979). This presents considerable difficulties for assessment of those patients with epilepsy who it is suspected may be exhibiting pseudoseizures consisting only of a viscerosensory aura, a subjective change as derealization, or brief twitching of one limb. The interpretation of a negative ictal EEG is therefore entirely dependent upon the concomitant clinical events. If the patient appears to be having any kind of seizure with loss of consciousness (tonic–clonic, absence or complex partial), the absence of ictal EEG change implies that the attack is not epileptic in origin. By contrast, the absence of ictal EEG changes during a simple partial seizure with psychic, viscerosensory or very limited motor symptoms, so far from being cause for suspicion, is the finding which was to be expected. Moreover, a complex partial seizure will occasionally be seen with very limited unilateral spread of the discharges and only minimal changes in the scalp EEG (Figure 2).

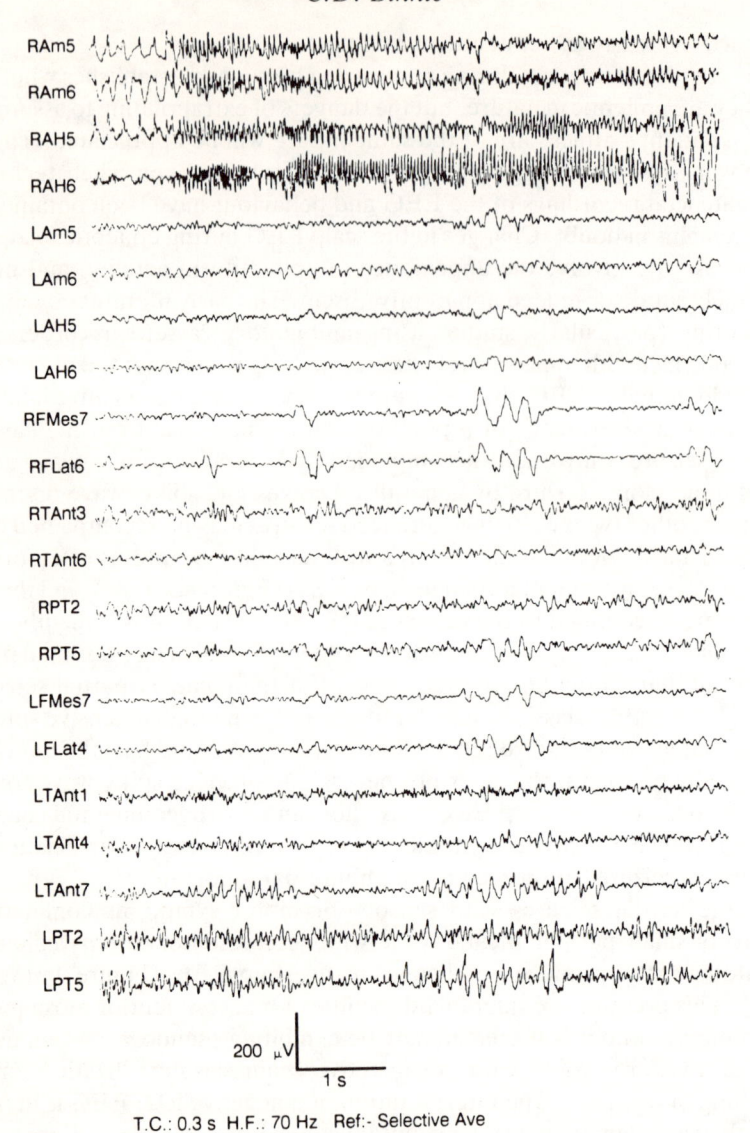

Figure 1. Simple partial seizure (rising epigastric sensation only), recorded with depth (channels 1–8) and subdural electrodes. Ictal discharges are virtually confined to deep right temporal contacts, are not recorded at subdural leads, and had not been detected in several previous ictal recordings with scalp electrodes

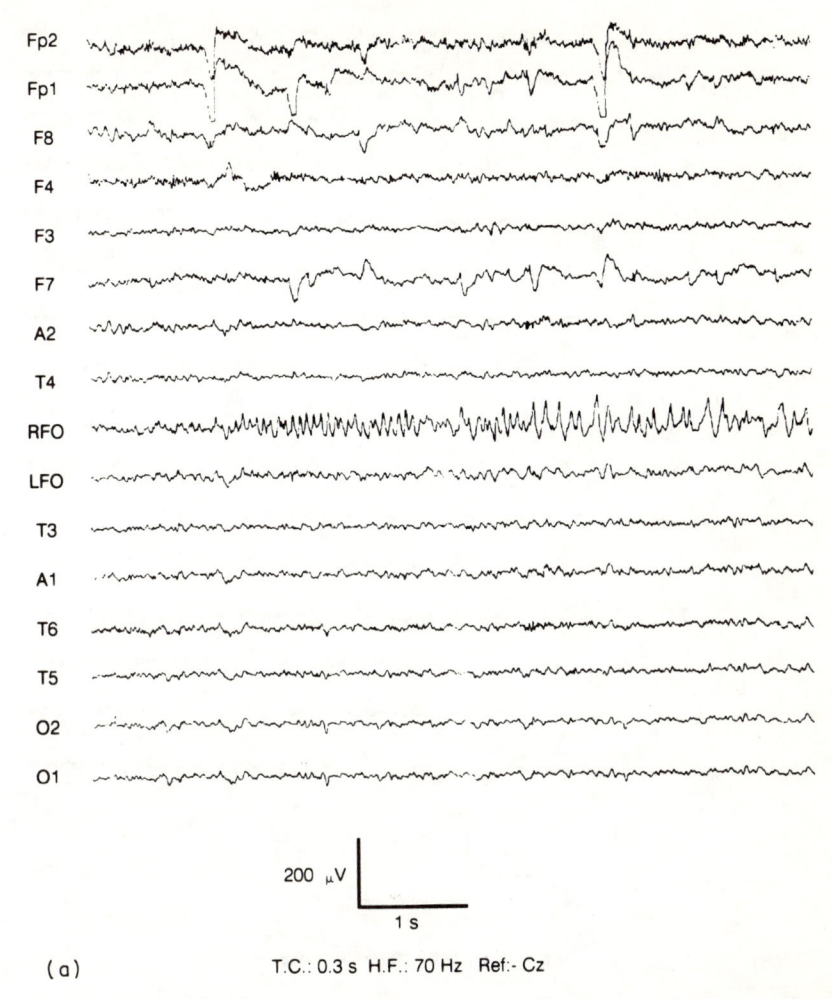

[EEG trace figure with channels: Fp2, Fp1, F8, F4, F3, F7, A2, T4, RFO, LFO, T3, A1, T6, T5, O2, O1; scale 200 μV, 1 s; T.C.: 0.3 s H.F.: 70 Hz Ref:- Cz]

(a)

Figure 2. Onset (a), middle (b), and late stage (c) of complex partial seizure with loss of consciousness, staring, and oroalimentary automatism, recorded with foramen ovale electrodes. Note that discharges are virtually confined to the right foramen ovale contact; they do not spread to the left and the changes at surface electrodes are minimal and not recognizable as ictal events

The above has implications for the choice of monitoring technology. Ambulatory monitoring without simultaneous video recording may safely be used to establish that a seizure is of epileptic origin, provided the ictal EEG phenomena are clearly distinguishable from artefact. However, if the EEG is apparently negative, its interpretation as evidence of a pseudoseizure is unsafe unless the time and nature of the attack are reliably established and it is known that the clinical symptoms were of a kind which, if of epileptic origin, should be

200 μV

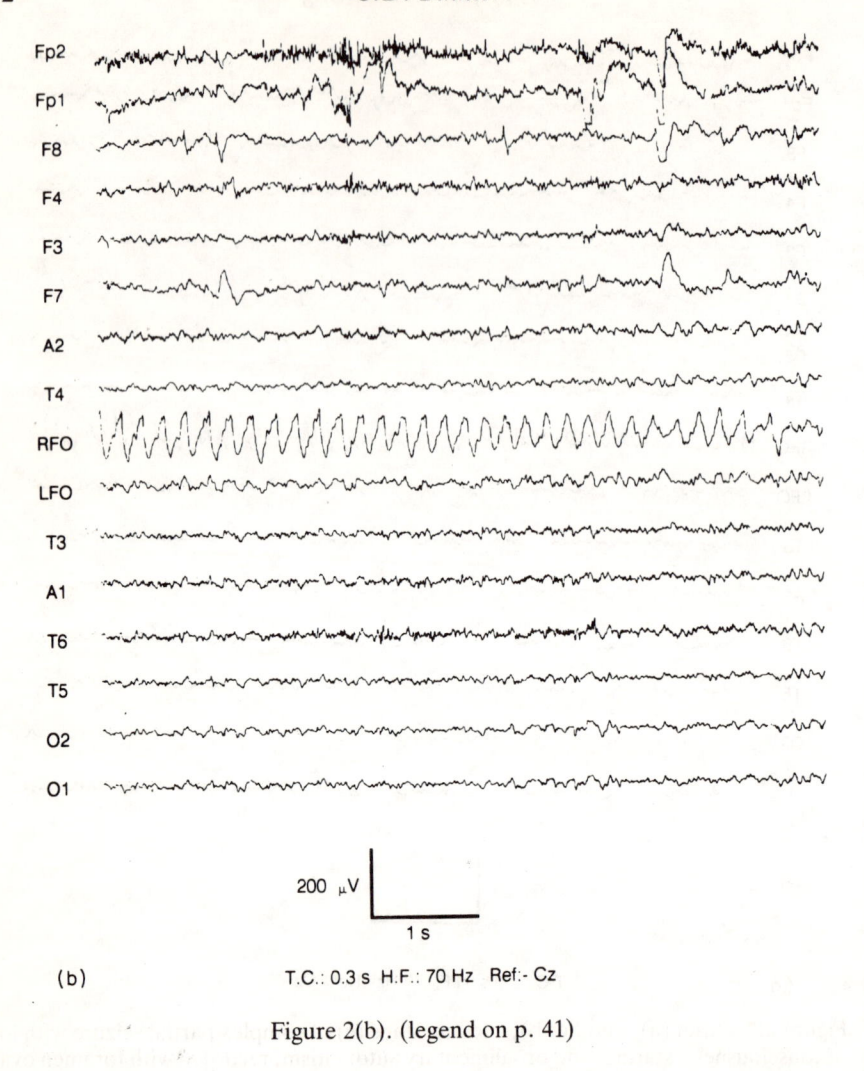

1 s

(b)   T.C.: 0.3 s H.F.: 70 Hz Ref:- Cz

Figure 2(b). (legend on p. 41)

accompanied by EEG changes. Often this is difficult to achieve without full EEG telemetry and video monitoring, and particular caution must be exercised in drawing conclusions from negative results of ambulatory cassette monitoring. Without a recording of high technical quality and video registration to determine the precise timing of the seizure, subtle changes in the scalp EEG will not be detected.

A further pitfall in the differential diagnosis of pseudoseizures by EEG monitoring arises in patients with attacks of frontal lobe origin, particularly those arising from foci in the orbital or mesial frontal region. Often 'bimanual–bipedal' seizures are seen: the patient exhibits symmetrical movements of

200 μV
1 s

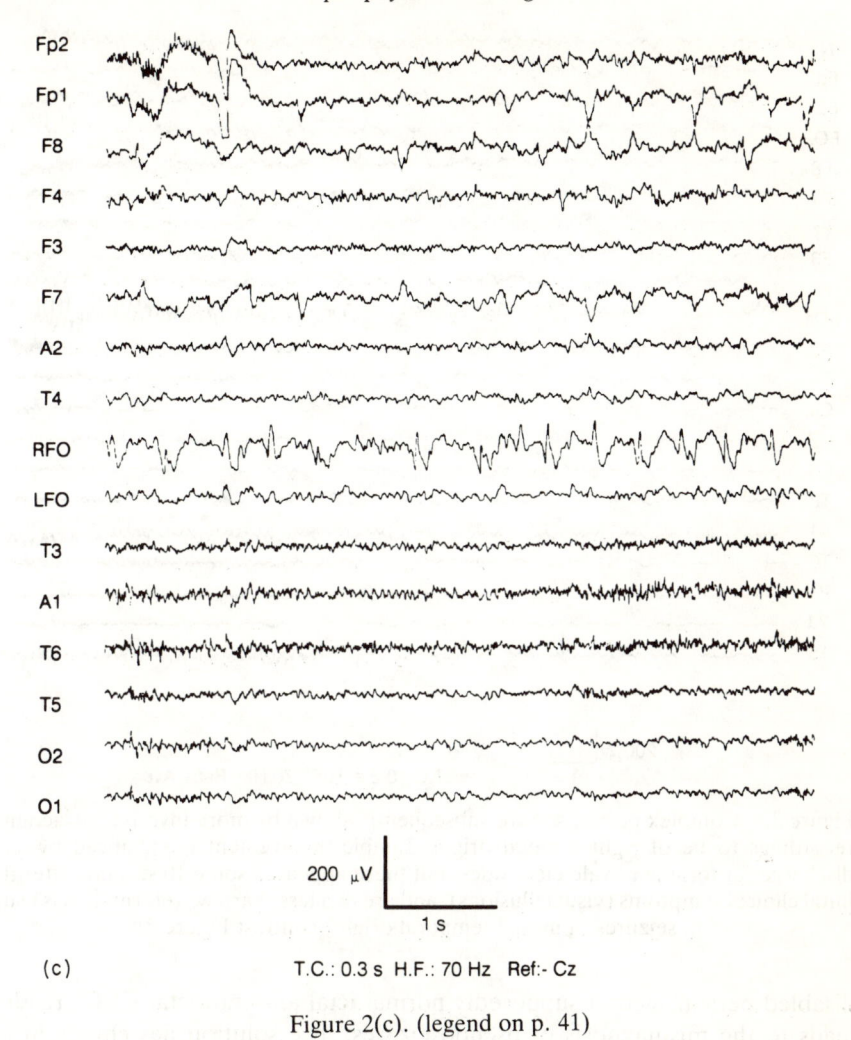

(c)   T.C.: 0.3 s H.F.: 70 Hz Ref:- Cz

Figure 2(c). (legend on p. 41)

limbs and trunk, may clap or play 'pat-a-cake' with the hands, stamp the feet, possibly run or sway backwards and forwards. The bizarre quality of the picture may be heightened by abusive or obscene utterances, and aggressive or overtly sexual behaviour. The interictal EEG is often unremarkable and ictal changes may be limited to bifrontal slow waves which are readily mistaken for eye movement artefacts. The patients are usually neurologically intact but may exhibit psychiatric abnormalities attributable in part to frontal lobe pathology or to the psychosocial consequences of the attacks and the uncertainties surrounding their diagnosis and management. This combination of attacks which lend themselves to a psychiatric interpretation, in a psychiatrically

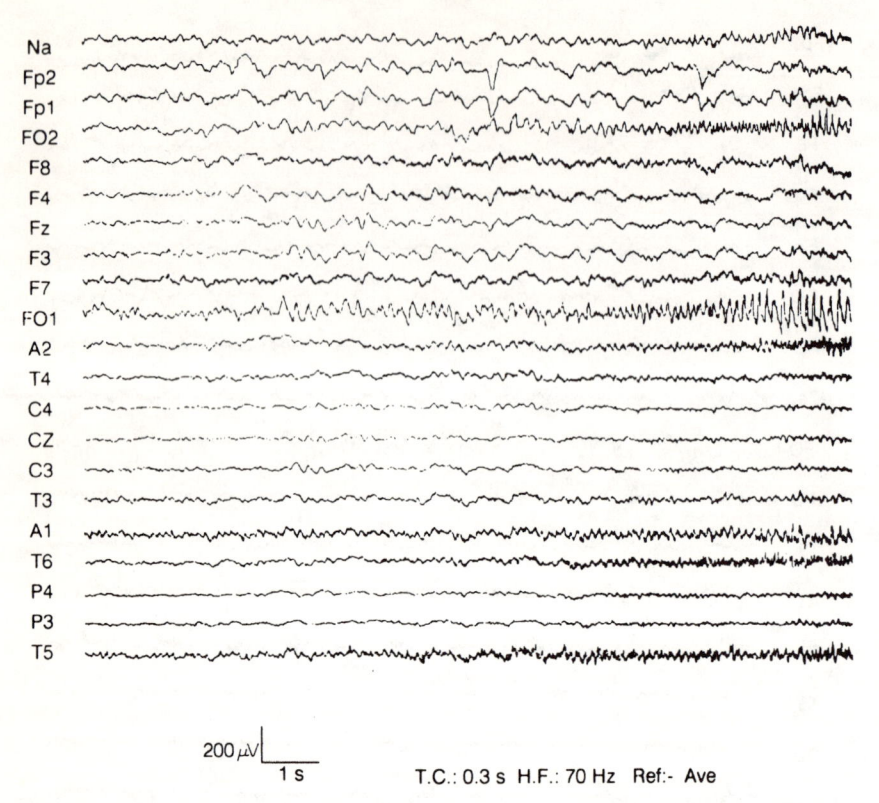

Figure 3. Complex partial seizure subsequently shown by more invasive intracranial recordings to be of right parietal origin. Limbic involvement is enhanced by ictal discharges at foramen ovale electrodes, but these appeared some 10 seconds after the inital clinical symptoms (visual illusions), and are of a less sharp waveform than is usual in seizures of mesial temporal origin (contrast Figure 2)

disabled person, with a supposedly normal ictal and interictal EEG, readily leads to the misdiagnosis of pseudoseizures. The solution lies chiefly in an awareness of the problem. The characteristic clinical pattern is easily recognizable by an experienced observer and should lead to a careful appraisal of the ictal EEG with particular reference to frontal slow waves.

In patients with possible simple partial seizures of temporal lobe origins or complex partial seizures in which ictal EEG change cannot confidently be excluded (e.g. on account of artefacts), a diagnostic solution may be provided by the use of foramen ovale electrodes (Wieser, Elger and Stodieck, 1985). In contrast to the long-established technique of sphenoidal recording from an electrode below the base of the skull, this method provides a true intracranial registration from single or multipolar electrodes inserted through the foramen ovale to lie alongside the medial aspect of the temporal lobe. The approach is familiar to every neurosurgeon who practises trigeminal thermocoagulation for neuralgia, and has thus far proved a relatively safe alternative to conventional implantation in the hands of its inventor and in our own series of some 70 cases. Even when a seizure arises elsewhere, if the limbic system is invaded (as is probably always the case in complex partial seizures) our experience to date suggests that changes are always detectable at one or both of the foramen ovale electrodes (Figure 3). Whilst there may be an understandable reluctance to use such invasive diagnostic techniques in possible pseudoseizures, they are not difficult to justify, as the degree of disability in these patients is no less than that in many of those undergoing assessment with a view to surgery.

Classification of Seizure Type

For didactic purposes it is taught that the various established antiepileptic drugs have a limited spectrum of action and that the choice of medication should be determined by the seizure type. Whilst there is indeed a degree of specificity which should determine the drug of first choice to be used in a newly diagnosed patient, the responses of the more refractory patients are unpredictable, and arguably the only specificity which exists concerns efficacy or otherwise in absences.

The differential diagnosis between absences and brief complex partial seizures is therefore most often chosen as the example to illustrate the use of monitoring for purposes of seizure classification as an aid to treatment of intractable epilepsy. A practical difficulty in making this distinction, even with the help of monitoring, is a certain vagueness in the International Classification of Epileptic Seizures. The entire range of clinical phenomenology seen in absences can also occur in complex partial seizures; thus by clinical criteria based on the seizure description alone, every absence could be a partial seizure. The distinction presumably rests on EEG findings; at any rate, the International Classification (Dreifuss, 1981) is described as 'clinical and electroencephalographic', but nowhere clearly states whether the EEG descriptions it contains are illustrative or essential criteria to be rigorously applied. Absences are accompanied by generalized symmetrical spike–wave activity; so also, however, are some complex partial seizures, and in practice the distinction often depends not on the clinical or electrographic features detected during monitoring, but on other considerations such as the age of the patient, the family history and the presence or absence of other features suggestive of local brain damage. In a series of patients with therapy-resistant 'absence-like attacks' (i.e. episodes of momentary impairment of consciousness with possibly some simple symmetrical automatisms), Binnie and Van der Wens (1986) found a range of ictal EEG phenomenology from stable foci through secondarily generalized discharges to symmetrical 3/s spike–wave activity. These findings were unrelated either to the detailed clinical features or to which medication proved most efficacious. In most patients this was a combination of drugs effective in absence seizures with those used in partial epilepsies (e.g. ethosuximide with phenytoin). Stefan and Burr (1986) and Henricksen (1986) found similar drug combinations to be most effective in therapy-resistant absence-like attacks. Except, therefore, in cases of obvious misdiagnosis where a proper history of an interictal EEG would indicate whether absences or complex partial seizures are more likely, it seems that monitoring as an aid to seizure classification may contribute little to the selection of treatment.

Determination of Seizure Frequency

Problems of drug control of resistant seizures may be exacerbated where the attacks themselves are frequent but are difficult to recognize. Estimates by patients, relatives and carers of the frequency of absences may be shown on monitoring to be very inaccurate (Sato et al., 1979). Similar considerations apply to brief partial seizures which may fall within the patient's normal behavioural repertoire. A momentary hesitation, a turning of the head to one side or an inappropriate smile, may be recognized as ictal events only by a consistent relationship to an EEG discharge. Difficulties may also be presented by brief, unrecognized nocturnal seizures, which may not cause any great inconvenience to the patient directly but have secondary consequences in disturbed sleep patterns and adverse effects on diurnal behaviour, particularly in children.

Thus in therapy-resistant patients with hard-to-recognize seizures, fine tuning of medication may be considerably helped by obtaining reliable estimates of seizure frequency from continuous monitoring (Rowan et al., 1979).

Preoperative Assessment

In that small group of therapy-resistant patients for whom surgery may offer a solution, the role of monitoring is often crucial. Surgical treatment of epilepsy follows three alternative strategies (see Polkey, Chapter 16):

(1) resection of a discrete focus of functionally and structurally abnormal brain from which the seizures arise,
(2) disconnection of pathways of seizure propagation (e.g. by callosotomy),
(3) removal of a large mass of dysfunctioning brain tissue (e.g. by hemispherectomy).

Various preoperative assessment programmes differ in the use which they make of monitoring and of more or less invasive methods of electrophysiological assessment (Engel, 1987). It clearly is possible to identify patients who may be successfully treated by surgery without the help of monitoring, much less the use of subacute intracranial recordings (Bloom, Jasper and Rasmussen, 1959; Polkey, 1981). Such patients will generally exhibit a discrete, usually temporal, lesion on radiological imaging at a site concordant with the clinical seizure pattern and interictal EEG findings. However, some surgical teams have successfully treated patients even without radiological abnormalities on the basis of a single, stable temporal EEG focus, and concordant clinical and neuropsychological findings (Polkey, 1981). Such patients typically have mesial temporal sclerosis, and it should be noted that successful treatment of epilepsy by resective surgery generally depends on removal of abnormal tissue: even where the structural abnormality is not demonstrable prior to operation, its presence is inferred from functional assessments.

However, to offer surgery only to these groups precludes a large portion of treatable patients, notably those without radiologically demonstrable lesions or in whom interictal EEG foci are multiple, extratemporal, absent, or at variance with other localizing evidence from clinical or neuropsychological assessment.

So rapid are the developments in this area that surgical protocols are continually changing; currently, the process of preoperative assessment at the Maudsley Hospital, London, proceeds as follows.

Phase Ia

Clinical evaluation Are the patient's attacks all epileptic in origin; are they resistant to appropriate medication in adequate dosage; do they represent a serious disability, having regard to the type and frequency of the seizures and the psychosocial status of the patient? One complex partial seizure in 6 months may be of more consequence for an actor than weekly tonic–clonic convulsions in a resident of a subnormality unit. An upper age limit of about 55 years is generally imposed, but there is no lower limit: continuous uncontrolled seizures may require surgery in an infant, and in a schoolchild 3 years therapeutic failure is ample to establish that complex partial seizures are intractable, and to justify surgery. Note that in deciding on admission to a preoperative assessment programme the presence of reported focal EEG abnormalities is not a requirement; if these are not found in conventional interictal records, alternative electrophysiological techniques are available for locating the site of seizure onset (see below).

At this point a choice can usually be made between the three possible surgical strategies:

(1) If the patient has partial epilepsy (with or without secondarily generalized seizures), has no evidence of extensive bilateral brain disease and has an IQ above 70, resective surgery is the first choice.
(2) Longstanding, preferably perinatal, gross, unilateral brain disease, with

seizures apparently arising only from the damaged hemisphere, suggests hemispherectomy to be appropriate.
(3) Generalized seizures, particularly if causing injury, and associated with bilateral brain disease, e.g. in secondary generalized epilepsy, may be relieved by callosotomy. Complete abolition of seizures is rare, but control of atonic or tonic–clonic attacks may greatly improve quality of life. EEG monitoring plays an important role only in the assessment for resective surgery, and the other strategies will not be considered further here.

Initial EEG assessment Wake and sleep EEGs are a minimum requirement. Most patients will have undergone previous examinations, but these will usually need to be repeated with particular attention paid to localization of any abnormalities. Non-standard, anterior temporal electrode placements may be required to determine topography of fronto-temporal discharges (Morris and Lüders, 1985). Except where the clinical and EEG findings clearly point to a non-temporal focus, sphenoidal recording with activation by intravenous barbiturates is required. If suitable surface placements have been used, sphenoidal recording as such will not reveal previously undetected foci, but may permit a distinction to be made between a mesial temporal and lateral temporal location (Binnie et al., 1989). Abnormalities of background activity, including asymmetry of barbiturate-induced fast activity, provide further clues to localization or lateralization of structural brain disease and may serve to support (or otherwise) focus localization, or to indicate which of two foci is more likely to be the source of the seizures.

It should perhaps at this point be explained that in patients with seizures of temporal lobe origin, precise localization of the focus has acquired a new significance since the introduction of selective amygdalo-hippocampectomy (Yasargil, Teddy and Roth, 1985). Traditional operations for en bloc or partial resection of the temporal lobe, which remove both the deep mesial structures and also neocortex, produce significant cognitive deficits. These are acceptable, provided the contralateral temporal lobe can adequately support memory function (this can be determined by the carotid amytal test). Amygdalo-hippocampectomy avoids or greatly reduces the deficits, and moreover offers the possibility of surgical treatment even in patients with bilateral damage. It thus appears to be the operation of choice in patients with a mesial temporal focus, without a gross lesion requiring more extensive resection and with evidence (e.g. from the carotid amytal test) of residual cognitive function worth preserving in the affected temporal lobe. It is the only operation which can be offered to patients in whom the contralateral hemisphere does not support memory. Except where there is radiological evidence of a small discrete mesial temporal lesion, selection of patients for amygdalo-hippocampectomy requires neurophysiological proof of a mesial temporal focus. This apparent digression may help to explain much of what follows.

Neuroradiology and Neuropsychology CT scans may reveal either lesions producing altered tissue density or atrophy manifest by increased CSF space, notably dilatation of one temporal horn in mesial temporal sclerosis (MTS). This last may be demonstrable only in scans taken with a gantry tilted 20°, along the axis of the temporal horns. MRI may detect more subtle structural abnormalities and PET scans may demonstrate extensive hypoperfusion, which is non-localizing but indicates the lobe or hemisphere from which the seizures most probably arise.

Neuropsychological assessment may indicate the side of pathology and warn of possible problems, due for instance to dysfunction of the hemisphere contralateral to the focus.

Preliminary assessment The presence of an operable, radiologically demonstrable lesion at a site concordant with the clinical, psychological and EEG findings will usually provide sufficient basis for operation.

Frequent (secondarily) generalized EEG discharges, or an overall EEG picture suggesting secondary generalized epilepsy, may indicate that a successful outcome is unlikely and that further preoperative assessment should be abandoned. In all other cases further investigations are required.

Phase Ib

Carotid amytal test In most patients with suspected temporal foci, and in some others, a carotid amytal test will be required to lateralize speech and to determine what deficits may result from operation. It may also help in other patients to lateralize the focus underlying secondarily generalized discharges, as these will be abolished when the side of the focus is anaesthetized.

EEG monitoring Ictal recordings obtained by monitoring using conventional electrode placements (including sphenoidal leads) may be of surprisingly little value in preoperative assessment. Whereas in partial epilepsies, particularly of temporal lobe origin, interictal discharges may be clearly focal and apparently stable, ictal changes in the scalp EEG during complex partial seizures are often ill-localized or bilateral. In seizures of temporal lobe origin, lateralization by ictal scalp EEGs is far from reliable, and in seizures of frontal lobe origin may be virtually random (Spencer et al., 1985).

As indicated above, the deficiencies of ictal scalp EEG recordings can now to some extent be overcome without recourse to conventional implantation of depth or subdural electrodes by the use of foramen ovale electrodes (Wieser, Elger and Stodieck, 1985). In patients with bitemporal interictal foci, the site of origin of the seizures can usually be lateralized by this method, and to meet the criteria for amygdalo-hippocampectomy, a mesial temporal origin of partial seizures can usually be reliably distinguished from a more lateral focus by ictal recordings with a combination of scalp and foramen ovale electrodes.

Even where a mesial temporal origin is not found, and possibly not expected, monitoring with scalp and foramen ovale electrodes may nevertheless be of value, providing justification for the use of more invasive techniques and offering some indication of the most likely site or side of origin of the seizures, to guide subsequent implantation. For instance, the appearance of epileptiform discharges at one foramen ovale contact some seconds after the onset of clinical ictal symptoms provides both a guide to lateralization and evidence that the attacks probably (but not necessarily) arise outside the temporal lobes. Conversely, generalized spike–wave activity at seizure onset may indicate that, even if a focus can be demonstrated by depth recording, a successful outcome of surgical treatment is rather unlikely (Lieb et al., 1981) and preoperative assessment should probably be abandoned.

Reassessment In patients with seizures of temporal origin, it will generally be possible at this point to choose between en bloc resection, amygdalohippocampectomy, or abandoning surgery (this last chiefly where there is a lateral temporal focus, and the contralateral temporal lobe does not support memory). Preoperative assessment may also be abandoned in patients with multifocal or generalized discharges at seizure onset, and in those considered unable to co-operate or to cope with further, more invasive investigations.

Phase II

Depth or subdural recording The technical details and clinical applications of intracranial recording are beyond the scope of the present discussion, but it may be noted that the need to map the location and consistency of onset within an electrode array which commonly includes upwards of 100 contacts demands prolonged monitoring and has created the requirement for systems with many more channels than the sixteen or so provided by most commercially available telemetry apparatus. Most groups employ either subdural electrode grids and strips or depth bundles, or sometimes first subdural electrodes and later depth if localization is still in doubt. In patients with complex partial seizures the Maudsley team employ a somewhat unorthodox technique developed by the Utrecht team (Van Veelen et al., 1979) which allows depth and subdural electrodes to be combined. The argument for this approach is that both depth and subdural electrodes alone can give misleading results. Depth electrodes sample only a very small volume of tissue and the number that can be implanted is necessarily limited; it is therefore possible to misinterpret as the site of seizure onset the first electrode to which ictal discharges spread from a focus which has not been implanted. Conversely, combined depth and subdural recordings (Figure 4) demonstrate that once discharges spread from deep structures they may first appear at surface contacts contralateral to the site of origin. In patients where a focus over the convexity, or high on the mesial

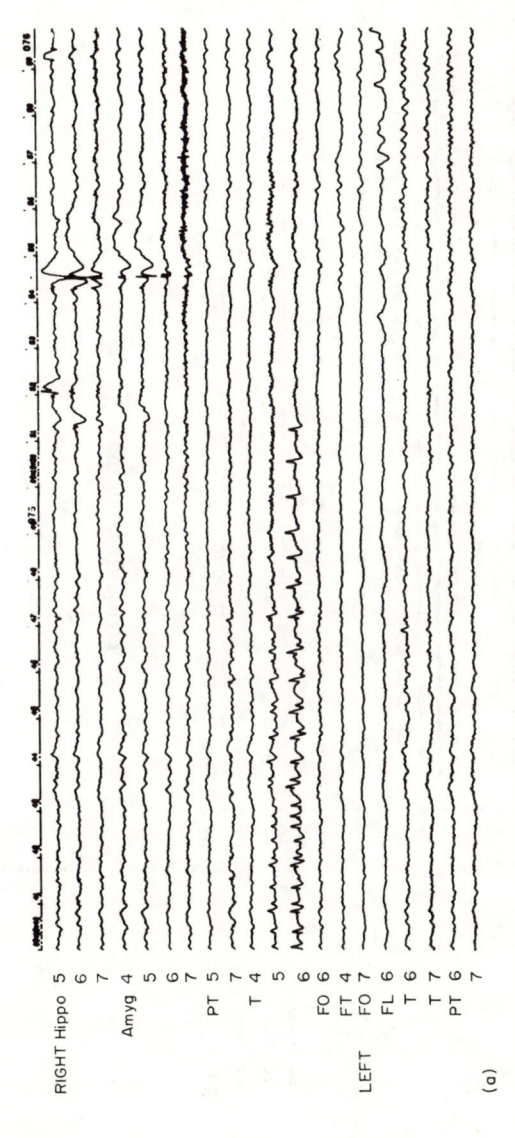

Figure 4. Depth and subdural recordings of a complex partial seizure arising in right amygdala. Patient is now seizure-free following right temporal lobectomy; pathology is mesial temporal sclerosis. Note onset with high-frequency multi-unit activity in right amygdala. When lateral neocortex is invaded, the most prominent changes are on the left, contralateral to the focus. Ictal recordings with scalp electrodes had understandably suggested incorrect lateralization. (Reproduced by permission of Binnie, CD. in Laidlaw J, Oxley J, Richen AJ (eds), A Textbook of Epilepsy, 3rd ed. Edinburgh: Livingstone, 1987)

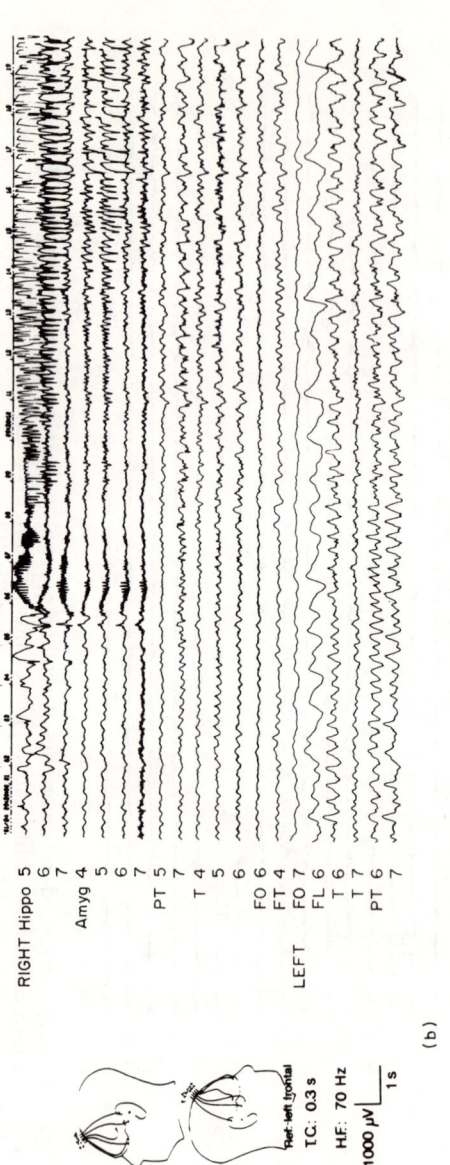

Figure 4(b). (legend on p. 51)

Figure 4(c). (legend on p. 51)

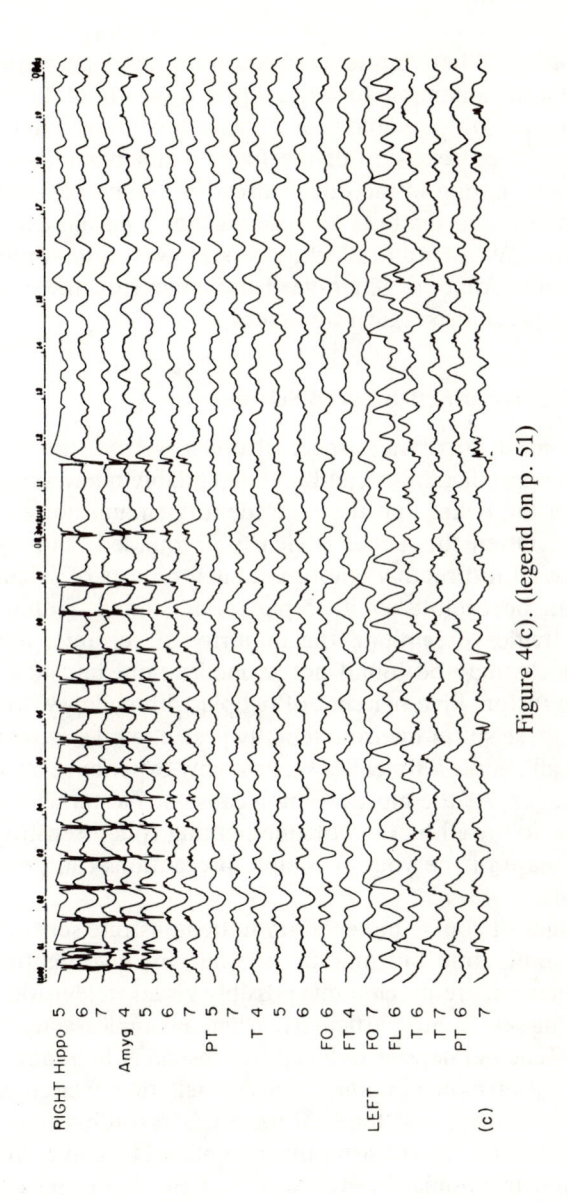

aspect of the hemisphere, is expected, subdural mats and strips are used, both for ictal recording and for functional mapping by evoked responses and by electrical stimulation.

Final assessment Where intracranial recording has demonstrated a consistent ictal onset at a site amenable to surgical removal without the risk of unacceptable neurological or psychological deficit, operation will now usually be offered. Even where excision of the focus is not possible, multiple subpial transection, preventing intracortical spread of discharges by a series of incisions, may be used instead of, or to supplement, partial excision, with good results (Morrell, Whisler and Bleck, 1989). However, multiple sites of seizure onset, or the appearance of generalized discharges from the start of the seizure, will generally preclude surgical treatment.

Detection of Reflex or Self-Induced Seizures

Perhaps the most horrifying aspect of epilepsy from the standpoint of the patient is its unpredictability, and understandably many sufferers take some comfort from the belief that they can identify circumstances which bring on their attacks. Often this belief is clearly ill-founded, and consequently the clinician may all too readily ignore patients' reports of seizure precipitants. Where it can be established that particular stimuli, situational factors or cognitive activities precipitate the majority of seizures, a solution to the patient's attacks may be found not in medication, but in avoidance of the precipitating factor. Five per cent of people with epilepsy are photosensitive and 70% of these suffer environmentally precipitated seizures; indeed, 50%, i.e. 2.5% of all people with epilepsy, probably experience exclusively visually triggered attacks. As the most common cause in Western society is television viewing, now followed by discotheque lighting (photosensitive epilepsy is in general a disease of the young), simple precautions can prevent seizures in many patients.

Monitoring is of course unnecessary to demonstrate sensitivity to intermittent photic stimulation but may be of value for investigating the role of a specific alleged seizure precipitant, possibly visual (television viewing, discotheque lighting, etc.), but particularly when a complex activity or situation is implicated. Reflex epilepsies induced, for instance, by reading, eating, chess playing, etc., often depend upon a total constellation of circumstances. Simply causing a patient to ingest food during EEG recording may be ineffectual, although seizures can be consistently precipitated by eating in a normal social context at table in a domestic environment. EEG recording during replication of circumstances alleged to induce seizures is greatly facilitated by the enhanced mobility offered by telemetry or ambulatory monitoring.

A category of reflex seizures of particular concern in the context of therapy resistance are those which are deliberately induced by the patient. By far the most common form of precipitation is visual, the patients being photosensitive. Some of these subjects are easily identified by a history of staring at bright lights whilst waving the spread fingers of one hand in front of the eyes (Andermann et al., 1962). However, a more common inducing manoeuvre involves slow eye closure with forced upward deviation of the eyes (Green, 1966), which telemetric studies suggest is carried out by some 25–30% of photosensitive subjects (Binnie et al., 1980). The phenomenon is easily recognizable but the history may give the impression that the reported eye movements are themselves ictal events or merely represent a nervous tic. Where there is any doubt this can be resolved by EEG and video monitoring of a few hours duration in a well-lit environment. Characteristically, the slow eyelid closures are followed often but not entirely consistently by generalized spike–wave activity. If the patient is stressed, e.g. by an interview with a doctor in a white coat, the frequency of the movements and discharges increases, sometimes to many dozens per hour. If the lighting is dimmed, the movements will continue, initially at least, but are no longer followed by discharges. Until one has gained the patient's confidence, any discussion of self-induction generally elicits an indignant denial, although later most patients will admit to a pleasurable sensation or relief of tension. Self-induced seizures are notoriously therapy resistant (Hutchinson, Stone and Davidson, 1958; Rail, 1973), and monitoring in a well-lit environment is indicated in any therapy-resistant photosensitive patient to determine whether or not self-induction occurs.

Conclusion

Porter, Penry and Lacy (1977) estimate that some 5% of people with epilepsy will require monitoring at some stage of their management. Sutula et al. (1981) showed that admission to an intensive reassessment programme greatly improved seizure control in previously resistant epilepsy and suggested that monitoring played a major role in such improvement. An evaluation study by Binnie in 1987 suggested that monitoring led to management decisions which resulted in sustained clinical improvement in 23% of a series of patients referred for intensive investigation. The advent of epilepsy monitoring has contributed significantly to improved management of previously therapy-resistant patients, and in centres where these techniques are routinely used, the incidence of eventual chronicity amongst newly diagnosed patients may be as low as 10% (Reynolds, personal communication).

References

Andermann K, Oaks G, Berman S et al. Self-induced epilepsy. Arch Neurol 1962; 6: 49–65.
Binnie CD. Ambulatory diagnostic monitoring of seizures in the adult. Adv Neurol 1987; 46: 169–182.

Binnie CD, Van der Wens P. Diagnostic re-evaluation by intensive monitoring of intractable absence seizures. In: Schmidt D, Morselli PL (eds) Intractable epilepsy: experimental and clinical aspects. New York: Raven Press, 1986; 99–107.

Binnie CD, Darby CE, De Korte RA, Wilkins AJ. Self-induction of epileptic seizures by eye closure: incidence and recognition. J Neurol Neurosurg Psychiatry 1980; 43: 386–9.

Binnie CD, Marston D, Polkey CE, Amin D. Distribution of temporal spikes in relation to the sphenoidal electrode. Electroencephalogr Clin Neurophysiol 1989; in press.

Bloom D, Jasper H, Rasmussen T. Surgical therapy in patients with temporal lobe seizures and bilateral EEG abnormality. Epilepsia 1959; 1: 351–65.

Blumhardt LD, Oozeer R. Simultaneous ambulatory monitoring of the EEG and ECG in patients with unexplained transient disturbances of consciousness. In: Stott FD, Raftery EB, Clement DL, Wright SL (eds) ISAM-GENT-1981: Proceedings of the Fourth International Symposium on Ambulatory Monitoring and Second Gent Workshop on Blood Pressure Variability. London: Academic Press, 1982: 172–82.

Blumhardt LD, Smith PEM, Owen L. Electrocardiographic accompaniments of temporal lobe epileptic seizures. Lancet 1986; i: 1051–6.

Callaghan N, McCarthy N. Ambulatory EEG monitoring in fainting attacks with normal routine and sleep EEG records. In: Stefan H, Burr W (eds) Mobile Long-Term EEG Monitoring: Proceedings of the MLE Symposium Bonn 1982. Stuttgart: Fischer, 1982: 61–5.

Desai BT, Porter RJ, Penry JK. Psychogenic seizures: a study of 42 attacks in six patients, with intensive monitoring. Arch Neurol 1982; 39: 202–9.

Dreifuss FE. Proposal for revised clinical and electroencephalographic classification of epileptic seizures. Epilepsia 1981; 22: 489–501.

Egli M, Mothersill I, O'Kane M, O'Kane F. The axial spasm—the predominant type of drop epilepsy in patients with secondary generalized epilepsy. Epilepsia 1985; 26: 401–5.

Elwes RDC, Johnson AL, Shorvon SD, Reynolds EH. The prognosis for seizure control in newly diagnosed epilepsy. N Engl J Med 1984; 311: 944–7.

Engel J. Approaches to localization of the epileptogenic lesion. In: Engel J (ed.) Surgical treatment of the epilepsies. New York: Raven Press, 1987: 75–100.

Gibson TC, Heitzman MR. Diagnostic efficacy of 24-hour electrocardiographic monitoring for syncope. Am J Cardiol 1984: 53: 1013–17.

Graf M, Brunner G, Weber H, Auinger C, Joskowicz G. Simultaneous long-term recording of EEG and ECG in 'syncope' patients. In: Stefan H, Burr W (eds) Mobile Long-Term EEG Monitoring: Proceedings of the MLE Symposium Bonn 1982. Stuttgart: Fischer 1982: 7–75.

Green JB. Self-induced seizures: clinical and electroencephalographic studies. Arch Neurol 1966; 15: 579–86.

Henricksen O. Absence seizures: multiple and reduction of multiple drug therapy. In: Schmidt D, Morselli P (eds). Intractable epilepsy: experimental and clinical aspects. New York: Raven Press, 1986: 187–93.

Hutchinson JH, Stone FH, Davidson JR. Photogenic epilepsy induced by the patient. Lancet 1958; i: 243–5.

Lieb JP, Engel J, Gevins A, Crandall PH. Surface and deep EEG correlates of surgical outcome in temporal lobe epilepsy. Epilepsia 1981; 22: 515–38.

Morrell F, Whisler WW, Bleck T. Multiple subpial transection: a new approach to the surgical treatment of focal epilepsy. J Neurosurg 1989; 70: 231–9.

Morris HH, Lüders H. Electrodes. Electroencephalogr Clin Neurophysiol 1985; 37 (suppl.): 3–25.

Polkey CE. Selection of patients with chronic drug-resistant epilepsy for resective surgery: 5 years' experience. J R Soc Med 1981; 74: 574–9.

Porter RJ, Penry JK, Lacy JR. Diagnostic and therapeutic reevaluation of patients with intractable epilepsy. Neurology (Minneap) 1977; 27: 1006–11.
Rail LR. The treatment of self-induced photic epilepsy. Proc Aust Assoc Neurol 1973; 9: 121–3.
Rowan AJ, Binnie CD, De Beer-Pawlikowski NKB, et al. Sodium Valproate: serial monitoring of EEG and serum levels. Neurology (Minneap) 1979; 29: 1450–9.
Roy A. Hysterical seizures. Arch Neurol 1979; 36: 447.
Sato S, Penry JK, White BG, Dreifuss FE, Sackellares JC. Double-blind crossover study of sodium valproate and ethosuximide in the treatment of absence seizures. Neurology (Minneap) 1979; 29: 603.
Schott GD, McLeod AA, Jewett DE. Cardiac arrythmias that masquerade as epilepsy. Br Med J 1977; 1: 1454–957.
Spencer SS, Williamson PD, Bridgers SL, Mattson RH, Ciccetti DV, Spencer DD. Reliability and accuracy of localization by scalp ictal EEG. Neurology 1985; 35: 1567–75.
Stefan H, Burr W. Absence signs: long term therapeutic monitoring. In: Schmidt D, Morselli P (eds) Intractable epilepsy. New York: Raven Press, 1986: 175–85.
Sutula TP, Sackellares JC, Miller JQ, Dreifuss FE. Intensive monitoring in refractory epilepsy. Neurology 1981; 31: 243–7.
Van Veelen CWM, Debets RMC, Van Huffelen AC, et al. Combined use of subdural and intracerebral electrodes in preoperative evaluation of epilepsy. J Neurosurg 1989; submitted.
Wieser HG. 'Psychische Anfalle' und deren stereoelektroenzephalographisches Korrelat. EEG EMG 1979; 10: 197–206.
Wieser HG, Elger CE, Stodieck SRG. The 'Foramen Ovale Electrode': a new recording method for the preoperative evaluation of patients suffering from mesiobasal temporal lobe epilepsy. Electroencephalogr Clin Neurophysiol 1985; 61: 314–22.
Yasargil MG, Teddy PG, Roth P. Selective amygdalo-hippocampectomy. Operative anatomy and surgical technique. In: Symon L (ed.) Advances and technical standards in neurosurgery. vol. 12. Wien: Springer-Verlag, 1985: 93–123.

5
CT and PET in Drug-resistant Epilepsy

D. Fish
Montreal Neurological Institute, Montreal, Canada

General Considerations

Most patients with drug-resistant epilepsy have partial seizures, with or without secondary generalization. Their prognosis and the possibility of surgical treatment are determined by the aetiology and localization of the epileptogenic process. Unfortunately it is rare for definitive information about either of these problems to be obtained from a single investigation. Clinical decisions are usually based upon an accumulation of data derived from different sources: clinical and neuropsychological assessments, neurophysiology and neuroimaging. These diverse investigations are not competitive but complementary, concordance between the findings of different modalities being an important factor in the identification of surgical candidates (Andermann, 1987).

CT provides information about structure, whereas PET may demonstrate functional abnormalities. Both techniques have made important contributions to the neuroimaging of patients with epilepsy, although each has limitations which may affect the interpretation of results.

The clinical value of these tests will be considered in relation to the following:

(1) the yield of abnormal results,
(2) technical and biological constraints,
(3) special techniques used to study epilepsy,
(4) the integration of findings with those derived from other modalities.

Chronic Epilepsy, Its Prognosis and Management
Edited by M.R. Trimble. © 1989 John Wiley & Sons

CT in Drug-resistant Epilepsy

Yield of Abnormal Results

CT scanning has been used to identify structural abnormalities in patients with epilepsy since the early 1970s (Gastaut and Gastaut, 1976). Several large series have demonstrated CT abnormalities in approximately 40–70% of patients with epilepsy (Angeleri et al., 1976; Caille et al., 1976; Collard, Dupont and Noel, 1976; Gall, Becker and Hacker, 1976; Gastaut and Gastaut, 1976; Guberman, 1983; Jabbari et al., 1978, 1980; Lagenstein et al., 1979; Mosely and Bull, 1976; Scollo-Lavizerri, Eichan and Wuthrich, 1976; Yang et al., 1979), with obvious fluctuations related to patient selection. However, these figures often include findings of uncertain clinical significance, such as generalized atrophy. The percentage of clinically relevant abnormalities may be much lower (Bachman, Hodger and Freeman, 1976; Jabbari et al., 1980).

Although it is well established that CT lesions are particularly frequent in patients with partial epilepsy (Angeleri et al., 1976; Gastaut and Gastaut, 1976; Guberman, 1983; McGahan, Dublin and Hill, 1979), it is difficult to determine the true incidence of useful CT abnormalities in drug-resistant epilepsy. These patients have usually been seen by several physicians since the onset of their seizures, and referral patterns will have been influenced by the previous clinical, EEG and radiological findings. However, it is clear that CT often provides important information in such cases. Spencer et al. (1984) reported clinically unsuspected focal CT abnormalities in 15% of 190 patients with drug-resistant epilepsy. In agreement with these results, Rich, Goldring and Gado (1985) found focal CT lesions in 22% of 137 patients with normal neurological examinations undergoing surgical treatment for epilepsy. Munari et al. (1987) reported a somewhat higher proportion of clinically relevant CT abnormalities (54%) in a group of 82 patients referred for stereotaxic EEG, possibly reflecting the method of patient selection.

Probably the most important CT abnormality in drug-resistant epilepsy is a hypodense lesion (Figure 1), which may contain calcification. In the absence of other diagnostic information, this is more likely to represent a glioma than other types of neoplasms, or benign conditions such as a hamartoma, cerebral infarction, arachnoid cyst or vascular malformation. Twenty-six out of the 32 lesions identified by Rich, Goldring and Gado (1985) in patients with intractable seizures were proven to be gliomas. Fifteen of them were hypodense, 12 were calcified, and 6 showed enhancement on CT. Thirty-two out of 35 hypodense CT lesions presenting as epilepsy that were biopsied by Wilden and Kelly (1987) were found to be gliomas. Even lesions which have remained static for many years should be treated with suspicion. Slowly growing tumours may cause seizures many years before other neurological sequelae become evident, and malignant change may occur in previously stable lesions (Rich, Goldring and Gado, 1985; Jabbari et al., 1980). Spencer et al. (1984) found a

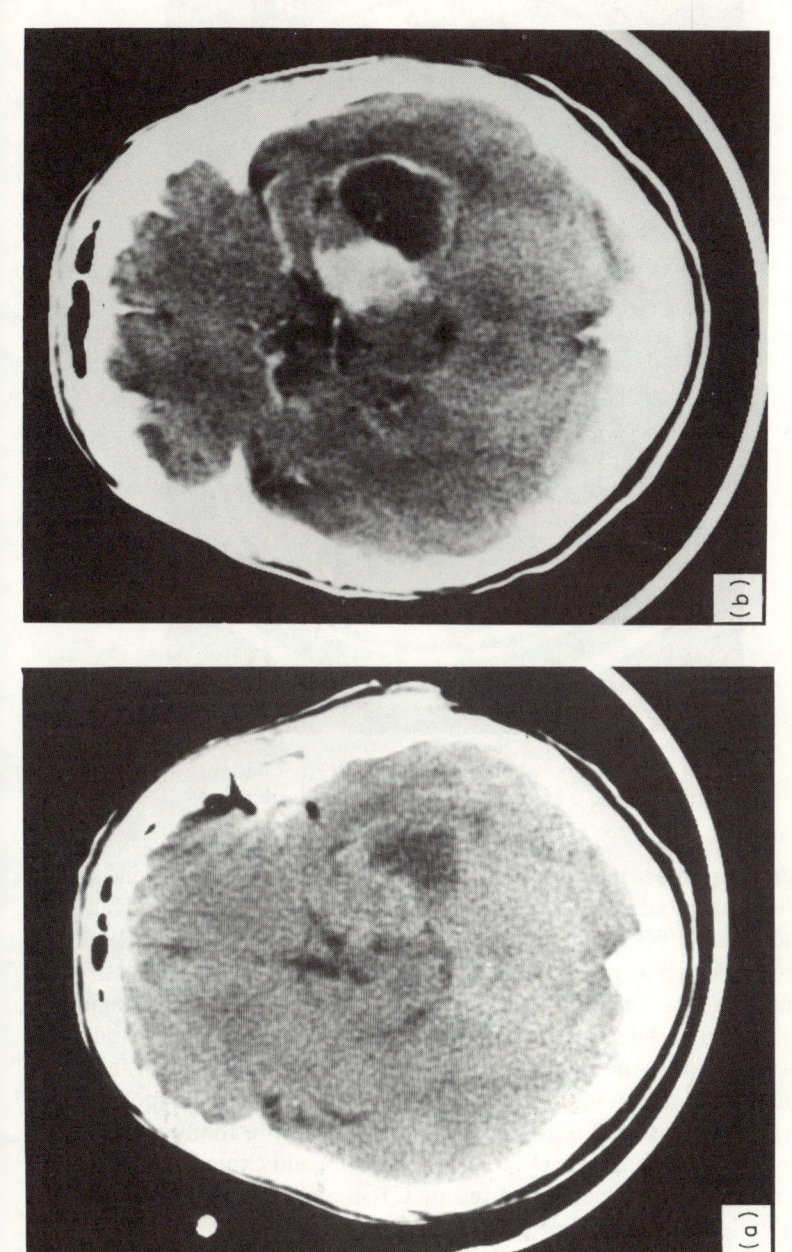

Figure 1. Plain CT scan (a) and following intravenous iodinated contrast (b) in a 52-year-old patient with a 28-year history of complex partial seizures, showing a left temporal hypodense contrast-enhancing lesion. Subsequent histology showed a glioma

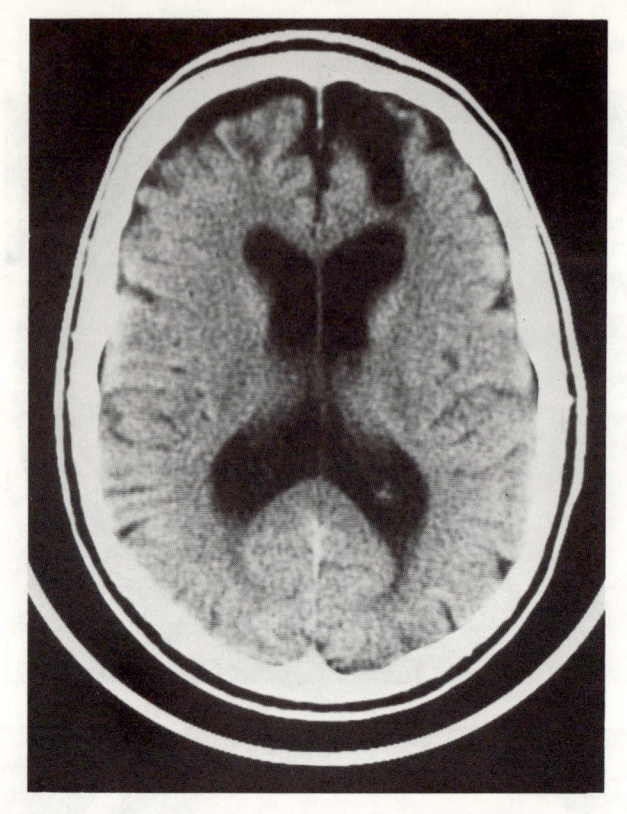

Figure 2. Bifrontal atrophy, more marked on the left, in a patient with frontal lobe epilepsy and a history of traumatic forceps delivery

mean interval from seizure onset to tumour detection of 11 years, and similar latent periods have been found by other workers (Blume, Girvin and Kaufman, 1982; Rasmussen, 1983; Rich, Goldring and Gado, 1985; Guberman, 1983).

Many conditions may present as drug-resistant epilepsy, and the possible CT findings are legion. These include focal atrophy (Figure 2), meningiomas, angiomas, tuberose sclerosis, and cerebral dysgenesis. The diagnostic probabilities will obviously be influenced by environmental and clinical factors as well as the radiological features. For example, ring-enhancing hypodense CT lesions in patients with epilepsy living in India are more likely to be due to tuberculosis than to neoplasia (Wadia et al., 1987), and clinically unsuspected cerebral infarcts may be demonstrated by CT in almost 10% of patients with late-onset epilepsy (Shorvon et al., 1984).

CT lesions are occasionally found in patients with drug-resistant generalized epilepsy (Gastaut and Gastaut, 1976), although the pathophysiological significance of these is uncertain.

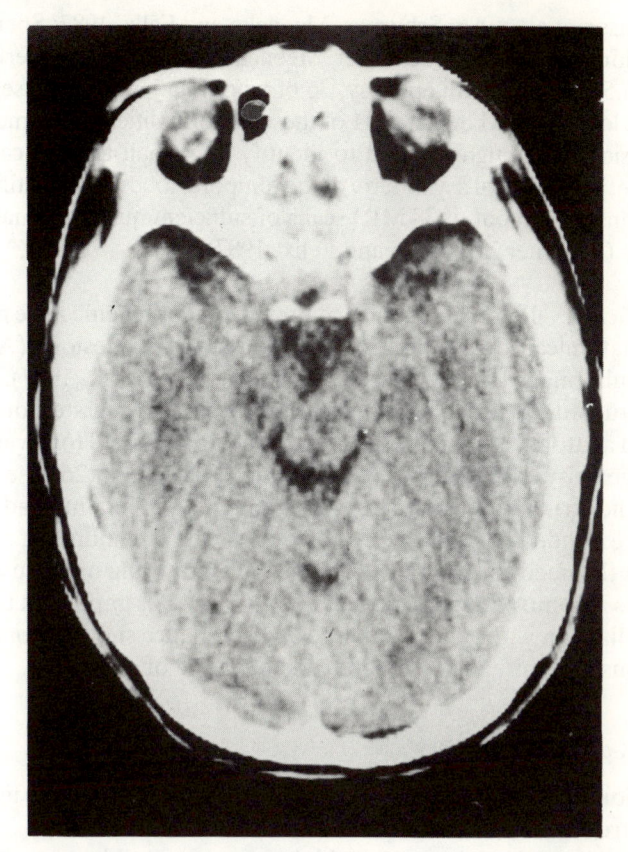

Figure 3. Plain CT scan showing mild beam hardening streak artefact in both temporal lobes due to the skull base

Limitations of CT in Drug-resistant Epilepsy

Technical factors Apparent asymmetry of the temporal horns is readily manufactured by slight head rotation. Therefore this CT finding is only reliable when gross changes are observed (Blom et al., 1984). Further difficulties in the assessment of the inferomesial temporal region result from beam hardening artefact due to the adjacent skull base (Blom et al., 1984; Guberman, 1983), as shown in Figure 3.

CT may fail to detect small or radiologically isodense lesions that do not have mass effect. Serial CT scans have revealed the presence of tumours that were not detected by previous examinations (Blume, Girvin and Kaufman, 1982; Guberman, 1983; Spencer et al., 1984), and focal gliosis is rarely demonstrated even by high-resolution CT (Schorner, Meencke and Felix, 1987). In recent years it has become clear that MRI is superior to CT in the detection of such lesions (Ormson et al., 1986; Schorner, Meencke and Felix, 1987; Sperling et al., 1986; Theodore et al., 1985b). Schorner, Meencke and Felix (1987) performed CT and MRI on 50 patients with epilepsy, 36 of whom had intractable seizures. CT identified 12 lesions. MRI detected 11 of these abnormalities and demonstrated a further 5 lesions, although it failed to identify one small area of calcification. Furthermore, unequivocal asymmetry of the temporal lobes was identified in 2 out of 35 CT scans and 15 out of 38 MRI scans of sufficient quality to make reliable comparisons (Schorner, Meencke and Felix, 1987).

Biological factors It is well established that the epileptogenic zone may have a different anatomical localization to identified structural lesions (Angeleri et al., 1976; Guberman, 1983; Munari et al., 1987; Wyllie et al., 1987). Munari et al. (1987) studied 75 patients with structural lesions using stereotaxic depth EEG. Good anatomical concordance was found in 37 cases. However, the zone of epileptogenicity extended well beyond the CT lesion in 26 cases, and was distinct to the structural lesion in 9. The remaining 3 patients had structural lesions that extended beyond the EEG focus. While the finding of a CT lesion may reduce the need for prolonged, intensive monitoring or the use of depth EEG studies in some patients (Spencer et al., 1984), it is important to correlate the CT localization with other modalities. Discordance should prompt further investigations and raise concern about the outcome of surgery.

Refinements of CT in Epilepsy

The limitations of standard CT have led to adaptations designed to improve the quality of structural information or to obtain functional data.

Better visualization of the temporal lobe may be possible using special scan planes or contrast studies. CT images may be obtained parallel to the long axis of the temporal lobe by tilting the gantry 5–20° from the orbito-meatal line as appropriate to each patient (Figure 4). This procedure increases the number of cuts through temporal lobe structures and may make an asymmetry of the temporal horns more evident (Figure 5), but the yield of new information is probably small (Blom et al., 1984). Herniation of the temporal horn, which is often associated with incisural sclerosis, may be identified following intrathecal metrizamide enhancement (Turner and Wyler, 1981; Wyler and Bolender, 1983), although this is an invasive procedure requiring a lumbar puncture prior to scanning.

CT is mainly used to provide structural information, but it may be adapted to provide functional data. Oakley et al. (1979) reported an increase in the amount of enhancement produced by intravenous iodinated contrast in the epileptogenic hemisphere compared to contralateral homologous regions in patients with partial seizures, although this difference was small relative to the background noise. Inhaled stable xenon-enhanced CT (XeCT) may be used to

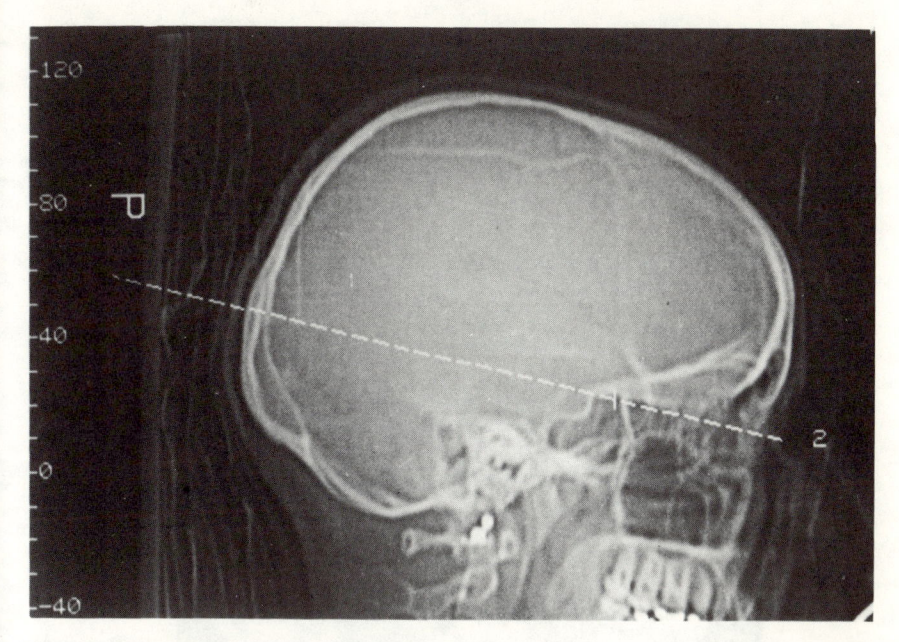

Figure 4. Plain skull X-ray showing the plane parallel to the long axis of the temporal lobes (dotted line)

determine regional cerebral blood flow (Gur et al., 1982). Following a non-enhanced baseline CT scan, serial images are taken in the same plane during xenon inhalation, with monitoring of the exhaled xenon concentration. Computation of cerebral blood flow from subtraction images is possible because xenon is radiodense and distributed according to blood flow. Using large fixed regions of interest, XeCT identified marked hypoperfusion, always corresponding to the side of the EEG focus, in 6 out of 12 patients with intractable seizures and unequivocal unilateral EEG abnormalities (Fish et al., 1987). Although this method has a poor signal to noise ratio and requires fully cooperative patients in order to avoid movement artefact, it may be of lateralizing value when PET is not available (Figure 6).

Integration of CT with Other Techniques

CT scanning provides clinically useful structural information in patients with drug-resistant epilepsy, but is probably inferior to MRI in the detection of small, non-calcified lesions, particularly when they involve the inferomesial temporal or orbito-frontal regions. XeCT allows relatively large asymmetries in regional cerebral blood flow to be identified, but with a lower signal to noise ratio than PET.

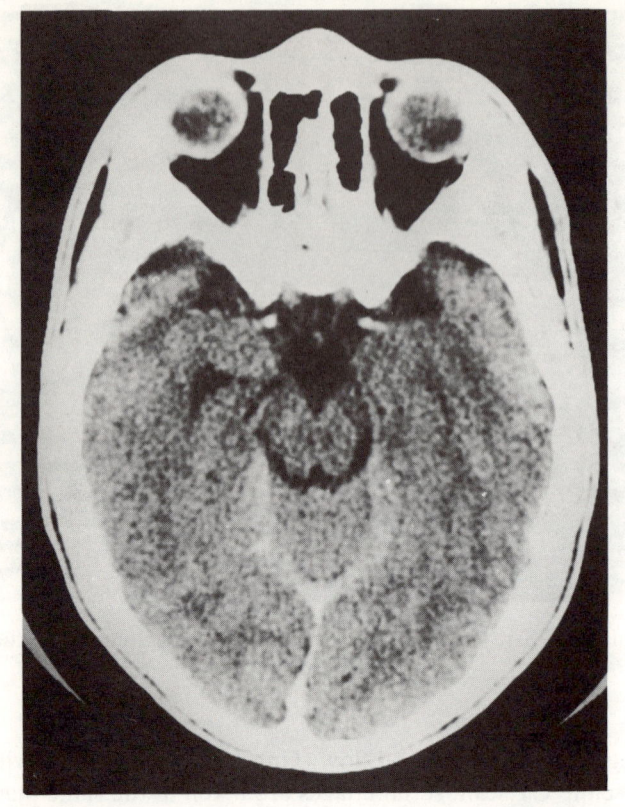

Figure 5. Plain CT scan showing an enlarged right temporal horn in a patient with a history of febrile seizures in childhood and subsequent complex partial seizures which were documented to be of right temporal lobe origin

In the future it may become more efficient to use CT as a screening procedure in patients with drug-resistant epilepsy, negative studies being followed up by more sensitive techniques.

PET in Drug-resistant Epilepsy

PET can measure regional cerebral blood flow (rCBF) and regional cerebral metabolic rate (rCMR). These parameters may be useful in the assessment of patients with drug-resistant epilepsy. Interictally, epileptic foci are associated with ipsilateral areas of hypoperfusion and hypometabolism. Conversely, during seizures these regions may show increased rCBF and rCMR.

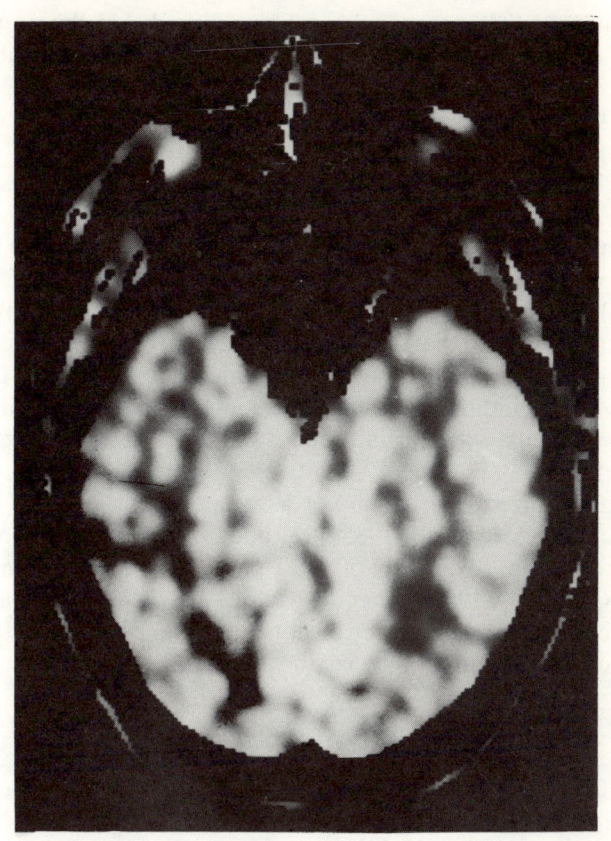

Figure 6. XeCT scans, showing reduced regional cerebral blood flow to the right temporal lobe, particularly the neocortex, in a 19-year-old patient with right temporal lobe epilepsy

Yield of Abnormal Results

Since the pioneering work of the UCLA group in the early 1980s (Engel et al., 1982a,b,c) it has become apparent that areas of reduced rCBF and rCMR may be identified interictally in approximately 60–80% of patients with partial epilepsy (Abou-Khalil et al., 1987; Bernardi et al., 1983; Frank et al., 1986; Theodore et al., 1983; Gloor et al., 1984). These functional changes are most often found in patients with mesial temporal foci, particularly those with structural lesions such as incisural sclerosis (Engel et al., 1982a, 1987). The extent of these abnormalities shows a wide variation from patient to patient, possibly in part due to variations in medication (Bernardi et al., 1983). More restricted changes in metabolism have been reported in patients not receiving phenytoin or phenobarbitone (Theodore et al., 1988). In spite of these intersubject differences, it is well established that the areas of hypometabolism or hypoperfusion correlate well with the sites of known epileptogenic foci (Abou-Khalil et al., 1987; Bernardi et al., 1983; Engel et al., 1982a,b,c, 1987; Gloor et al., 1984; Frank et al., 1986; Theodore et al., 1983, 1985b, 1988).

The severity of the reduction in rCBF or rCMR within the areas of function change also shows substantial intersubject variability, and of course is also related to the choice of regions of interest. However, in 26 cases Engel et al. (1982c) reported that these areas showed a mean reduction in rCMR of 24% (range 8–56), compared to contralateral homologous brain regions. Similarly, Frank et al. (1986) found that the areas of functional change in 21 patients with partial epilepsy and normal CT showed a mean reduction of 23% in rCBF and 21% in rCMR. In addition they reported much larger changes in rCBF and rCMR in 4 patients with partial epilepsy and CT lesions (69% and 79% respectively).

Primary generalized epilepsy is not associated with areas of focal hypometabolism (Theodore et al., 1985a), although this type of abnormality has been reported in approximately 50% of patients with the Lennox–Gastaut syndrome (Gur et al., 1982b; Theodore et al., 1987; Chuangi et al., 1987). It remains to be established whether or not the presence of such abnormalities will be clinically useful in the subclassification of this syndrome.

Limitations of PET in Drug-resistant Epilepsy

Technical constraints   The assessment of functional PET images is impeded by the following factors:

(1) It may be difficult to determine the anatomical localization of abnormalities demonstrated by a purely functional PET scan.
(2) Although PET is a quantitative technique, it is difficult to define a suitable region of interest for the study of patients with partial seizures, because of the variable localization of metabolic or perfusion abnormalities.
(3) The most commonly used isotope ([^{18}F]fluorodeoxyglucose) requires a scanning time of about 30–45 min.

The first problem may be overcome by the use of matched PET and CT or MRI scans taken in the same planes. Superimposition of the two images allows the anatomical localization of functional abnormalities.

The definition of regions of interest (ROIs) is fundamental to the quantitative analysis of functional images. Two types are in common use: fixed and variable. Fixed ROIs study the same regions in each patient, thereby allowing easy intersubject comparisons and reducing observer bias. However, small fixed ROIs may miss discrete foci of marked functional change, while these may be diluted out by the use of large ROIs. Unfortunately, the use of variable ROIs, placed so as to fit visually identified foci of altered function, makes intersubject comparisons difficult for statistical reasons, and may introduce observer bias. To date, quantitative analyses of PET scans have failed to significantly improve on qualitative visual assessments (Theodore et al., 1988).

Scanning time is important in epilepsy because of the need to study the patient under constant conditions. The longer the scan time, the more chance of a paroxysmal event occurring. Subclinical or unreported seizures during scanning could lead to negative or misleading findings in view of the opposite changes observed ictally and interictally.

Ictal PET scans showing focal increased perfusion or metabolism have been performed on a few patients (Engel et al., 1983; Newmark et al., 1982; Frank et al., 1986). However, the obvious physical difficulties preclude this type of investigation from being used in routine clinical practice. Ictal function images are much more readily obtained using single photon emission computerized tomography (SPECT), because only the isotope injection needs to be done during or soon after the ictus. This is fixed in the brain on a first-pass basis, and scans may be performed in the following hour (Lee, Markland and Siddiqui, 1986).

The most important constraint on PET is still financial. The cost of PET equipment, and the need for access to a cyclotron unit, necessitate centralization of this resource.

Biological constraints The preoperative identification of epileptic foci involves lateralization and localization. The lateralizing effectiveness of PET has been well established. Localization is less certain. Areas of hypometabolism may be much more widespread than the focus. For example, limbic foci are usually associated with neocortical areas of reduced rCMR (Abou-Khalil et al., 1985), and restricted epileptogenic lesions are often associated with PET changes that involve other cerebral lobes, sometimes even bilaterally (Gloor et al., 1984; Bernardi et al., 1983; Engel et al., 1982c, 1987). Holmes, Kelly and Theodore (1988) found a poor correlation between the localization of interictal metabolic abnormalities demonstrated by PET and the ictal EEG and clinical findings. This difficulty may reflect the effect of the focus on associated cortical areas. Given this biological constraint, it seems unlikely that metabolic PET scanning will be able to reliably solve the clinically important differentiation of temporal and frontal lobe epilepsy.

Future Adaptations of PET in Epilepsy

rCBF and rCMR provide only indirect information about the epileptic process. The real value of PET may be in the identification of receptor changes associated with epileptic foci. Neurochemical studies in surgically removed epileptogenic tissue have shown changes in the levels of excitatory amino acids (Sherwin et al., 1988). Unfortunately this type of PET work is currently limited by the lack of suitable ligands, although modifications to some of the recently developed antiepileptic drugs may allow such receptor studies to be performed.

Integration of PET with Other Studies

PET provides lateralizing information in patients with partial seizures. This information is particularly useful in the following three situations. Firstly, it may reduce the need for intracranial studies when it is concordant with other investigations that have been strongly suggestive, but not quite conclusive, about the lateralization of temporal lobe seizures. Secondly, it may allow a predominantly unilateral depth EEG implantation in patients with suspected extratemporal foci that have not been adequately identified by non-invasive techniques. Thirdly, a PET result that is discordant with the surface ictal EEG studies or other lateralizing data should prompt further investigation, probably including depth studies, and raise concern about the outcome of surgical treatment.

References

Abou-Khalil BW, Siegel GJ, Hichwa RD et al. Topography of glucose hypometabolism in epilepsy of medial temporal origin. Ann Neurol 1985; 18: 151–2.

Abou-Khalil BW, Siegal GJ, Sackellares JC et al. Positron emission tomography studies of cerebral glucose metabolism in partial epilepsy. Ann Neurol 1987; 22: 480–6.

Andermann F. Identification of candidates for surgical treatment of epilepsy. In: Engel J (ed.) Surgical treatment of the epilepsies. New York: Raven Press, 1987: 51–70.

Angeleri F, Amici F, Marchesi GF et al. Summary: computerised transverse axial tomography in epilepsy. Epilepsia 1976; 17: 342.

Bachman DS, Hodger FJ, Freeman JM. Computerised axial tomography in chronic seizure disorders of childhood. Paediatrics 1976; 58: 828–32.

Bernardi S, Trimble MR, Frackoviak RSJ et al. An interictal study of partial epilepsy using positron emission tomography and the oxygen-15 inhalation technique. J Neurol Neurosurg Psychiatry 1983; 46: 473–7.

Blom RJ, Vinuela F, Fox AJ et al. Computed tomography in temporal lobe epilepsy. J Comput Assist Tomogr 1984; 8: 401–5.

Blume WT, Girvin JP, Kaufman JCE. Childhood brain tumours presenting as chronic uncontrolled focal seizure disorders. Ann Neurol 1982; 12: 538–41.

Caille JM, Cohadron F, Loiseau P, Constant PH, Summary: computerised transverse axial tomography in epilepsy. Epilepsia 1976; 17: 341.

Chuangi HT, Mazziotta JC, Engel JP, Phelps ME. The Lennox Gastaut syndrome: metabolic subtypes determined by 2-deoxy-2-^{18}F-fluoro-D-glucose positron emission tomography. Ann Neurol 1987; 21: 4–13.

Collard M, Dupont H, Noel G. Summary: computerised transverse axial tomography in epilepsy. Epilepsia 1976; 17: 340–1.

Engel JP, Brown WJ, Kuhl DE, Phelps ME, Mazziotta JC, Crandall PH. Pathological

findings underlying focal temporal lobe hypometabolism in partial epilepsy. Ann Neurol 1982a; 12: 518–28.
Engel JP, Kuhl DE, Phelps ME et al. Comparative localisation of epileptic foci in partial epilepsy by PCT and EEG. Ann Neurol 1982b; 12: 529–37.
Engel JP, Kuhl DE, Phelps ME et al. Interictal cerebral glucose metabolism in partial epilepsy and its relation to EEG changes. Ann Neurol 1982c; 12: 510–17.
Engel JP, Kuhl DE, Phelps ME et al. Local cerebral metabolism during partial seizures. Neurology 1983; 33: 440–3.
Engel J, Cahan LD, Sutherland WW, Crandall PH, Phelps ME. The use of positron emission tomography in the surgical treatment of epilepsy. In: Wieser HG, Elger CE (eds) Presurgical evaluation of epileptics. Berlin: Springer-Verlag, 1987: 136–40.
Fish DR, Lewis TT, Brooks DJ et al. Regional cerebral blood flow in patients with focal epilepsy studied using xenon enhanced CT brain scanning. J Neurol Neurosurg Psychiatry 1987; 50: 1584–8.
Frank G, Sadzot B, Salmon E et al. Regional cerebral blood flow and metabolism in human focal epilepsy and status epilepticus. In: Delgado-Escueta AV, Ward AA, Woodbury DM et al. (eds). Basic mechanisms of the epilepsies: Molecular and cellular approaches. New York: Raven Press, 1986: 935–48.
Gall MV, Becker H, Hacker H. Computerised transverse axial tomography in epilepsy. Epilepsia 1976; 17: 340–1.
Gastaut H. Conclusions: computerised transverse axial tomography in epilepsy. Epilepsia 1976; 17: 337–8.
Gastaut H, Gastaut JL. Computerised transverse axial tomography in epilepsy. Epilepsia 1976; 17: 325–36.
Gloor P, Yamamoto Y, Ochs R et al. Regional cerebral metabolism measured by positron emission tomography in patients with partial epilepsy: Correlation with EEG findings. In: Porter RJ, Mattson RH, Ward AA et al. (eds) Advances in Epileptology, 15th International Symposium. New York: Raven Press, 1984: 45–22.
Guberman A. The role of computed cranial tomography in epilepsy. Can J Neurol Sci 1983; 10: 16–24.
Gur RC, Sussman NM, Alavi A et al. Positron emission tomography in two cases of childhood epileptic encephalopathy (Lennox Gastaut syndrome). Neurology 1982a; 32: 1191–5.
Gur D, Wolfson SK, Yonas H et al. Local cerebral blood flow by xenon enhanced CT. Stroke 1982b; 13: 750–8.
Holmes MD, Kelly K, Theodore WH. Complex partial seizures. Correlation of clinical and metabolic features. Arch Neurol 1988; 45: 1191–3.
Jabbari B, Huott AD, DiChiro G et al. Surgically correctable lesions detected by CT in 143 patients with chronic epilepsy. Surg Neurol 1978; 10: 319–22.
Jabbari B, Huott AD, DiChiro G et al. Surgically correctable lesions solely detected by CT scan in adult-onset chronic epilepsy. Ann Neurol 1980; 17: 344–7.
Lagenstein I, Kuhne D, Sternowiky HJ, Rothe M. Computerised cranial transverse tomography (CTAT) in 145 patients with primary and secondary generalised epilepsies, West syndrome, myoclonic-astatic petit mal absence epilepsy. Neuropaediatrie 1979; 10: 15–28.
Lee BI, Markland ON, Siddiqui AR. Single photon emission tomography brain image using N,N,N'-3-propanediamine-2HCl (HIPDM): Intractable complex partial seizures. Neurology 1986; 36: 1471–7.
McGahan JD, Dublin AB, Hill RP. Evaluation of seizure disorders by computed tomography. J Neurosurg 1979; 50: 328–32.
Mosely IF, Bull JWD. Computerised transverse axial tomography in epilepsy. Epilepsia 1976; 17: 339.

Munari C, Giallonardo AT, Musolino et al. Specific neuroradiological examinations necessary for stereotactic procedures. In: Wieser HG, Elger CE (eds) Presurgical evaluation of epileptics. Berlin: Springer-Verlag, 1987: 141–5.

Newmark ME, Brooks R, De la Paz R et al. The effect of clinical seizures on positron emission tomography (PECT). In: Akimoto H, Kazamatsuri H, Seino M, Ward AA (eds) Advances in Epileptology: xiiith Epilepsy International Symposium. New York: Raven Press, 1982: 195–7.

Oakley J, Ojemann GA, Ojemann LM et al. Identifying epileptic foci on contrast enhanced computerised tomographic scans. Arch Neurol 1979; 36: 669–71.

Ormson MJ, Kispert DB, Sharbrought FW et al. MRI and CT imaging of cryptic structural lesions in refractory partial epilepsy. Radiology 1986; 157: 212.

Rasmussen TB. Surgical treatment of complex partial seizures. Results, lessons and problems. Epilepsia 1983; 245: 565–76.

Rich KM, Goldring S, Gado M. Computed tomography in chronic seizure disorder caused by glioma. Arch Neurol 1985; 42: 26–7.

Schorner W, Meencke HJ, Felix R. Temporal lobe epilepsy. Comparison of CT and magnetic resonance imaging. Amer J Radiol 1987; 149: 1231–9.

Scollo-Lavizerri G, Eichan K, Wuthrich R. Summary: computerised transverse axial tomography in epilepsy. Epilepsia 1976; 17: 342.

Sherwin A, Robitaille Y, Quesney et al. Excitatory amino acids are elevated in human epileptic cerebral cortex. Neurology 1988; 38: 920–3.

Shorvon SD, Gilliatt RW, Cox TCS et al. Evidence of vascular disease from CT scans in late onset epilepsy. J Neurol Neurosurg Psychiatry 1984; 47: 225–30.

Spencer DD, Spencer SS, Mattson RH et al. Intracerebral masses in patients with intractable partial epilepsy. Neurology 1984; 34: 432–6.

Sperling MR, Wilson G, Engel J, Babb TL, Phelps M, Bradley W. Magnetic resonance imaging in intractable partial epilepsy. Correlative studies. Ann Neurol 1986; 20: 57–62.

Theodore WH, Newmark ME, Sato S et al. ^{18}F-Fluorodeoxyglucose positron emission tomography in refractory complex partial seizures. Ann Neurol 1983; 14: 429–37.

Theodore WH, Brooks R, Margolin R et al. Positron emission tomography in generalised seizures. Neurology 1985a; 35: 684–90.

Theodore WH, Dorwart R, Holmes M, Porter RJ, DiChiro G. Neuroimaging in epilepsy: Comparison of PET, CT and MRI. Neurology 1985b; 35S: 13.

Theodore WH, Rose D, Patronas N et al. Cerebral metabolism in the Lennox Gastaut syndrome. Ann Neurol 1987; 14–21.

Theodore WH, Fishbein D, Dubinsky R et al. Patterns of cerebral glucose metabolism in patients with partial seizures. Neurology 1988; 38: 1201–6.

Turner DA, Wyler AR. Temporal lobectomy for epilepsy: mesial temporal herniation as an operative and prognostic finding. Epilepsia 1981; 22: 623–9.

Wadia RS, Makhale CN, Kelkar AV, Grant KB. Focal epilepsy in India with special reference to lesions showing ring or disc like enhancement on contrast computed tomography. J Neurol Neurosurg Psychiatry 1987; 50: 1298–301.

Wilden JN, Kelly PJ. CT computerised stereotaxic biopsy for low density CT lesions presenting with epilepsy. J Neurol Neurosurg Psychiatry 1987; 1302–5.

Wyler AR, Bolender NF. Preoperative CT diagnosis of mesial temporal sclerosis for surgical treatment of epilepsy. Ann Neurol 1983; 13: 59–64.

Wyllie E, Luders H, Morris HH III et al. Clinical outcome after a complete or partial cortical resection for intractable epilepsy. Neurology 1987; 37: 1634–41.

Yang PJ, Berger MD, Cohen ME, Duffer PK. Computed tomography and childhood seizure disorders. Neurology 1979; 29: 1084–8.

6
Syndromes of Chronic Epilepsy in Children

John M. Pellock
Medical College of Virginia, Richmond, USA

The definition of chronic epilepsy varies among investigators. For the objective of this discussion I define chronic epilepsy in children as a group of disorders which do not go into remission after a few years. As shown in Figure 1, some will be controlled while others are intractable to antiepileptic drug (AED) therapy. Furthermore, in both categories the majority will be associated with other neurological deficits or may exist as the sole abnormality, with recurrent seizures being the primary disability. Although most cases of chronic epilepsy are of the intractable type, certain syndromes have seizures controlled by AEDs but need treatment throughout life or may have rare exacerbations if the appropriate risk factors are present, as in juvenile myoclonic epilepsy (JME). Intractable epilepsy is defined as epilepsy with seizures that remain uncontrolled for years despite appropriate therapy.

The epidemiology of both chronic and intractable epilepsy in children is difficult to ascertain. Although previously stated to represent a higher percentage, only about 50% of all cases of epilepsy start in childhood (Hauser and Nelson, 1989). A cumulative incidence of one or more unprovoked seizures of 1.1% by age 10 years in the population of Rochester, Minnesota, has been noted for non-febrile seizures (Hauser, Annegers and Kurland, 1984). This number is escalated significantly when considering the relationship between mental retardation (MR), cerebral palsy (CP) and the occurrence of epilepsy. The frequency of epilepsy in neurologically handicapped children was 10% in children with MR alone or CP alone; when both CP and MR were present, approximately 50% developed epilepsy.

Overall remission rates following the diagnosis of epilepsy from longitudinal

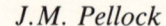

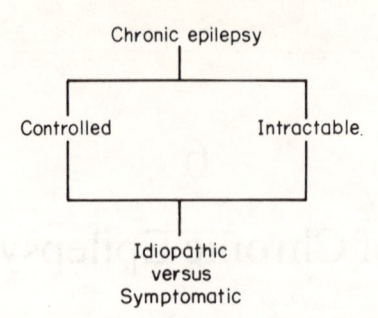

```
                    Chronic epilepsy
                           |
              ┌────────────┴────────────┐
         Controlled                Intractable
              └────────────┬────────────┘
                           |
                      Idiopathic
                       versus
                     Symptomatic
```

Figure 1. Chronic epilepsy: approach to the diagnosis of syndromes

population studies suggest a figure of 70% (Annegers, Hauser and Elveback, 1979; Brorson and Wranne, 1987; Shafer et al., 1988). In addition, there is a higher likelihood of remission in children than in adults, although children with other encephalopathies such as MR and CP have lower rates of remission. Two factors significantly predict poor prognosis, which is defined as failure to achieve a 5-year remission: (1) a generalized spike–wave EEG pattern, and (2) a generalized major motor seizure (primary or secondarily generalized convulsion) (Shafer et al., 1988). Shinnar et al. (1985) predict successful medication withdrawal after a 2-year seizure-free interval in about 75% of children. Lower relapse rates were seen in those with normal EEG at the time of withdrawal, improvement in EEG pattern over time, early age at onset of seizures, and partial complex seizures. Worsening or no change of EEG represented a higher risk of relapse. Children with MR, CP, or spikes on EEG and neonatal seizures, represent a special category; these are markers for high risk of death, chronic motor disability and chronic epilepsy (Hauser and Nelson, 1989).

Survivors after neonatal seizures develop subsequent epilepsy in early childhood 20–25% of the time. Thus association with other neurological disabilities and pathologies seems to be highly indicative of those more likely to proceed to chronic epilepsy.

Classification of Seizures

For purposes of communication it is important that there is a single terminology for seizures. Syndromes of chronic epilepsy in childhood therefore cannot be approached before a thorough understanding of seizure classification is accepted. The seizure is the event, the symptom, with which the patient presents to the physician. A seizure is a symptom of epilepsy and is defined by the behavior during the event and the ictal electroencephalogram correlation. Seizure types are separated into partial, generalized and unclassified types by the 1981 International Classification of Epileptic Seizures, as shown in Table 1 (Commission on Classification and Terminology of the International League

Table 1. International Classification of Epileptic Seizures. From Dreifuss (1989a)

I. Partial (focal, local) seizures
   A. Simple partial seizures (consciousness not impaired)
      1. With motor symptoms
      2. With somatosensory or special sensory symptoms
      3. With autonomic symptoms
      4. With psychic symptoms
   B. Complex partial seizures (with impairment of consciousness)
      1. Beginning as simple partial seizures and progressing to impairment of consciousness
         a. With no other features
         b. With features as in I.A.1–I.A.4
         c. With automatisms
      2. With impairment of consciousness at onset
         a. With no other features
         b. With features as in I.A.1–I.A.4
         c. With automatisms
   C. Partial seizures evolving to secondarily generalized seizures
      1. Simple partial seizures evolving to generalized seizures
      2. Complex partial seizures evolving to generalized seizures
      3. Simple partial seizures evolving to complex partial seizures to generalized seizures

II. Generalized seizures (convulsive or non-convulsive)
   A. Absence seizures
      1. Absence seizures
      2. Atypical absence seizures
   B. Myoclonic seizures
   C. Clonic seizures
   D. Tonic seizures
   E. Tonic–clonic seizures
   F. Atonic seizures (astatic seizures)

III. Unclassified epileptic seizures
   Includes all seizures that cannot be classified because of inadequate or incomplete data and some that defy classification in hitherto described categories. This includes some neonatal seizures, e.g. rhythmic eye movements, chewing, and swimming movements

Against Epilepsy, 1981). Partial seizures are classified primarily on the basis of whether or not consciousness is impaired during the attack, with simple partial seizures having no impairment and complex partial seizures revealing impaired consciousness. All partial seizures may secondarily generalize.

Generalized seizures can be convulsive or non-convulsive. The first clinical changes indicate involvement of both hemispheres from the onset. Ictal EEG patterns are bilateral in generalized convulsions whereas those of partial seizures are typically unilateral. Generalized seizures involve large volumes of brain from the outset and are typically associated with early impairment of consciousness. They range from absence, characterized only by impaired consciousness, to generalized tonic–clonic convulsions. The reader is referred elsewhere for more complete discussions of seizure classification (Commission on Classification and Terminology of the International League Against Epilepsy, 1981; Dreifuss, 1989a).

Epileptic Syndromes

Whereas seizures are classified on the basis of clinical and EEG characteristics, the epilepsies and epilepsy syndromes have been defined by clusters of signs and symptoms that customarily occur together. As initially proposed in 1985 in the International Classification of Epilepsies and Epileptic Syndromes (Commission on Classification and Terminology of the International League Against Epilepsy, 1985) and subsequently modified (Dreifuss, 1989a), this classification considers such features as the predominant seizure type(s), age of onset, natural history, EEG (ictal and interictal), response to AEDs, etiology, family history, and prognosis. A secondary classification of the epilepsies is based on the etiology of the seizures: idiopathic (primary) versus symptomatic (secondary). Symptomatic epilepsies are typically due to identifiable causes such as tumors, stroke, arteriovenous malformation, trauma, identifiable metabolic disorders and other associated diseases or injuries.

A number of epilepsy syndromes have been identified in childhood. In general the idiopathic or primary epilepsies are more often generalized than partial and tend to be more favorable in prognosis. However, benign types of epilepsy can be found in children with both symptomatic and idiopathic epilepsy syndromes. Table 2 lists the 1985 International League Against Epilepsy classification of the epilepsies and epileptic syndromes. The major categories include localization-related, generalized, those epilepsies and syndromes that are undetermined as to whether they are focal or generalized, and special syndromes such as benign febrile seizures and chronic epilepsia partialis continua.

Among the localization-related syndromes, benign childhood epilepsy with centro-temporal spikes (Beaussart, 1972; Dreifuss, 1989a; Loiseau and Duche, 1989) and childhood epilepsy with occipital paroxysms are thought to be relatively benign and typically do not become chronic epilepsy. However, the prognosis of the latter group is not definitive (Dreifuss, 1989b). The rare syndromes of benign neonatal familial convulsions and benign neonatal convulsions (third- and fifth-day fits) are examples of early-onset benign epilepsy forms, as is the syndrome of benign myoclonic epilepsy in infancy. The absence syndromes, including childhood absence (pyknolepsy), juvenile absence epilepsy and JME (impulsive petit mal), are considered benign because of the usual ability to successfully treat these patients, but some will go on to have a tendency to have lifelong seizures unless they remain on AEDs, making them

Table 2. International Classification of Epilepsies and Epileptic Syndromes. From Commission on Classification and Terminology of the International League Against Epilepsy (1985)

1. Localization-related (focal, local, partial) epilepsies and syndromes
    1.1. Idiopathic (with age-related onset). At present two syndromes are established:
       benign childhood epilepsy with centrotemporal spike
       childhood epilepsy with occipital paroxysms
    1.2. Symptomatic. This category comprises syndromes of great individual variability and types are characterized by:
       simple partial seizures
       complex partial seizures
       secondarily generalized seizures
    1.3. Unknown as to whether syndrome is idiopathic or symptomatic
2. Generalized epilepsies and syndromes
    2.1. Idiopathic (with age-related onset, in order of age appearance)
       benign neonatal familial convulsions
       benign neonatal convulsions
       benign myoclonic epilepsy in infancy
       childhood absence epilepsy (pyknolepsy, petit mal)
       juvenile absence epilepsy
       juvenile myoclonic epilepsy (impulsive petit mal)
       epilepsy with grand mal seizures (GTCS) on awakening
    2.2. Idiopathic and/or symptomatic (in order of age of appearance)
       West's syndrome (infantile spasms, Blitz–Nick–Salaam–Krampfe)
       Lennox–Gastaut syndrome
       epilepsy with myoclonic–astatic seizures
       epilepsy with myoclonic absences
    2.3. Symptomatic
       2.3.1 non-specific etiology
          early myoclonic encephalopathy
       2.3.2 specific syndromes: epileptic seizures may complicate many disease states. Under this heading are included those diseases in which seizures are the presenting or predominant feature
3. Epilepsies and syndromes undetermined as to whether they are focal or generalized
    3.1. With both generalized and focal seizures
       neonatal seizures
       severe myoclonic epilepsy in infancy
       epilepsy with continuous spikes and waves during slow-wave sleep
       acquired epileptic aphasia (Landau–Kleffner syndrome)
    3.2. Without unequivocal generalized or focal features
4. Special syndromes
    4.1. Situation-related seizures (Gelegenheitsanfalle)
       febrile convulsions
       seizures related to other identifiable situations, such as stress, hormones, drugs, alcohol, or sleep deprivation
    4.2. Isolated, apparently unprovoked epileptic events
    4.3. Epilepsies characterized by specific modes of seizures precipitated
    4.4. Chronic progressive epilepsia partialis continua of childhood

more chronic. The reader is referred elsewhere for further discussion of these relatively benign forms of epilepsy (Aicardi, 1988a,b; Dreifuss, 1989b; Roger et al., 1985).

Childhood Syndromes of Chronic Epilepsy

Juvenile Myoclonic Epilepsy

Janz's syndrome (Janz and Christian, 1957) or impulsive petit mal, now referred to as juvenile myoclonic epilepsy (JME) (Asconape and Penry, 1984; Delgado-Escueta and Enrile Bascal, 1984; Tsuboi, 1977), typically presents during puberty, with the patient experiencing their first 'grand mal' or clonic–tonic seizure. Only with repeated questioning is the full syndrome realized. Seizures with bilateral single or repetitive arrhythmic irregular myoclonic jerks predominantly in the arms, and absences, are also noted with patients having all seizure types or just partial expression. Sudden falls may be caused by the jerks, and both myoclonic and generalized tonic–clonic seizures are more common in the morning. No disturbance of consciousness is noticed with myoclonic jerks. Later in the course, seizures are precipitated by sleep deprivation or alcohol use. Ictal and interictal EEGs have variable types of generalized spike and wave activity, often rapid irregular spike–waves and polyspikes. The patients are frequently photosensitive. Although sex distribution is equal, the disorder seems to be inherited and has been provisionally linked to a locus on the short arm of chromosome 6 (Greenburg, Delgado-Escueta and Widelitz, 1988). Treatment is usually successful with valproate but relapses are quite common unless medication is continued. In uncontrolled cases, primidone or polytherapy may be necessary.

Although JME is thought to be a benign syndrome related to the absences, its chronicity and relapsing nature upon medication discontinuation qualifies it as a chronic form of epilepsy. Other forms of absence, such as juvenile absence epilepsy or even the childhood form when accompanied by tonic–clonic seizures and/or myoclonic jerks, overlap with this syndrome, although their age of onset may vary slightly. Similarly, patients with absence syndromes with atypical absence seizures and/or slow spike–wave EEG paroxysms may be more resistant to therapy and express a more chronic form of epilepsy. These entities also overlap with the syndrome of generalized tonic–clonic seizures on awakening (Dreifuss, 1989a,b).

West Syndrome (Infantile Spasms, Blitz–Nick–Salaam–Krampfe)

West syndrome is characterized by infantile spasms, arrested psychomotor development and hypsarrhythmia (Jeavons and Bower, 1964; Kellaway et al., 1979; Lacy and Penry, 1976; West, 1841). This triad may not be fully expressed but the syndrome is more common in boys, with an onset between 4 and 7 months, nearly always beginning before 1 year. Infantile spasms may clinically present as flexor, extensor or nods, and are most commonly mixed (Kellaway et al., 1979).

The prognosis is generally poor but the syndrome has been separated into two groups. The symptomatic group is characterized by previous evidence of encephalopathy (tuberose sclerosis, hypoxic–ischemic encephalopathy), while a smaller cryptogenic group has no evidence of prior abnormality. The absolute prognosis is based on this differentiation, with a better response to ACTH being seen in those in the cryptogenic group (Hrachovy, 1989). The ultimate prognosis, however, depends upon the etiology and perhaps early discovery and treatment (Dreifuss, 1989b); this is especially true of the cryptogenic cases. In symptomatic cases the prognosis is typically poor for normal development and for control of infantile spasms or later epilepsy.

Lennox–Gastaut Syndrome

This syndrome, like the previous one, is listed under the category allowing for either idiopathic or symptomatic cases. Many children with uncontrolled and intractable epilepsy are said to be in this group but a more restricted definition is required to truly define the disorder (Aicardi, 1988b; Roger, Dravet and Bureau, 1989). Typical age of onset is from 1 to 8 years, but onset is most commonly seen in preschool children. Seizure types most commonly seen include tonic axial, atonic and absence seizures (atypical). Other frequently noted seizure types such as myoclonic, generalized tonic–clonic and partial seizures are also noted. The EEG is typically characterized by an abnormal background and slow spike–wave paroxysms of 2.5 Hz or slower in a generalized or multifocal distribution. With sleep, fast rhythmic bursts may appear. Seizure frequency is quite high and difficult to control. MR is common. More than half the children suffer from a prior encephalopathy. Poor prognosis is especially true with those in the symptomatic group with early onset of seizures before age 3 years, a high seizure frequency and a constantly slow EEG background rhythm without periods of improvement and association of focal changes with diffuse slow spike–waves (Roger, Dravet and Bureau, 1989).

Epilepsy with Myoclonic–Astatic Seizures

One of several childhood syndromes characterized by myoclonic seizures, this syndrome begins between 7 months and 6 years, most often from 2 to 5 years. With a hereditary predisposition and normal development, boys are twice as often affected as girls (Doose et al., 1970; Doose and Gundel, 1982). Seizures are myoclonic–astatic absences, with both clonic and tonic components and tonic–clonic seizures. Idiopathic and symptomatic in origin, the course and outcome is somewhat variable. Tonic seizures develop late in those with an unfavorable prognosis, and status epilepticus frequently occurs. The EEG with irregular fast spike and wave or polyspike and wave activity may be normal initially (Doose and Gundel, 1982).

Epilepsy with Myoclonic Absences

The prognosis for this idiopathic or symptomatic absence syndrome is less favorable than that for childhood absence because of mental deterioration, resistance to therapy and possible evolution to other types of epilepsy such as Lennox–Gastaut. Characteristic seizures are absences accompanied by severe bilateral rhythmical clonic jerks often associated with tonic contraction (Tassinari and Bureau, 1985). Its bilateral synchronous and symmetrical EEG discharge of 3 Hz spike and wave does not distinguish it from more benign types. Seizures occur many times daily and children are aware of the jerks. Associated seizures are relatively rare. The age at onset is approximately seven years and there is somewhat of a male predominance (Dreifuss, 1989b; Roger et al., 1985).

Early Myoclonic Encephalopathy

This symptomatic myoclonic syndrome is characterized by three principal features: onset before 3 months of age; initial fragmentary myoclonus followed by erratic partial seizures and massive myoclonia and tonic spasms; and an EEG characterized by suppression burst activity which may evolve to hypsarrhythmia (Dreifuss, 1989b; Roger et al., 1985). Following severe psychomotor retardation, death may occur during the first year. Familial cases have been reported, suggesting an underlying metabolic disorder. The relationship to the syndrome described by Ohtahara et al. (1976) is unclear.

Severe Myoclonic Epilepsy in Infancy

This recently defined syndrome is characterized by a family history of epilepsy or febrile convulsions, normal development before onset, seizures beginning during the first year of life as generalized or bilateral febrile clonic seizures, a secondary appearance of myoclonic jerks, and partial seizures (Dravet, Bureau and Roger, 1985). The EEG shows generalized spike–wave and polyspike–wave, early photosensitivity, and focal abnormalities. Psychomotor retardation is apparent from the second year of life and ataxia, pyramidal signs and interictal myoclonus appear. Children with this epileptic syndrome are very resistant to all forms of treatment.

Progressive Myoclonic Epilepsy

This syndrome actually combines several disease entities with their own distinct clinical and pathological findings (Berkovic et al., 1986). It includes juvenile Gaucher's disease, cherry red spot myoclonus syndrome, juvenile ceroid lipofuscinosis and Lafora body disease. In these progressive conditions, myoclonus is prominent. The onset is in childhood or adolescence, and neurological deficits involve cerebellar, pyramidal and extrapyramidal systems. Though MR may occur, it is not inevitable.

Neonatal Seizures

Except for the rare and benign third- and fifth-day neonatal seizures or those related to transient metabolic abnormalities, neonatal seizures may lead to a number of other neurological syndromes as the child develops (Hauser and Nelson, 1989). Many of these are quite devastating as significant neurological disease and injury is already present, with neonatal seizures representing only one symptom of the entire complex. Neonatal seizures are most frequently noted to have subtle clinical manifestations (Volpe, 1987), including tonic, horizontal deviation of the eyes with or without jerking, eyelid blinking or fluttering, sucking, smacking or other buccal lingual oral movements, swimming or pedaling movements and occasionally apneic spells. Spells of tonic extension of the limbs, mimicking decerebrate or decorticate posturing, have also been noted in prematures. Multifocal clonic seizures are also noted, with spread to other body parts. Myoclonic seizures occur rarely but carry a poor prognosis.

Neonatal seizure types, however, require further definition, as EEG correlates have not been as precise as those for epilepsy in older children and adults (Mizrahi and Kellaway, 1987; Scher et al., 1989). Characterization and classification of neonatal seizure types, including subtle activities called seizures, continue to evolve. Some may not represent true cortical seizures and may represent subcortical phenomena. Therefore their exact link to other epileptic occurrences is unknown.

Epilepsy with Continuous Spike–Waves During Slow-wave Sleep

Patients with various seizure types, partial and generalized, occurring during sleep, and atypical absences when awake, make up this syndrome (Tassinari et al., 1985). Tonic seizures do not occur. Characteristic EEG patterns consist of continuous, diffuse, spike–waves during slow-wave sleep seen after the onset of seizures. Duration may be from months to years and the prognosis is guarded because of the appearance of neuropathological disorders despite what is usually a benign evolution of seizures.

Kojewnikow's Syndrome

Two distinct types of this syndrome are now recognized (Dreifuss, 1989b; Kojewnikow, 1895; Rasmussen, Olszewsik and Lloyd-Smith, 1958; Roger et al., 1985). The first represents a form of rolandic partial epilepsy in both adults and children associated with variable lesions of the motor cortex. Diagnostic features include motor partial seizures, frequent late appearance of myoclonia originating from the same site, EEG with normal background and focal paroxysmal abnormality (spike and slow waves), with demonstrable etiology and no progression except that expected on the basis of the causal relationship. The second, more specific, childhood disorder is of suspected viral etiology and has an onset between 2 and 10 years with a peak at 6 years. Primarily partial motor seizures progress to other seizure types (which persist during sleep), progressive motor deficit and ultimately MR. The EEG background shows asymmetric slow diffuse delta waves and numerous ictal and interictal spike and sharp wave discharges not strictly limited to the rolandic area. Early surgical therapy is a growing consideration in these patients.

Considerations Beyond Specific Syndromes

Only a small group of children can be definitely classified into specific syndromes early in the course of their epilepsy. Careful evaluation and follow-up will ultimately define the patient's own 'syndrome'. The identification of specific epilepsy syndromes in childhood allows one to differentiate between those more likely to be associated with chronic epilepsy and/or chronic encephalopathy and those with a more benign outcome although the seizure type may be quite threatening at onset. Nevertheless, there are limitations to the concept of epileptic syndromes (Aicardi, 1988b). Patients should not be forcibly placed into syndromic classification groupings when they only have part of the requisite factors. Others may have localization-related epilepsy or have a more diffuse cerebral disturbance without a specific syndromic or etiologic diagnosis.

Multiple factors are responsible for chronicity and inadequate control of seizures. These include patient errors of poor compliance and erratic lifestyle, physician diagnostic errors in classification, or a failure to uncover precipitating factors, and treatment errors when improper or inadequate drugs are prescribed (Aicardi, 1988a). As epilepsy frequently represents only one manifestation of further brain dysfunction, other symptoms should be considered. Some authors have suggested that onset during early infancy associated with organic brain damage with mental impairment and neurological signs disposes patients to be in poor prognostic categories of epilepsy (Aicardi, 1988a; Chevrie and Aicardi, 1978). Partial seizures with complex motor phenomena, especially beginning at a young age, are extremely difficult to control and typically evolve to other forms of epilepsy (Duchowny, 1987). Although prior

Table 3. Factors predictive of chronic epilepsy

Syndrome of chronic epilepsy
Onset as neonate/infant (?)
Organic brain damage
Mental impairment
Neurological signs
Specific encephalopathy
Seizure type
Tonic
Atonic
Spasms
Myoclonic
Multiple seizure types
Multiple seizure recurrences
Recurrent status epilepticus
Long duration/failure of previous AEDs
Abnormal EEG (background or paroxysmal)
Poor psychological and/or socio-economic background

studies of status epilepticus (SE) in children predicted a poor outcome, recent evidence suggests a more benign outcome unless SE is associated with other significant encephalopathy (Maytal et al., 1989). Multiple seizures or recurrent SE are more often associated with chronic epilepsy (Towne et al., 1988). In general, an unfavorable prognosis in childhood epilepsies and therefore chronicity might be considered in children who share a list of factors associated with an unfavorable prognosis as shown in Table 3.

As noted in the descriptions above, even when patients are classified within a syndrome more specific factors may permit a greater predictive power and decide a favorable or unfavorable outcome.

Epileptic syndromes are not disease entities. As noted, most have varied causes and diverse outcomes. Syndrome classification can definitely help predict the chronicity of epilepsy but may not be as complete a predictor as one would optimally desire. It is this author's opinion that attempting to appropriately place children and adults into specific epilepsy syndromes allows for the greatest estimation of all related factors and will allow the best treatment of their disorder and eventual prediction of outcome.

References

Aicardi J. Epilepsy in children. New York: Raven Press, 1986: 17–182.
Aicardi J. Clinical approach to the management of intractable epilepsy. Dev Med Child Neurol 1988a; 30: 429–40.
Aicardi J. Epileptic syndromes in childhood. Epilepsia 1988b; 29 (suppl. 3): S1–S5.

Annegers JF, Hauser WA, Elveback LR. Remission of seizures and relapse in patients with epilepsy. Epilepsia 1979; 20: 729–37.
Asconape J, Penry JK. Some clinical and EEG aspects of benign juvenile myoclonic epilepsy. Epilepsia 1984; 25: 108–114.
Beaussart M. Benign epilepsy of children with rolandic (centrotemporal) paroxysmal foci: A clinical entity. Study of 221 cases. Epilepsia 1972; 13: 795–811.
Berkovic SF, Andermann F, Carpenter S et al. Progressive myoclonus epilepsies: Specific cases and diagnosis. N Engl J Med 1986; 315: 296–305.
Brorson LO, Wranne L. Long-term prognosis in childhood epilepsy: Survival and seizure prognosis. Epilepsia 1987; 28: 324–30.
Chevrie JJ, Aicardi J. Convulsive disorders in the first year of life: Neurology and mental outcome and mortality. Epilepsia 1978; 19: 67–74.
Commission on Classification and Terminology of the International League Against Epilepsy. Proposal for revised clinical and electroencephalographic classification of epileptic seizures. Epilepsia 1981; 22: 489–501.
Commission on Classification and Terminology of the International League Against Epilepsy. Proposal for the classification of the epilepsies and epileptic syndromes. Epilepsia 1985; 26: 268–78.
Delgado-Escueta AV, Enrile Bacsal F. Juvenile myoclonic epilepsy of Janz. Neurology 1984; 34: 285–94.
Doose H, Gundel A. 4–7 cps rhythms in the childhood EEG. In: Anderson VE, Hauser WA, Penry JK et al. (eds) Genetic basis of the epilepsies. New York: Raven Press, 1982: 82–3.
Doose H, Gerken H, Leonhardt R et al. Centrencephalic myoclonic–astatic petit mal. Neuropediatrics 1970; 2: 59–78.
Dravet C, Bureau M, Roger J. Severe myoclonic epilepsy in infants. In: Roger J, Dravet C, Bureau M, Dreifuss FE, Wolf P (eds) Epileptic syndromes in infancy, childhood and adolescence. London: John Libbey, 1985.
Dreifuss, FE. Classification of epileptic seizures and the epilepsies. Pediatr Clin North Am 1989a; 36: 1–15.
Dreifuss, FE. Pediatric epilepsy syndromes: an overview. Cleve Clin J Med 1989b; 56 (suppl. part 2): S166–71.
Duchowny MS. Complex partial seizures of infancy. Arch Neurol 1987; 44: 911–14.
Greenburg DA, Delgado-Escueta AV, Widelitz H. Juvenile myoclonic epilepsy (JME) may be linked to the BF and HLA loci on human chromosome 6. Am J Med Genet 1988; 31: 185–92.
Hauser WA, Annegers JF, Kurland LT. The incidence of epilepsy in Rochester, Minnesota 1935–79. 1984; Epilepsia 25: 666.
Hauser WA, Nelson KB. Epidemiology of epilepsy in children. Cleve Clin J Med 1989; 56 (suppl. part 2): S185–94.
Hrachovy RA. Infantile spasms. Pediatr Clin North Am 1989; 31: 311–29.
Janz D, Christian W. Impulsiv-Petit mal. Dtsch Z Nervenheilk 1957; 176: 346–86.
Jeavons PM, Bower BD. Infantile spasms: A review of the literature and a study of 112 cases. In: Clinics in developmental medicine, No. 15. London: Spastics Society and Heinemann, 1964.
Kellaway P, Hrachovy RA, Frost JD et al. Precise characteristics and quantification of infantile spasms. Ann Neurol 1979; 6: 214–18.
Kojewnikow L. Eine besondere Form von corticaler Epilepsie. Neurologisches Centralblatt 1895; 14: 47–8.
Lacy JR, Penry JK. Infantile spasms. New York: Raven Press, 1976.
Loiseau P, Duché B. Benign childhood epilepsy with centrotemporal spikes. Cleve Clin J Med 1989; 56 (suppl. part 1): S17–S22.

Maytal J, Shinnar S, Moshe SL et al. Low morbidity and mortality of status epilepticus in children. Pediatrics 1989; 83: 323–31.
Mizrahi EM, Kellaway P. Characterization and classification of neonatal seizures. Neurology 1987; 37: 1837–44.
Ohtahara S, Ishida T, Oka E et al. On the age-dependent epileptic syndromes: the early infantile encephalopathy with suppression-burst. Brain Dev 1976; 8: 270–88.
Rasmussen TE, Olszewsik J, Lloyd-Smith D. Focal cortical seizures due to chronic localized encephalitides. Neurology 1958; 8: 435–45.
Roger J, Dravet C, Bureau M. The Lennox–Gastaut syndrome. Cleve Clin J Med 1989; 56 (suppl. part 2): S172–80.
Roger J, Dravet C, Bureau M, Dreifuss FE, Wolf P (eds) Epileptic syndromes in infancy, childhood and adolescence. London: John Libbey, 1985: 325–41.
Scher MS, Painter MJ, Bergman I et al. EEG diagnoses of neonatal seizures: Clinical correlates and outcome. Pediatr Neurol 1989; 5: 17–24.
Shafer S, Hauser WA, Annegers JF, Klass DW. EEG and other early predictors of later epilepsy remission: A community study. Epilepsia 1988; 29: 590–600.
Shinnar S, Vining EPG, Mellitz ED et al. Discontinuing antiepileptic medication in children with epilepsy after two years without seizures: A prospective study. N Engl J Med 1985; 313: 976–80.
Tassinari CA, Bureau M. Epilepsy with myoclonic absences. In: Roger J, Dravet C, Bureau M, Dreifuss FE, Wolf P (eds) Epileptic syndromes in infancy, childhood and adolescence. London: John Libbey, 1985: 121–9.
Tassinari CA, Bureau M, Dravet C et al. Epilepsy with continuous spike and waves during slow sleep. In: Roger J, Dravet C, Bureau M, Dreifuss FE, Wolf P (eds) Epileptic syndromes in infancy, childhood and adolescence. London: John Libbey, 1985.
Towne AR, Ko D, Driscoll S SM et al. Age distribution and mortality in status epilepticus. Ann Neurol 1988; 24: 135–6.
Tsuboi T, Primary generalized epilepsy with sporadic myoclonias of myoclonic petit mal type. Stuttgart: Thieme, 1977: 19–35.
Volpe JJ, Neonatal seizures Clin Pediatrics 1987; 22: 129–44.
West WJ, On a peculiar form of infantile convulsion. Lancet 1841 i: 724–5.

7
Prognosis and Prophylaxis of Traumatic Epilepsy

D. Janz
Free University of Berlin, Berlin, West Germany

Introduction

The state of knowledge concerning epileptic seizures and epilepsies following brain traumas has altered during recent years in many respects. The question that has concerned us more than any other is whether prophylactic therapy is possible, necessary and how it should best be carried out. It therefore seems appropriate to deal with post-traumatic epilepsy particularly in this light, i.e. causes and course should be considered in relationship to the advantages and risks of prophylactic treatment.

Post-traumatic Early Seizures

On the basis of the latency period between trauma and first seizure, a distinction is made between epileptic seizures of early and late onset. (Many authors call this traumatic early and traumatic late epilepsy. But since the term epilepsy implies an illness with recurring epileptic seizures and since, from a prophylactic standpoint, the question is whether it is an acute reaction or a chronic process, caution in the choice of terms is necessary in order not to draw premature conclusions.) This distinction is prognostically useful, since the earlier the seizures occur the less they tend to recur, i.e. to become the first seizure of post-traumatic epilepsy; similarly, the longer this interval, the greater the probability of traumatic late epilepsy (Wessely, 1981) (Table 1). Since early seizures are definitely the expression of a direct effect of the

Table 1. Time of first fit in 131 cases of traumatic early seizures within 4 weeks of injury (TLS = traumatic late seizures). From Wessely (1981)

	1st day	2nd day	1st week	2nd week	4th week	Total
Without TLS	21	20	10	3	3	57
With TLS	17	15	16	12	14	74
Total	38	35	26	15	17	131
	29%	26.6%	19.8%	11.4%	13%	100%

trauma, in other words a pathological reaction, which cannot be timed accurately, there has been up to now no agreement about the maximum length of time allowed—whether 1, 2 or even 4 weeks—in order to define the term 'early'.

Wessely (1981) records about the same number of seizures in each of the first 2 days, and thereafter a gradual decrease for up to 4 weeks (Table 1). Jennett (1980, 1981) finds—with regard to the incidence per week—a sharp decline between the first and the following weeks, from which observation he derives the pragmatic suggestion that only those seizures occurring during the first week should be defined as early seizures (Figure 1). The fact that he, along with other authors (Stöwsand, 1971; Ritz et al., 1980, 1981), and in contrast to Wessely (1981), records early seizures most frequently in the first 24 h, and particularly within the first hour after the trauma, suggests differences in the population under observation.

As regards the type of seizure in the case of early seizures, focal motor seizures are often encountered (Jennett (1975), 41%; Ketz (1980, 1981), 21 of 42 cases) as well as major seizures, whereas psychomotor seizures were not observed before the second week (Jennett, 1975). A third of patients with early seizures have only one seizure. Status epilepticus occurs in between 3% (Ketz, 1980, 1981) and 10% (Jennett, 1980, 1981) of cases and predominantly in children under 5 years of age (Jennett, 1980, 1981); indeed, traumatic early seizures are considered to occur on the whole more frequently in children and particularly after minor head trauma (Jennett, 1980, 1981; Ritz, 1980, 1981). In a study of 35 children with mainly severe head injuries, however, Lange-Cosack et al. (1979) found 16 with early epileptic seizures, mainly in the form of unilateral convulsions or focal major seizures.

The following factors tend to favour the occurrence of early seizures: the length of unconsciousness or of post-traumatic amnesia. This seems to be even more important in the case of children, since 7 out of 8 cases of Lange-Cosack et al. (1979) who were unconscious for more than 24 h had early seizures; as opposed to this, only 18 out of 154 cases of Jennett and Lewin (1960) with amnesia lasting longer than one day developed early seizures (12% as opposed to 2.7% of those whose amnesia was of shorter duration). Moreover, early seizures also occur more frequently in the case of injuries with depressed

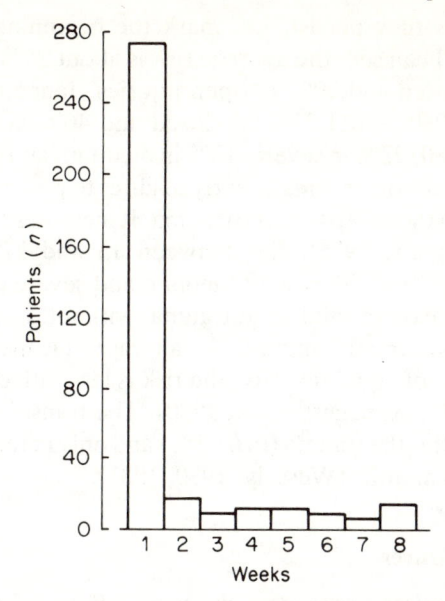

Figure 1. Time of first fit within 8 weeks of injury

fractures or intracranial haematomas. With the possible exception of children in whom early seizures even after minor trauma have been observed (Jennett, 1980, 1981; Ritz et al., 1980, 1981) (so that the interpretation as to the seizures occurring as a result of the trauma is open to question), early seizures as a rule seem to indicate the presence of severe contusion. According to Wessely (1980, 1981), they should be regarded as 'alarm signs' of the presence of an intracranial complication (e.g. a space-occupying haemorrhage).

Although the incidence is correlated with the severity of brain trauma, it will also vary to a great extent with the age composition and diagnostic criteria of the medical institutions to which the patients are admitted. Whilst Jennett (1980, 1981) maintains that 5% of all patients who are admitted to hospital with a brain trauma develop one or several early seizures, this is a figure more than double that reported in a very carefully conducted field study of the Mayo Clinic, i.e. 2.1% (Annegers et al., 1980), which approximately corresponds to the results of the investigations of Elvidge (1939) (1.9%) and Kollevold (1976) (2.9%). The greater incidence is probably due to the selection of more severe cases than those meeting only the minimal requirements of head injury with post-traumatic amnesia and to the fact that the seizures and not the brain trauma were the reason for admission (Annegers et al., 1980).

Apart from the fact that early epileptic seizures can be indicative of intracranial bleeding or, as in the case of an early epileptic status epilepticus, may become the reason for urgent therapy, it is important to know how often and in what circumstances they persist, i.e. mark the beginning of post-traumatic epilepsy. As far as I can see, the average risk is about 25%; Ketz (1980, 1981) found 25.9% in closed and 20% in open injuries, Jennett and Lewin (1960) 28.5%, Jennett (1980, 1981) 27% in closed and 46% in open injuries, and Annegers et al. (1980) 22% in severe, 13% in medium, and 0% in mild injuries. The risk of transition from traumatic early seizures to post-traumatic epilepsy is also correlated with the severity of the trauma. It increases to 45% in the case of open injuries (Jennett, 1975), lies between 13 and 27% (Jennett, 1975; Annegers et al., 1980) in the case of medium and severe closed injuries, and drops to 0% in the case of mild head trauma, without, however, the minimal condition of post-traumatic amnesia in all cases (Annegers et al., 1980). Considering trauma of equal severity, the risk is less with children than adults (Jennett, 1980, 1981; Annegers et al., 1980). The transition occurs mainly in the first 3 months after the trauma (in 63.5%) and only in rare cases (26%) does it still occur after 6 months (Wessely, 1980, 1981).

Traumatic Late Seizures

When epileptic seizures occur after the acute effects of the skull and brain trauma have subsided, they are called traumatic late seizures, and when occurring repeatedly, traumatic late epilepsy. Just as with early seizures, which tend to cease spontaneously, the prognosis of late seizures is not necessarily unfavourable, so that epilepsy does not develop in all cases. Out of 51 cases in the Mayo Clinic study (Annegers et al., 1980) whose course had been followed for at least 6 years, 19 only suffered one seizure. Of the 28 cases of Jennett and Lewin (1960) with late seizures, 7 cases had only one seizure, and only 9 cases had had more than three seizures after a 7-year follow-up investigation. The question as to whether early treatment may have had a favourable effect cannot be judged in either of these studies, but Evans (1962) also showed a tendency to natural remission on the basis of a 7–11-year follow-up of 55 cases of post-traumatic epilepsy, and this has also been confirmed by other authors (Wessely, 1980, 1981; Russell and Whitty, 1952; Walker, 1957). In only 18 out of 75 cases of Evans (1962) did more than one major seizure still occur per year; 32 were free of seizures, 19 of whom were no longer taking antiepileptic drugs. Traumatic late epilepsies do not become chronic in approximately one-quarter of cases, with a variability of between 13% for closed, and 45% for open injuries, follow-up investigations giving the impression of a 'generally favourable course' (Wessely, 1980, 1981). Wessely (1980, 1981) reports that 109 out of 348 cases, i.e. one-third, remained free from seizures for more than 5 years.

Looking at the latency period between trauma and seizures, it can be assumed that two-thirds of the late seizures which occur after early seizures have become manifest within the first 6 months. Of cases with primarily late seizures, however, only 30–45% have become manifest within the same period

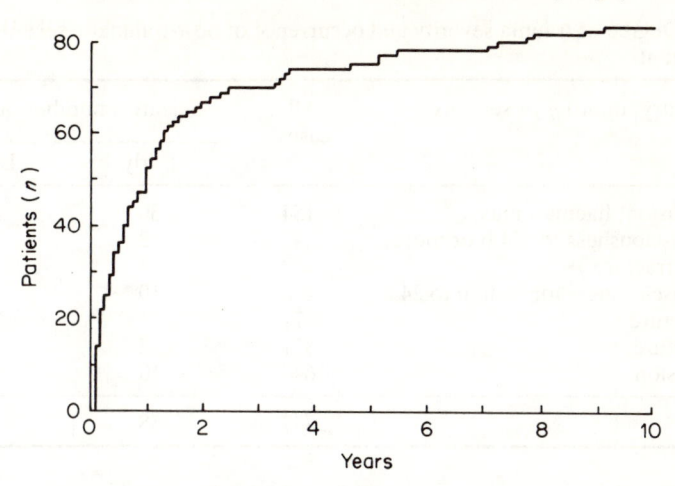

Figure 2. Time of onset of seizures expressed as a cumulative graph showing the current number of patients who had developed seizures after injury

of time (Wessely, 1980, 1981; Caveness et al, 1979; Walker and Jablon, 1959), as can be seen from the diagram of Evans (1962) (Figure 2). In the course of the first year, 50–60% have become manifest, and after 2 years 65–80% (Wessely, 1980, 1981).

The interval during which a causal relationship between seizures and preceding trauma can still be considered possible is still the subject of much discussion. Taking into account that the incidence curve clearly flattens out after about the third year, only strict criteria for a causal relationship after this period of time should be employed—such as a definite correlation between initial and paroxysmal focal signs and symptoms. The dubiety of a relationship after an interval of more than 4 years has been clearly demonstrated in the Mayo Clinic investigation using epidemiological methods. The authors of this study are able to show that, in comparison with the known rate of incidence for epilepsy in each age group of the population, epileptic seizures which developed later than 4 years after closed head trauma did not occur for the first time statistically more frequently than would be expected in the absence of trauma (Annegers et al., 1980).

The risk of traumatic epilepsy depends on the type of injury, its location, severity of trauma and complications. Thus we know from war injuries that bullet wounds which have at least penetrated the dura lead to traumatic epilepsies in 36–53% of cases (Russell and Whitty, 1952; Walker and Jablon, 1959; Ashcroft, 1941; Weiss et al., 1983). The risk increases to about 70% when wound infections have occurred (Evans, 1962) or in cases of brain abscess (Legg et al., 1973). It is greater, i.e. around 42–44%, when the injury involved the parietal and temporal region; it is less, i.e. 17–24%, in injuries of frontal

Table 2. Degree of trauma severity and occurrence of post-traumatic seizures. From Annegers et al.

Type of injury, in order of severity	All cases	Seizures, number of cases	
		Early	Late
Brain contusion, haematomas	154	30	21
Loss of consciousness for 24 h or more	41	2	2
Depressed fracture	52	3	1
Loss of consciousness for 30 min to 24 h	418	10	8
Basilar fracture	71	1	0
Linear fracture	371	2	7
Mild contusion	1640	10	12
Total	2747	58	51

and occipital poles. Not only does the frequency of traumatic epilepsies apparently decrease the further away the traumatic focus is from the motor cortex, but also the more distant foci require correspondingly more time to become epileptogenic, e.g. whilst it can take years for temporal lesions to lead to seizures it takes still longer with frontal and occipital foci (Paillas et al., 1970). The relative risk of developing epilepsy after penetrating head injuries dropped according to the Vietnam Study from about 580 times higher than the general age-matched population in the first year to 25 times higher after 10 years (Salazar et al., 1985). Although such patients remain at some increased risk for seizures even 10–15 years post-injury, most can be 95% certain of avoiding epilepsy if they have been seizure-free for 3 years post-trauma (Weiss et al., 1986).

In the case of skull and brain traumas which have not been caused by bullet injuries, an increase in epilepsy risk of up to 35% has been observed in the case of intracranial haematomas; of up to 17% in the case of a depressed fracture (Jennett, 1980, 1981); and, depending on the length of unconsciousness, of 1.7% when post-traumatic amnesia was less than 1 hour, and up to 12% when it continued for longer than 7 days (Jennett and Lewin, 1960). Annegers et al. (1980) demonstrated very clearly the relationship between different degrees of trauma and risks for early and late post-traumatic seizures (Table 2). The risk increases when several risk factors coincide, and Jennett (1975) has developed an empirical risk scale, whereby the statistically expected risk, which lies between 3 and 70%, can be assessed in each case according to the particular combination of factors involved (Figure 3). Similar risk tables, which include the interval between trauma and the occurrence of seizures, have been worked out by Feeney and Walker (1953) and Weiss et al. (1986).

In the assessment of epilepsy risk, the EEG, strangely enough, plays a surprisingly small part. In this respect, Jennett (1980, 1981) is in agreement

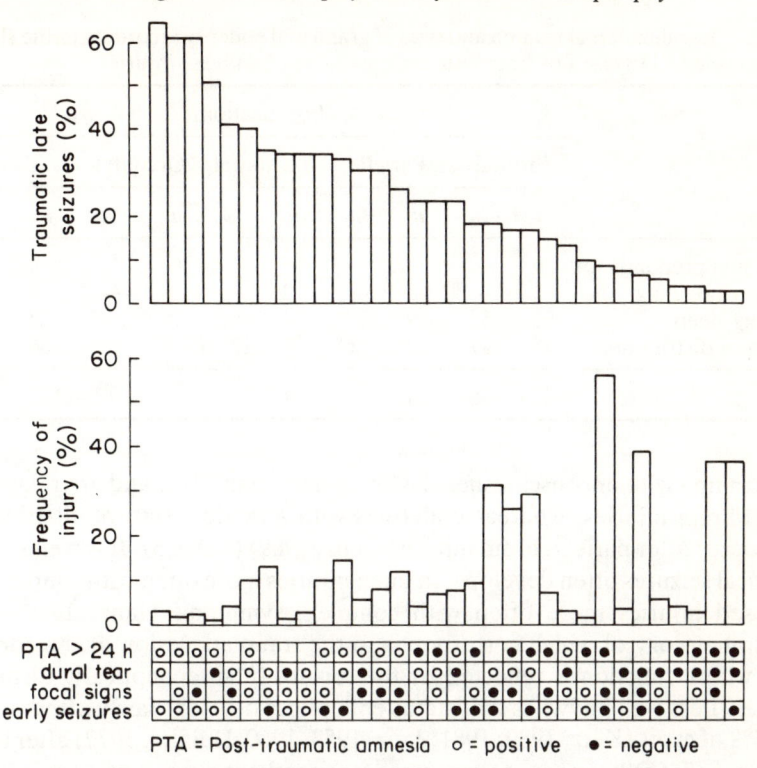

Figure 3. Risk of traumatic epilepsy according to different combinations of risk factors. The frequency with which different combinations of factors occurred is displayed below the incidence of late traumatic seizures associated with each combination. From Jennet (1975)

with other authors (Ritz et al., 1980; Courjon, 1970; Scherzer and Wessely, 1978) that the 'EEG (offers) little help in answering the question as to whether a late epilepsy will develop'. With penetrating head injuries, however, all patients with anterior temporal or central spike foci experienced post-traumatic seizures (Jabbari et al., 1986).

Seizure type and the natural history of traumatic epilepsies differ from those of idiopathic epilepsies in that age-dependent minor seizures, such as astatic seizures, absences and myoclonic seizures of the impulsive petit mal types, are entirely absent; major seizures often occur spread over the day in a randomly distributed manner and less often in the form of an epilepsy on awakening which, when it does occur, more often has an evening (after work) peak (Janz, 1953, 1960). With regard to the relationship between type and localization of injuries and dependency of major seizures to the sleeping–waking cycle, little attention has been paid to the fact that traumatic sleep epilepsies often occur

Table 3. Localization of trauma and type of grand mal epilepsy according to the sleep–waking cycle in 118 cases of traumatic epilepsy after open head injuries

	Localization									
	Frontal		Parietal		Temporal		Occipital		Total	
	n	%	n	%	n	%	n	%	n	%
Grand mal predominantly										
after awakening	3	—	8	—	2	—	1	—	14	—
during sleep	21	55	9	24	4	10.5	4	10.5	28	100
random distribution	18	27	37	56	8	12	3	5	66	100
Total	42	35	54	46	14	12	8	7	118	100

after trauma with unconsciousness lasting longer than 24 h, and are related to frontal brain injuries, whereas epilepsies with a random seizure distribution often occur after parietal brain injuries (Janz, 1969) (Table 3). It is well known that focal seizures often develop—in open injuries more often with simple, and in closed injuries more often with complex, symptoms (Janz, 1969)—the symptomatology of which corresponds to the traumatic lesion of the cortical area, whose function is reflected by the seizure in an epileptically distorted manner. Less well known is that status epilepticus develops fairly often, i.e. in 11–17% of cases (Ketz, 1980, 1981; Janz, 1953, 1960; Heintel, 1972) after brain trauma, and, furthermore, occurs more frequently as a result of open injuries than after closed injuries (Ketz, 1980, 1981; Janz, 1960; Heintel, 1972; Oxbury and Whitty, 1971). Peculiar to these traumatic status attacks is that they mainly develop after injury of the frontal brain—and specifically in open injuries after a unilateral extensive injury of the frontal lobe (Figure 4)—and that they often, either singularly or repeatedly, represent the only epileptic symptom in such cases (isolated or iterated grand mal status) (Janz, 1960; Heintel, 1972; Oxbury and Whitty, 1971; Janz, 1974).

Prophylactic Medication

Now that we know something of the conditions whereby seizure expectancy can be assessed statistically in any given case and have an impression of the time aspects, the form and frequency of the expected seizures—in other words, of their spontaneous prognosis—it is useful to consider the means and prospects of prophylactic treatment. The most favourable reports on prophylactic medication, using 160–240 mg phenytoin and 30–60 mg phenobarbitone daily over a period of at least 3 years, were carried out in a very disciplined manner in Czechoslovakia before the pharmacokinetic era of epilepsy treatment (Servit, 1977; Servit and Musil, 1974), and could not now be replicated. The co-workers

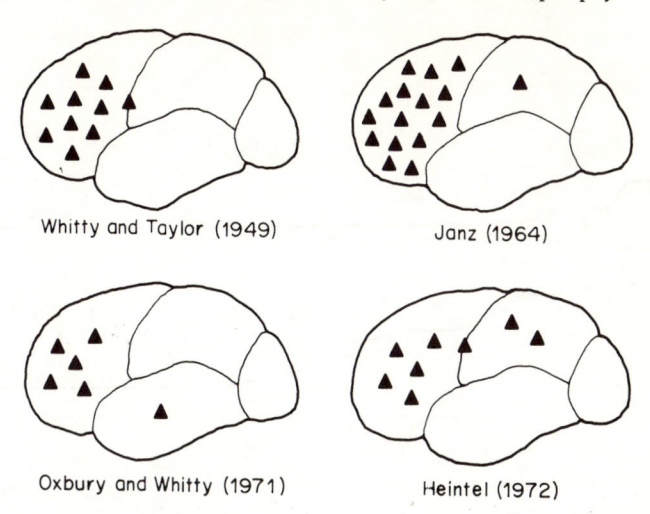

Figure 4. Site of lesions in cases of open head injuries and grand mal status

of Servit (1960), who had previously demonstrated experimentally the possibility of the medical prevention of epileptic seizures after brain trauma, have seen epileptic seizures after at least 3 and in most cases 5 years of follow-up in 3 out of 143 treated patients; in 2 of the 3 cases the seizures occurred only after termination of medication during the fourth and fifth year, and in 6 of 24 untreated patients, 4 had already had attacks in the first year after the trauma (Servit and Musil, 1981). Because the number of cases was thought to be too small, and the protocol of the investigation without placebo medication and double-blind controls unsatisfactory, a large prospective study was instigated in America using the aforementioned conditions and with the same medication and dosage (Rapport and Penry, 1973); the results were not published, apparently because it was concluded that a therapeutically effective serum level was generally not achieved (US-Plan: Head Injury, 1977) and seizures tended to appear more often in the untreated group than in the non-treated group (Penry, personal communication). The results of a second study with an alteration of medication have not yet been reported. In the meantime a number of studies of prophylactic treatment have been published using a variety of drugs—carbamazepine (Glötzner, 1983), phenytoin (Wohns and Wyler, 1979; Young et al., 1979; North et al., 1980; Salazar et al., 1985), phenobarbitone (Jennett and Lewin, 1960), valproic acid (Leviel and Naquet, 1977; Price, 1980)—in varying doses, in different forms of application, i.e. oral, i.v. and i.m., injections and infusions, and with different treatment periods. In none of the studies could the favourable results of the Czechoslovakian authors be reproduced. Out of 24 patients who were treated for 6 months or longer with

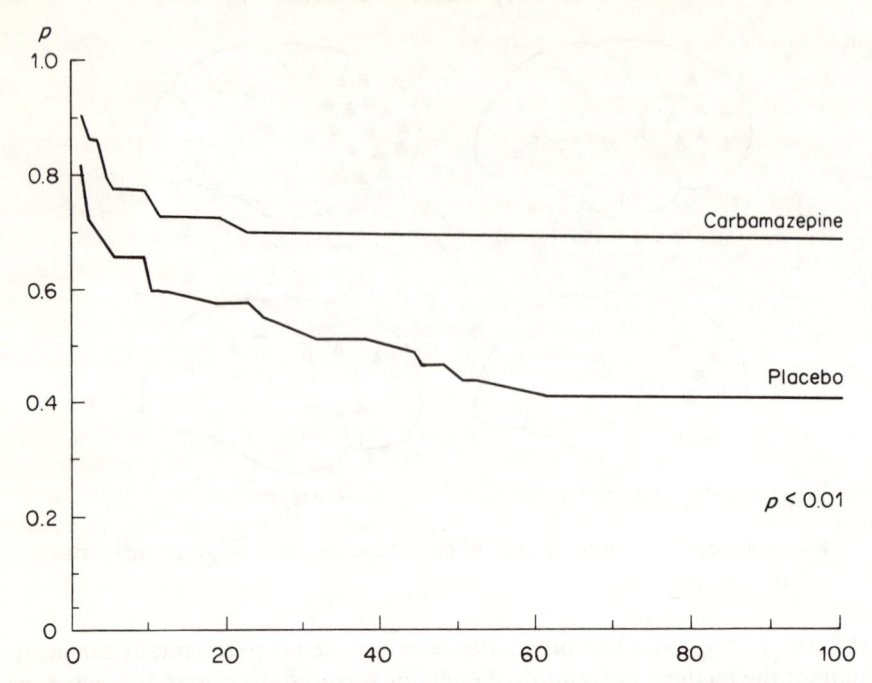

Figure 5. Effectiveness of prophylactic medication or carbamazepine in 108 patients with brain trauma. Cumulative probability (p) of remaining free of seizures until week indicated

phenobarbitone, 6 developed seizures, 5 of them after termination of medication. Six out of 12 untreated patients with approximately equally severe trauma developed seizures (Jennett and Lewin, 1960). Eight out of 101 patients who were treated with phenytoin after brain surgery developed seizures, as opposed to 17 out of 102 patients who were treated with placebo (North et al., 1980). In a group of 84 patients in whom a therapeutic level of 10–20 µg/mg was rapidly achieved by means of i.v. and i.m. injections of phenytoin immediately after the trauma, 5 cases developed a seizure between the 2nd and 52nd week, which is less frequently than would be expected on the basis of findings in the literature, but only 30 patients were still under observation after 3 months (Young et al., 1979). In a retrospective study of 50 patients who were also 'loaded' with 1000 mg phenytoin i.v. shortly after the trauma and generally received 400 mg daily thereafter, seizures were recorded in 5 cases, and out of 12 untreated patients in 6 cases (Wohns and Wyler, 1979). According to the Vietnam Head Injury Study, phenytoin therapy in the first year after penetrating head injuries did not prevent later seizures (Weiss et al., 1986). Glötzner (1983), in a methodologically satisfactory study, was recently able to show that the administration of carbamazepine beginning on the day of the trauma, whilst not being able to reduce the frequency of early seizures with certainty, led to a significant reduction in late seizures. A transition from early to late seizures occurred, moreover, as in Jennett's study (Jennett, 1975), in 28% of cases; Glötzner (1983) has demonstrated the effectiveness of prophylaxis in graphs of cumulative probability (Figure 5). Whereas new seizures were still appearing in the placebo group up to the 60th week, no new cases of post-traumatic seizures appeared after the 20th week in the treatment group, who were matched with the control group according to severity of trauma and other variables; the degree of effectiveness, with approximately 50% less seizures than in the placebo group, is not very impressive.

In almost all studies the complaint is made that, whilst the level of risk can be reasonably assessed according to the investigations of Jennett (1975, 1980, 1981) and others (Feeney and Walker, 1979; Weiss et al., 1983, 1986), and whilst the avoidability of post-traumatic seizures with prophylactic medication is experimentally well substantiated, the practical realization meets insurmountable barriers. Only about 6% of patients take their drugs for longer than 1 year (Jennett, 1980, 1981). Even in the case of studies which were motivated by scientific interest, therapeutic levels could still only be determined in 55–60% of cases after 6 months. To what extent results prove to be much poorer when medical prophylaxis becomes routine has been seen in the Vietnam war. For the first time, postoperative exhibition of prophylactic medication was made obligatory in the American group. In 75% of cases it consisted of 300–400 mg phenytoin daily, and in a further 20% an additional 96 mg of phenobarbitone. The incidence of traumatic epileptic seizures was somewhat greater in the case of the treated persons (177 out of 453) than in those who had discontinued treatment or were not treated (167 out of 577) (Caveness et al., 1979).

On the basis of these reports, the following comments can be made. Routine prevention of post-traumatic seizures with drugs is not indicated, since the benefit bears no relationship to the effort involved. The attempt to prevent early seizures medically does not seem to be appropriate even in the case of increased risk, since the measures that need to be taken to achieve a therapeutically effective serum concentration in a very short time are only justified in status epilepticus. In all those cases with a high risk of epilepsy it is worthwhile considering conventional initiation of prophylactic medication, i.e. gradually increasing dosage. One should discuss with the patient the possibility of beginning drug treatment only after a first seizure has occurred, especially since the Czechoslovakian authors report that they were still able to prevent the recurrence of seizures, and thereby its chronicity, when treatment was started only after the first seizure (Popek and Musil, 1969). Since the occurrence of one seizure after brain trauma still does not signify epilepsy, I am of the opinion that treatment should not be initiated until two seizures have occurred in a brief interval, and then given according to the usual rules. For the treatment of manifest epilepsy, the well-known rules of blood-level-controlled medication of the drug of choice according to type of seizures, course and expected side-effects, are valid (Schmidt, 1981).

The question as to whether the rules of treatment are also valid in the case of prophylactic medication is unclear. Phenobarbitone and valproic acid were found effective in the prevention of febrile convulsions, but carbamazepine and phenytoin were ineffective (Schmidt, 1981). If the development of traumatic epilepsy were comparable with a kindling effect, then phenobarbitone would presumably be the drug of choice—to the extent that animal experiments allow conclusions—whereas phenytoin would be useless and carbamazepine and valproic acid probably effective (Leviel and Naquet, 1977; Wada et al., 1976; Wauquier et al., 1979). On the other hand, phenytoin has proved effective in the suppression of seizures in experimentally induced cortical lesions. Apart from the choice of drug, the question as to what dosage or plasma concentration is prophylactically effective remains unanswered. Servit and Musil (1981) feel that their theoretical assumption, based on practical results, that even relatively small doses, 'which perhaps exert no noteworthy therapeutic effect' are prophylactically effective during the 'incubation period', is valid. The unsuccessful major experiment on the treatment of brain-damaged subjects of the Vietnam war with much higher doses cannot serve as an argument to the contrary, since it was hardly conducted systematically. A controlled comparison of medical regimens differing in type and dosage has so far not been done.

Last but not least there is controversy about the necessary duration of treatment. Young et al. (1979) pleaded for continuation for at least a number of months. Wohns and Wyler (1979) have terminated medication after 1 year but, when specific activity was still evident in the EEG, continued medication for at least 5 years even in the absence of seizures. Servit and Musil (1981) treated for a period of at least 2 years and report that even after treatment lasting 3 or 4 years, seizures occurred for the first time, though in their series, as in Jennett and Lewin's study (Jennett and Lewin, 1960), it is not clear whether they were in fact withdrawal seizures—which is, moreover, an additional risk of treatment. Whoever initiates treatment should have a well-founded idea of how long it should last, but the literature provides no clear guidelines for this decision.

Unless the patient himself insists, I see no necessity, either on grounds of the risk involved, or on grounds of the EEG, or of other circumstances, for prophylactic treatment. Also, in the case of a first seizure there are no criteria for the likelihood that it will recur. There is not really any social complication that could be prevented by premature or early medical treatment. For example, patients with particularly risky professions—Jennett (1980, 1981) mentions surgeons and pilots in this respect—will hardly remain capable of employment after brain injury involving such a high risk of epilepsy that prophylactic treatment is worthy of consideration. Finally, a strong motive which is repeatedly cited in favour of prophylactic medication is the worry that the patient may lose his driving licence after a first post-traumatic seizure. The question as to whether, even with a high risk, half of all patients should receive a laborious, and in the final analysis, risky, treatment is, for those who have reservations regarding prophylactic medication (Evans, 1962; Caveness et al., 1979; Janz, 1976; Rish and Caveness, 1973; Wolf, 1980), decisive.

Conclusions

The watershed between early and late seizures is the first week after the trauma. The development of both correlates with the severity of the trauma as does the risk of a late epilepsy after early seizures. Early seizures do not recur in three-quarters of the cases, late seizures do not recur in one-quarter of the cases, with a span between closed and open brain injuries, with and without complications. Up to 60% become manifest within the first year and up to 80% within the second year after the trauma. The incidence of seizures occurring more than 4 years after closed head injuries is not greater than would be expected without trauma. The risk of epileptic seizures is greatest (approximately 70%) in the case of open wounds with wound infections and brain abscesses. It is about 30–50% in the case of bullet wounds and about 10–20% in the case of closed brain injuries. It is greater in the case of localized injuries of the central region than in lesions of the frontal and occipital poles. In the case of blunt skull trauma, factors which increase the risk are: depressed fracture, intracranial haematoma, long period of unconsciousness. Early and late seizures are mainly of the focal type, in the case of early seizures with primarily simple, in the case of late seizures with primarily complex, symptomatology. The course of major seizures is mainly independent of the sleep–waking cycle. Status epilepticus occurs fairly often, particularly after open frontal brain injuries. EEG investigations seem to be uninformative with regard to both prognosis and course.

The experimental, and most of the clinical, studies suggest that prophylactic antiepileptic medication reduces the incidence of traumatic late seizures. The questions as to which drug, in which dosage and plasma concentration, is sufficiently effective and reliable, and how long treatment should last, have not been answered. Even with the higher risk of epilepsy, the usefulness and risks of treatment should be weighed up with the patient and consideration should be given to the fact that, even in the case of epileptic seizures without trauma, one does not begin treatment after the first fit but only after a repetition of seizures.

References

Annegers JF, Grabow JD, Groover RV, et al. Seizures after head trauma: a population study. Neurology (Minneap) 1980; 30: 683–689.
Ashcroft PB. Traumatic epilepsy after gunshot wounds of the head. Br Med J 1941; 1: 739–744.
Caveness WF, Meirowski AM, Rish BL, et al. The nature of post-traumatic epilepsy. J Neurosurg 1979; 50: 545–553.
Courjon J. A longitudinal electro-clinical study of 80 cases of post-traumatic epilepsy. Epilepsia 1970; 11: 29–36.
Elvidge AR. Remarks on post-traumatic convulsive state. Trans Am Neurol Assoc 1939; 65: 125–129.
Evans JH. Post traumatic epilepsy. Neurology (Minneap) 1962; 12: 665–674.
Feeney DM, Walker AE. The prediction of posttraumatic epilepsy. A mathematical approach. Arch Neurol 1979; 36: 8–72.
Glötzner FL. Ansfallsprophylaxe mit Carbamazepin nach schweren Schädelhirnverletrungen. Neurochirurgia 1983; 26: 66–79.
Heintel H. Der Status Epilepticus. Stuttgart: Fischer, 1972.
Jabbari B, Vengrow MI, Salazar AM, et al. Clinical and radiological correlates of EEG in the late phase of head injury: A study of 515 Vietnam Veterans. Electroencephalogr Clin Neurophysiol 1986; 64: 285–293.
Janz D. 'Diffuse' Epilepsien. Dtsch Z Nervenheilk 1953; 170: 486–513.
Janz D. Status epilepticus und Stirnhirn. Dtsch Z Nervenheilk 1960; 180: 562–594.
Janz D. Die Epilepsien. Stuttgart: Thieme, 1969.
Janz D. In: Vinken PJ, Bruyn GW (eds). Handbook of Clinical Neurology. The Epilepsies 1974; 15: 311. Amsterdam: North-Holland Publishing Co.
Janz D. Problems encountered in the treatment of epilepsy. In: Birkmayer W (ed) Epileptic Seizures—Behaviour—Pain. Bern, Stuttgart, Wien: Hans Huber Publications, 1976: 65–75.
Janz D. Prognosis and prophylaxis of traumatic epilepsy. In: Rose FC (ed) Research Progress in Epilepsy. London: Pitman, 1983: 161–74.
Jennett B. Early traumatic epilepsy. Lancet 1969; i: 1023–1025.
Jennett B. Epilepsy after Non-missile Head Injuries. London: Heinemann Medical Books, 1975.
Jennett WB. Die Vorhersage von posttraumatischen Epilepsien. In: Remschmidt H, Rentz R, Jungmann J (eds) Epilepsie. Stuttgart: Thieme, 1980, 1981: 98–105.
Jennett WB, Lewin WS. Traumatic epilepsy after closed head injuries. J Neurol Neurosurg Psychiat 1960; 23: 295–301.
Ketz E. Erkennung und Wertung pathoplastischer Faktoren bei posttraumatischen Epilepsien. In: Remschmidt H, Rentz R, Jungmann J (eds) Epilepsie. Stuttgart: Thieme, 1980, 1981.
Kollevold T. Immediate and early cerebral seizures after head injury. J Oslo City Hosp 1976; 26: 99–114.
Lange-Cosack H, Wider B, Schlessener JH, et al. Spätfolgen nach Schädelhirntraumen im Säuglings- und Kindesalte. Neuropädiatrie 1979; 10: 105–127.
Legg NJ, Gupta PC, Scott DF. Epilepsy following cerebral abscess. Brain 1973; 96: 259–268.
Leviel V, Naquet R. A study of the action of valproic acid on the kindling effect. Epilepsia 1977; 18: 229–234.
North JB, Ponhall RK, Hanieh A, et al. Postoperative epilepsy: a double-blind trial of phenytoin after craniotomy. Lancet 1980; i: 384–386.

Oxbury JM, Whitty CWM. Causes and consequences of status epilepticus in adults. Brain 1971; 94: 733–744.
Oxbury JM, Whitty CWM. The syndrome of isolated status epilepticus. J Neurol Neurosurg Psychiat 1971; 34: 182–184.
Paillas JE, Paillas N, Bureau M. Post-traumatic epilepsy. Epilepsia 1970; 11: 5–15.
Popek K, Musil F. Klinický pokus a prevenci posttraumatické epilepsie potezkých zranénich mozku u dospelých. Cas Lek Cesk 1969; 108: 133–147.
Price DJ. In: Parsonage MF, Caldwell ADS (eds) The Place of Sodium Valproate in the Treatment of Epilepsy. London: Academic Press, 1980: 23–30.
Rapport RL, Penry KJ. A survey of attitudes towards the pharmacological prophylaxis of post-traumatic epilepsy. J Neurosurg 1973; 38: 159–166.
Rish BL, Caveness WF. Relation of prophylactic medication to the occurrence of early seizures following cranio-cerebral trauma. J Neurosurg 1973; 38: 155–158.
Ritz, ER, Jacobi G, Thorbecke R. Die posttraumatische Epilepsie im Kindersalter. In: Remschmidt H, Rentz R, Jungmann J (eds) Epilepsie. Stuttgart: Thieme, 1980, 1981.
Russell WR, Whitty CWM. Studies in traumatic epilepsy. J Neurol Neurosurg Psychiat 1952; 15: 93–98.
Salazar AM, Jabbari B, Vance SC, et al. Epilepsy after penetrating head injury. I. Clinical correlates: A report of the Vietnam Head Injury Study. Neurology 1985; 35: 1406–1414.
Scherzer E, Wessely P. EEG in post-traumatic epilepsy. Eur Neurol 1978; 17: 38–42.
Schmidt D. Die Behandlung der Epilepsien. Stuttgart: Thieme, 1981.
Servit Z. Prophylactic treatment of post-traumatic audiogenic epilepsy. Nature 1960; 188: 669–670.
Servit Z. Prophylactic treatment of posttraumatic epilepsy—clinical results and theoretical interpretations. In: Majkowski J (ed) Posttraumatic epilepsy and pharmacological prophylaxis. Warsaw: Polish Chapter of the ILAE, 1977: 182–191.
Servit Z. Musil F. Prophylactic treatment of post-traumatic epilepsy. Epilepsia 1974; 15: 640.
Servit Z, Musil F. Prophylactic treatment of posttraumatic epilepsy. Experimental and clinical studies in Czechoslovakia (1960–1972). Epilepsia 1981; 22: 315–320.
Stöwsand D. Paresen und epileptische Reaktionen im Initial-Stadium des Hirntraumas. Stuttgart: Thieme, 1971.
US-Plan: Head Injury. In: Plan for Nationwide Action on Epilepsy. US Department of Health, Education and Welfare. DHEW Publication No. (NIH) 78–311 Vol II Part I 1977: 245–255.
Wada JA, Osawa T, Sato M, et al. Acute anticonvulsant effects of DPH, phenobarbital and carbamazepine. Epilepsia 1976; 17: 77–88.
Walker AE. Prognosis of post-traumatic epilepsy. J Am Med Assoc 1957; 164: 1636–1641.
Walker AE, Jablon S. A follow up of head injured men of World War 2. J Neurosurg 1959; 16: 600–610.
Wauquier A, Ashton D, Melis W. Behavioural analysis of amygdaloid kindling in beagle dogs. Exp Neurol 1979; 64: 579–586.
Weiss GH, Feeney DM, Caveness WF, et al. Prognostic factors for the occurrence of posttraumatic epilepsy. Arch Neurol 1983; 40: 7–10.
Weiss GH, Salazar AM, Vance SC et al. Predicting posttraumatic epilepsy in penetrating head injury. Arch Neurol 1986; 43: 771–773.
Wessely P. Zur Bedeutung von Zeitfaktoren bei posttraumatischen Anfällen. In:

Remschmidt H, Rentz R, Jungmann J (eds) Epilepsie. Stuttgart: Thieme, 1980, 1981: 138–143.

Wohns RNW, Wyler AR. Prophylactic phenytoin in severe head injuries. J Neurosurg 1979; 51: 507–509.

Wolf P. Discussion remark. In: Parsonage MJ, Caldwell ADS (eds) The Place of Sodium Valproate in the Treatment of Epilepsy. London: Academic Press, 1980: 31–32.

Young B, Rapp R, Brooks W, et al. Post-traumatic epilepsy prophylaxis. Epilepsia 1979; 20: 671–681.

8
Cognitive Hazards of Seizure Disorders*

Michael R. Trimble
Institute of Neurology, London, UK

Epilepsy is a chronic disorder in which the main clinical characteristic is a liability to have recurrent seizures. In the majority of cases, the disorder begins in childhood, and it is usual for sufferers to take long-term anticonvulsant therapy. Although it is true that many patients with epilepsy retain their keenness of intellect and are able to lead a normal lifestyle, patients with resistant epilepsy are often not so fortunate.

Impairment of cognitive abilities and a decline of intellectual functions have been commented on as a complication of epilepsy for many years. An early study was performed by Reynolds (1861), who attempted to assess the mental state of epileptic patients between their seizures by dividing them into four different groups. The first were those that were considered normal, the second had 'slight defect of memory', the third had 'in addition to the defective attention or loss of memory, diminution of the faculty of apprehension', and the fourth were those who 'exhibit also more or less confusion of ideas'. He found that 38% of his patients were free from 'mental failure', but two-thirds were in some way affected, 'a notable degree of mental incapacity existed in but one-seventh of the total number of cases'. Likewise, Gowers (1881) stated 'the mental state of epileptics, as is well known, frequently presents deterioration, and this constitutes one of the consequences of the disease which is much dreaded, and is often most serious. In its slightest form there is merely defective memory, especially for recent acquisitions. In more severe degree there is greater imperfection of intellectual power, weakened capacity for attention, and often defective moral control'.

* This chapter was previously published in Epilepsia 1988; 29, suppl I: S19–S24, and is reproduced by permission of Raven Press, New York.

Chronic Epilepsy, Its Prognosis and Management
Edited by M.R. Trimble. 1989 Published by John Wiley & Sons Ltd

Curiously, this aspect of epilepsy has received little attention until recently, and it became assumed that any relationships between epilepsy and alteration of the mental state were of an indirect nature. This belief is summed up by the writings of Lennox (1941), who said 'mental impairment does not necessarily or usually accompany seizures or result from them'. In his large series of over 1600 patients, only 1% were 'markedly deteriorated'.

Of the many possible factors that may lead to alteration of the mental state, the ones that have received the most attention related to underlying organic factors, in particular brain damage and seizure variables. A brief review of the literature will be given prior to a summary of two studies that have been carried out, one in children and one in adults, that have attempted to analyse some of the variables that may be related to cognitive deterioration in patients with severe epilepsy.

Organic Factors Underlying Neuropsychological Deficits

Brain Damage

Several investigators have noted that patients with symptomatic epilepsy are more likely to have impaired intellect than those with epilepsy and no known cause (Lennox, 1942; Bourgeois et al., 1983). Kløve and Matthews (1966) examined four groups of patients. Normal controls were compared to patients with epilepsy and identifiable brain pathology, to those with epilepsy and no brain damage, and to patients with brain damage but no epilepsy. In the majority of their comparisons, normal subjects were superior to the other three groups, and generally the scoring was worse in the brain-damaged groups. The performance of those with epilepsy and brain damage was inferior to those who had epilepsy and no brain damage, while the performance of the brain-damaged group without epilepsy was superior to that of the brain-damaged group with epilepsy. Thus, pre-existing brain damage, although obviously a factor, does not completely explain the neuropsychological deficits observed in patients with epilepsy, and when patients with brain damage are excluded from analyses, or brain-damage effects are controlled for, neuropsychological deficits are still found.

Seizure Variables

Age of onset of seizures, duration of epilepsy, seizure type, and seizure frequency have been examined. Most investigators have found that an early age of onset of seizures has a poorer prognosis with regard to intellectual abilities, although few studies specifically control for seizure type and duration of epilepsy. Dickmen, Matthews and Harley (1975) compared two groups of patients matched for duration and frequency of tonic–clonic seizures but differing with regard to age of onset, and noted that patients with epilepsy that started before the age of 5 years were more impaired in the majority of tasks than those with later onset seizures.

O'Leary et al. (1981) also examined children with tonic–clonic seizures, and in their statistical analysis covaried for illness duration. Again, children with early-onset seizures were more significantly impaired.

There is less agreement about seizure type, but much of the confusion arises from the difficulty of classifying seizures in the clinical setting. It is clear that patients with generalized absence seizures have impaired cognitive performance for the duration of their EEG spike–wave abnormality, although generally patients with this form of seizure show minimal interictal problems. However, if the absences are frequent, impairment of performance in the classroom setting may lead to educational underachievement.

In one recent study, Giordani et al. (1985) assessed a large number of patients, used the International Seizure Classification, and in analysis of covariance used age of onset of seizures, duration of seizures, frequency of seizures, and drug variables as covariants. Patients with partial seizures were found to perform significantly better on the majority of subtests of the WAIS when compared to those with generalized seizures.

Several recent studies have explored seizure frequency, and note a relationship to intellectual performance. Dickmen and Matthews (1977), looking at patients with major motor seizures, noted that a group with high seizure frequency performed more poorly than those with low seizure frequency on a variety of cognitive tasks, mainly from the WAIS and Halstead neuropsychological test battery. The worst scores were in patients with a long seizure history and an early age of onset. Seidenberg et al. (1981) used a longitudinal design and compared the test–retest performance on the WAIS of two groups of adult patients. For one group, seizure frequency had decreased during the test–retest interval, and for the other it had increased or remained unchanged. The former group showed significantly more improvements on the intelligence quotients (IQ) tests.

Dodrill (1986) examined relationships between the frequency of generalized tonic–clonic seizures and a variety of psychological variables in a large number of patients with epilepsy who had exceptionally clear seizure histories. He noted that an episode of status epilepticus or more than 100 individual convulsions were associated with decreased functioning in a variety of areas. Wilkus and Dodrill (1976) noted on a battery of psychological tests that a group of patients with generalized discharges on the EEG performed the poorest, and in general patients with discharges occurring at a rate of more than 1/min did worse than those with fewer discharges. These data suggest that in patients with generalized seizures, seizure frequency is an important variable for cognitive processing, and that the rate of interictal EEG activity may also correlate with cognitive impairment. Similar data have been suggested for partial seizures by Binnie (1986). He pointed out that so-called 'subclinical' discharges may indeed have clinical significance, since his group could show transitory cognitive impairment on some selective cognitive tasks that correlated with brief interictal EEG focal discharges.

Anticonvulsant Drugs

Another important variable in relation to cognitive change in epilepsy is the prescription of anticonvulsant drugs. Extensive reviews of this are available elsewhere (Trimble and Thompson, 1986) and a summary of the current state of information would be as follows. Detrimental effects on neuropsychological abilities have been reported for the majority of existing anticonvulsants, although the nature of the deficits observed differs between different studies and different prescriptions. In general, phenytoin is the one that is most often implicated and carbamazepine the least. Another finding that emerges from recent studies is that a relationship exists between anticonvulsant serum level concentration and cognitive impairments, with high but not necessarily toxic levels being associated with deficits.

In studies in which patients on polytherapy have had their medication rationalized, with a diminishing burden of anticonvulsant prescription, improvements in cognitive function have been demonstrated that take place over several months, and affect a wide spectrum of cognitive abilities (Thompson and Trimble, 1982a). In patients on monotherapy, differences in the profile of impairment of cognitive abilities have been examined by comparing patients on high and low serum levels of phenytoin, carbamazepine, and valproate, and have been complemented by studies in healthy volunteers taking anticonvulsant medication for 2 weeks in a series of investigations using a double-blind, controlled crossover design. The data from these studies (Thompson, Huppert and Trimble, 1981; Thompson and Trimble, 1982b; Thompson and Trimble, 1981) demonstrated that the drugs exerted different cognitive impairments, although there was consistency between the patient and volunteer studies. Carbamazepine exerted the least effect, while phenytoin, both in volunteers and in patients, led to widespread disruption of cognitive ability, with valproate holding an intermediate position. Two benzodiazepine anticonvulsants were also examined in the volunteers, namely clonazepam and the 1,5-benzodiazepine, clobazam. Clonazepam, at an oral dose of 0.5 mg t.d.s., produced a general impairment of abilities, and appeared to impair new learning, patients failing to demonstrate practice effects on a number of tasks that were noted with clobazam. Cognitive impairments with clobazam were minimal, in keeping with the other literature on this drug, which emphasizes its non-sedative and psychotropic properties (Cull and Trimble, 1985).

Although these effects are important, they should not be confused with an alternative proposition, namely that anticonvulsant drugs play a role in the development of a chronic insidious encephalopathy in patients with epilepsy, which leads to a decline of intellectual functions, a dementia syndrome, which in many cases is irreversible. Thus, the effects shown in volunteers in the above studies (Thompson, Huppert and Trimble, 1981) seem to occur in most people to whom the drugs are given, irrespective of whether epilepsy is present or not. In patients with epilepsy, the anticonvulsants become an additional burden to the cognitive handicaps that are already derived from underlying seizure and brain-damage-related variables as discussed above. In the majority of cases, these effects seem reversible, as shown in the studies of rationalization of patients' medications (Thompson and Trimble, 1982a).

The Dementia of Epilepsy

As suggested above, the fact that a certain number of patients with epilepsy show relentless cognitive deterioration has been recognized for some time. A number of the variables that may be related to this have been presented, and it would seem obvious that in any patient the clinical picture may arise from several compounding variables. We have carried out two investigations that have specifically attempted to assess differences between patients with epilepsy who have acquired intellectual deterioration in comparison with a group who do not. The first of these was at the Lingfield Hospital School for Epilepsy (Trimble and Corbett, 1980), and the second at the Chalfont Centre for Epilepsy in a collaborative study with Dr P. Bittencourt, Dr P. Lorenzo, Dr J. Oxley, Dr I. Reider, Dr P. Thompson, Dr E. Valentine and Prof. A. Richens.

In the Lingfield Hospital School study, 312 children with epilepsy had a complete neuropsychiatric examination carried out; the medications that patients were receiving were recorded from their charts, and their seizure frequency taken from their case records. Psychological tests were provided, and those children who had received two or more estimates of their IQ while they were at the school were selected to detect a group whose IQ had deteriorated over time. The criteria for deterioration was a fall of IQ greater than 10 points in two estimates of IQ done over 1 year apart.

Of the total sample, 204 fulfilled the requirements, and 15% of these showed a deterioration of IQ. The mean fall was 21.3 points, with a range of -10 to -48. A number of variables were then examined, comparing the group with IQ fall to those who did not show an IQ fall. The children who had deteriorated showed significantly higher serum levels of phenytoin and primidone and lower serum folic acid levels than those without an IQ fall, and even when only children having less than ten seizures a month were examined, to minimize the impact of seizure frequency, the findings still pertained for phenytoin and serum folic acid. Interestingly, in this investigation, no relationship was seen between seizure frequency and fall of IQ.

In the study carried out in collaboration with the Chalfont Centre, 40 patients were selected, all of whom had chronic epilepsy and were resident at the centre. Detailed seizure and drug charts were studied for every patient covering a period of 10 years prior to the investigation. As reliable a history as possible of seizure variables and total anticonvulsant intake was therefore available for a considerable period of time prior to the investigation, and, further, any head injury associated with seizures was recorded.

Table 1. Total intake of drugs over 10 years ($N = 40$)

	Mean (g)	SD	Range
Phenytoin	1009	312	0–1460
Phenobartitone	241	239	1–624
Carbamazepine	526	860	0–3650
Primidone	1402	1316	0–3923
Valproate	446	732	0–2336
Ethosuximide	607	1162	0–4562

Table 2. Seizure frequencies in patients under study ($N = 40$)

	Mean	SD	Range
Tonic–clonic	172	154	0–508
Complex partial	246	503	0–1894
Spike–wave	335	700	0–2589
Others	172	429	0–2113

Seizures were classified into four types, namely tonic–clonic, complex partial, seizures associated with clear spike–wave activity on the EEG, and others. Head injury was recorded by noting when the patients required nursing, medical, or surgical attention for head injury, and the total drug intake was calculated by adding up the actual prescriptions that patients received over a 10-year period.

Patients underwent psychological testing (Dr Thompson) in which an estimated premorbid IQ was obtained and a modified form of the WAIS given. Patients who had deteriorated by greater than 15 points were then compared to those where there was no deterioration.

Of the 40 patients, 30 were male and the age range was 20–57 years. Twenty-one were rated as deteriorated. The total drug intake over 10 years is given in Table 1, and the total seizure frequencies in Table 2. Table 3 shows the significant relationships between seizure factors, head injury, and drug intake when the group with deterioration was compared to those with no deterioration. It can be seen that three variables seemed of the most importance: generalized tonic–clonic seizures, medical attention for head injury, and anticonvulsant drugs, notably phenytoin and primidone.

Both of the above studies, one in children and one in adults, have concentrated on a small group of patients who have undergone cognitive deterioration in the setting of epilepsy. This may be appropriately referred to as dementia, although others use the term encephalopathy. Both studies investigated the relative role of a number of variables in relation to cognitive decline, and some consistency does emerge. Further, the data provided are in keeping with other

Table 3. Significance values (one-tailed) for seizure factors, head injury, and drug intake—demented versus non-demented

	p value
Seizures	
Generalized tonic–clonic	<0.005
Generalized spike–wave	NS
Complex partial	NS
Others	NS
Age of onset	NS
Duration of epilepsy	NS
Anticonvulsant drugs	
Phenobarbitone	NS
Carbamazepine	NS
Valproate	NS
Phenytoin	<0.05
Primidone	<0.05
Medical attention for head injury	<0.002

literature. In both studies, drugs are implicated, particularly phenytoin. The association between this drug and a deteriorated cognitive state, sometimes referred to as a dementia or an encephalopathy, but associated with neurological signs of toxicity, has been well recognized, the syndrome being well reviewed by Roseman (1961) and being referred to by Rosen (1966) as dilantin dementia. The latter author described 20 patients in whom school performance improved rapidly when phenytoin was discontinued for various reasons, improvement being associated with corresponding changes in psychological tests. However, this picture is not always associated with toxic serum levels of the drug, and the encephalopathy may be associated with involuntary movements and a modest rise of cerebrospinal fluid (CSF) protein.

Reynolds and Travers (1974) noted, in a series of 57 adult epileptic outpatients on chronic anticonvulsant therapy, that intellectual deterioration and psychomotor slowing were associated with significantly higher concentrations of both phenobarbitone and phenytoin compared with patients without such changes, an effect that did not seem to relate to seizure frequency. These data in adults were thus similar to those in our study of children, and lend weight to the importance of anticonvulsants in provoking such clinical pictures. Whether it is a direct effect of some of these drugs or a secondary effect of intermediate metabolic disturbances such as the disruption of folic acid metabolism is unclear. Nonetheless, it is interesting that folate deficiency is related to the taking of phenobarbitone and phenytoin. Carbamazepine and valproate have only minimal effects on serum folate levels (Dellaportas et al., 1982; Turnbull et al., 1982), these two drugs also being less related to impairment of cognitive function, and, certainly with regard to carbamazepine, to date have not been implicated in progressive cognitive decline.

Summary and Conclusions

To suffer from epilepsy and to have recurrent seizures is a major social handicap. In recent years it has become clear that with skilful use of clinical and electroencephalographic investigation techniques, and serum level monitoring, it is possible to control seizures in the majority of patients, allowing them to lead as full a life as possible. However, there are a group of patients whose seizures are intractable, and as a consequence receive anticonvulsant drugs over many years. It is a clinical tragedy when patients in this group begin to show cognitive and intellectual decline, which happens in a subgroup. To date, it has not been possible to identify those patients that develop this clinical picture, although attempts should be made in future research to do so. Thus, if patients at risk may be identified, the factors that put them at risk may also be identified, and attempts to prevent intellectual deterioration occurring can then be made.

In this chapter I have reviewed a number of factors that may be related to progressive intellectual decline, and highlighted seizure- and treatment-related variables. It would seem that patients most at risk are those who have continuing seizures, mainly of a generalized tonic–clonic type, during which they fall and suffer recurrent head injuries. These patients are more likely to have taken long-term prescriptions of the older barbiturate drugs or phenytoin, and in several studies the role of phenytoin in exacerbating the clinical picture emerges. Polytherapy in itself is a continuous hazard for these patients, since polytherapy may not only be noxious in its own right, but also will certainly compound any existing deterioration from other organic factors.

For those of us who manage patients with chronic epilepsy, assessment and management of cognitive disabilities assume increasing importance the more we recognize their presence. We seek the continued development of more effective anticonvulsant drugs that have minimal sedative properties and can be safely given to our patients over many years.

References

Binnie CD. Monitoring seizures. In: Trimble MR, Reynolds EH (eds) What is epilepsy? Edinburgh: Churchill Livingstone, 1986: 82–7.

Bourgeois BFD, Prensky AL, Palkes HS, Talent BK, Busch SG. Intelligence in epilepsy: a prospective study in children. Ann Neurol 1983; 14: 438–44.

Cull CA, Trimble MR. Anticonvulsant benzodiazepines and performance. In: Royal Society of Medicine International Congress and Symposium, Series 74. London: Royal Society of Medicine, 1985: 121–8.

Dellaportas CI, Shorvon SD, Galbraith AW, Laundy M, Reynolds EH. Chronic toxicity in epileptic patients receiving single drug treatment. Br Med J 1982; 285: 409–10.

Dickmen S, Matthews CG. Effect of major motor seizure frequency on cognitive–intellectual function in adults. Epilepsia 1977; 18: 21–9.
Dickmen S, Matthews CG, Harley JP. The effect of early versus late onset of major motor epilepsy upon cognitive intellectual function. Epilepsia 1975; 16: 73–81.
Dodrill CB. Correlates of generalised tonic–clonic seizures with intellectual, neuropsychological, emotional and social function in patients with epilepsy. Epilepsia 1986; 27: 399–411.
Giordani B, Berent S, Sackellares JC, Rourke D, Seidenberg M, O'Leary DS, Dreifuss FE, Ball TJ. Intelligence test performance of patients with partial and generalised seizures. Epilepsia 1985; 26: 37–42.
Gowers WE. Epilepsy and other chronic convulsive diseases. London: Churchill, 1881.
Kløve H, Matthews CG. Psychometric and adaptive abilities in epilepsy with different aetiology. Epilepsia 1966; 7: 330–8.
Lennox WG. Science and seizures. New York: Harper and Brothers, 1941.
Lennox WG. Brain injury, drugs and environment as causes of mental decay in epilepsy. Am J Psychiatr 1942; 99: 174–80.
O'Leary DS, Seidenberg M, Berent S, Boll TJ. Effects of age of onset of tonic–clonic seizures on neuropsychological performance in children. Epilepsia 1981; 22: 197–204.
Reynolds EH, Travers RD. Serum anticonvulsant concentrations in epileptic patients with mental symptoms. Br J Psychiatry 1974; 124: 440–5.
Reynolds JR. Epilepsy: its symptoms, treatment and relation to other chronic convulsive diseases. London: Churchill, 1861.
Roseman E. Dilantin toxicity. Neurology 1961; 11: 912–21.
Rosen JA. Dilantin dementia. Trans Am Neurol Assoc 1966; 93: 273.
Seidenberg M, O'Leary DS, Berent S, Boll T. Changes in seizure frequency and test re-test scores on the WAIS. Epilepsia 1981; 22: 75–83.
Thompson PJ, Huppert F, Trimble MR. Phenytoin and cognitive functions: effects on normal volunteers and implications for epilepsy. Br J Clin Psychol 1981; 20: 151–62.
Thompson PJ, Trimble MR. In: Clobazam and cognitive functions. Effects in healthy volunteers. Royal Society of Medicine International Congress and Symposium, Series 43. London: Royal Society of Medicine, 1981: 33–8.
Thompson PJ, Trimble MR. Anticonvulsant drugs and cognitive functions. Epilepsia 1982a; 23: 531–44.
Thompson PJ, Trimble MR. Comparative effects of anticonvulsant drugs on cognitive functioning. Br J Clin Practice 1982b; 18 (suppl.): 154–6.
Trimble MR, Corbett JA. Behavioural and cognitive disturbances in epileptic children. Irish Med J 1980; 73 (suppl.): 21–8.
Trimble MR, Thompson PJ. Neuropsychological aspects of epilepsy. In: Grant I, Adams KM (eds) Neuropsychological assessment of neuropsychiatric disorders. New York: Oxford University Press, 1986: 321–46.
Turnbull DM, Rawlings MD, Weightman D, Chadwick DW. A comparison of phenytoin and valproate in previously untreated epileptic patients. J Neurol Neurosurg Psychiatry 1982; 45: 55–9.
Wilkus RJ, Dodrill CB. Neuropsychological correlates of the EEG in epileptics. Epilepsia 1976; 17: 89–100.

9
Social Difficulties and Severe Epilepsy: Survey Results and Recommendations

Pamela J. Thompson and Jolyon Oxley
National Society for Epilepsy, Chalfont St Peter, UK

Introduction

Having epilepsy is more than coping with a medical diagnosis. It can influence many aspects of an individual's life. In recent years there has been evidence of increasing awareness of the social dimensions of this disorder and their importance to the medical profession. In the UK a leading pharmaceutical company has sponsored meetings devoted to specific social problems, covering topics such as driving (Godwin-Austen and Espir, 1983), employment (Edwards, Espir and Oxley, 1986), the criminal law (Fenwick and Fenwick, 1985), education (Oxley and Stores, 1987), and, most recently, the family (Hoare, 1988). Review chapters in major textbooks have also appeared (Craig and Oxley, 1988; Scambler, 1987).

Research into social aspects of epilepsy is also on the increase. Generally speaking, however, research studies have sampled groups that are heterogeneous with respect to seizure frequency and severity. Investigators report a wide range of social difficulties which are more frequently to be found in patients with poorly controlled seizures, multiple seizure types or associated problems (Rodin, 1987; Dodrill, 1986; Beran and Flanagan, 1987). Patients falling into this category, while being identified as an at-risk group, are seldom the target for more thorough investigation. Consequently, little is known about the nature and extent of the difficulties they experience. More detailed information of this kind is essential for planning appropriate services, thus helping to reduce the level of social difficulties encountered and the impact of the disability.

Chronic Epilepsy, Its Prognosis and Management
Edited by M.R. Trimble. © 1989 John Wiley & Sons Ltd

The present study aimed to explore more systematically the social difficulties experienced by individuals with difficult-to-control seizures. The results presented here are an extension of a previously published survey (Thompson and Oxley, 1988). The main study group were patients admitted to a residential assessment centre for epilepsy, a group that has been enlarged since the previous report. A second group of patients who were referred for consideration for surgical treatment of their seizures is also now included. Patients of this type also have poorly controlled seizures but some interesting differences emerged in comparison with the assessment centre referrals.

This chapter also discusses the social problems found in these patients and points to some effective strategies for prevention and remedy.

Patients Studied

Assessment Centre Group

The assessment unit at the Chalfont Centre for Epilepsy provides a thorough medical assessment as well as an evaluation of an individual's employment and independent living potential. Assessment takes on average 3 months. One hundred and twelve patients admitted to the unit during the period January 1986 to January 1988 were included in the study. Patients were excluded if a diagnosis of epilepsy was unconfirmed or if they were unable to cope with the intellectual demands of the study. Medico-demographic details of the group are given in Table 1. From this it can be seen that the patients are a relatively young group with intellectual skills biased towards the below-average ability ranges. The majority of the sample have complex partial seizures with or without secondarily generalized seizures. The onset of epilepsy was mostly in childhood with a few patients experiencing significant periods of remission. Most patients were experiencing at least weekly seizures at the time of admission.

Surgical Evaluation Group

The 32 patients who were surveyed were referred for an assessment of their suitability for neurosurgical intervention to the National Hospital for Nervous Diseases during the period September 1985 to August 1988. Details of this group are given in Table 1. They too are a relatively young group. However, a wide range of intellectual ability was represented, the majority of the sample falling within the average range. Not surprisingly, the majority of the patients had complex partial seizures, but fewer than the assessment centre sample experienced secondary generalization. Three patients in addition to experiencing complex partial seizures had atonic attacks. These three patients were being considered for possible corpus callosotomy. The age of onset of epilepsy was later than the assessment centre sample, although the duration of epilepsy

Table 1. Medico-demographic details of the patient samples

	Assessment centre	Surgical evaluation
Number	112	32
Males	56	16
Age (years)		
Mean	27.1	29.6
Range	16–55	17–51
IQ		
Mean	84.1	100
Range	61–124	75–120
Type of epilepsy		
Generalized	10%	0%
Complex partial	21%	56%
Complex partial with secondary generalized	69%	44%
Age of onset		
Mean	8.6	11.7
Range	0–49	3–40
Duration		
Mean	18.5	17.6
Range	2–52	3–44
Seizure frequency		
<monthly	3%	0%
monthly	8%	9%
weekly	53%	66%
daily	36%	25%

was comparable. The majority of the sample experienced seizures on a weekly basis and are therefore also a group with refractory seizures.

Methods Used

Every participant completed the Social Problems Questionnaire (SPQ) (Corney and Clare, 1985). This is a short self-report measure which assesses an individual's personal satisfaction with social aspects of their life, including housing, occupation, finances, social and leisure activities, and family relationships. Patients rate their level of satisfaction on a 4-point scale with a rating of 'moderate' or 'marked' dissatisfaction in response to any question constituting a significant social problem. The SPQ is therefore not an objective measure but it was felt that patients' perception of their social situation was a valid and often undervalued method of assessment. The questionnaire has been employed with a range of other groups with data available for comparison (Corney and

Table 2. Percentage of samples reporting moderate or severe dissatisfaction on the Social Problems Questionnaire (SPQ)

	Work	Social contacts	Marriage/ relation- ship	Fin- ance	Hous- ing	Rela- tives
Assessment centre Samples ($N = 112$)	71	67	49	34	27	26
Surgical evaluation sample ($N = 32$)	34	22	28	22	6	16
Epilepsy outpatients ($N = 23$)	22	17	22	22	13	13
Social work referrals ($N = 65$)	19	35	31	29	35	20
GP attenders Inner London	12	21	19	26	17	11

Clare, 1985). Furthermore, it is easy to understand and is short, taking 5–10 minutes to complete.

Results and Discussion

The percentage of our two samples reporting dissatisfaction with various aspects of their lives is given in Table 2. In addition, the findings reported by Corney and Clare (1985) with three other groups, namely GP attenders, social work referrals and epilepsy outpatients, are presented for comparison. Each area will now be considered separately.

Daily Occupation

Survey results It was the area of daily occupation that caused both of our groups greatest dissatisfaction, with 71% of the assessment unit group and 34% of the surgical evaluation group reporting moderate to severe dissatisfaction. This level is higher than for the other patient groups surveyed by Corney and Clare (1985), including the epilepsy outpatient group. The majority of the assessment centre sample reporting dissatisfaction were those who were currently out of work with no daily occupation, or those who were attending day centres (see Table 3). Only 10% of the sample were working and all but two of these reported significant dissatisfaction. The main reason for this dissatisfaction was that they believed their jobs to be undemanding and without respon-

Table 3. Daily occupation of the patients at the time of admission

	Assessment centre (%)	Surgical evaluation (%)
Open employment	10	56
At home	69	44
Day centre	12	0
Full-time education	3	0
Other	6	0

sibility. Indeed, the majority were in unskilled jobs, despite the fact that a number had academic and vocational qualifications which suggested that they would be capable of at least semi-skilled work.

The surgical evaluation sample were more likely to be working. Fifty-six per cent of the sample were in full-time employment at the time of referral, with just under half in unskilled work. Indeed, a number of individuals in the sample had high-level jobs involving managerial responsibility. Two patients were self-employed, one as a carpenter and the other providing a secretarial service. The majority of patients reporting dissatisfaction with daily occupation were those who were out of work at the time of the assessment.

Discussion It is not surprising that people with complicated epilepsy have difficulties with employment, and a great deal has been written about this (Edwards, Espir and Oxley, 1986; Scambler, 1987; Craig and Oxley, 1988). Unemployment and underemployment are reported in patients whose seizure control must be considered better than that of the individuals in our sample. Indeed, McClelland (1987), referring to an American survey, writes 'Experimental employment officers . . . have a 40 per cent success rate in placing people with epilepsy in jobs if they have six seizures a year. If they have 20 a year the success rate is 11 per cent but for those who have more than one seizure a week, only one in every 165 people would be placed in competitive employment'. It is of interest that many of our surgical referral sample were holding down jobs despite poor seizure control.

In our previous report we argued that poor seizure control alone was probably insufficient to account for the high level of unemployment in our assessment centre sample. The basis for this was that there were individual cases who had relatively poor seizure control but yet were in employment (Thompson and Oxley, 1988). The results obtained from the patients considered for surgery would seem to endorse this view. Of course, the nature of the attacks rather than the frequency might be a factor influencing employment (McClelland, 1987). This was not systematically explored in our two samples, but in the group referred for possible surgical intervention a number had partial seizures that were embarrassing in content and less easily recognizable as seizures. Seizures of this type might be less acceptable to employers and work colleagues.

It becomes necessary, therefore, to consider other factors that may contribute to the employment chances of people with uncontrolled seizures. Naturally, an individual's ability and qualifications must influence their job prospects. Sixty-two per cent of the assessment centre referrals had received mainstream education and 52% had achieved some form of qualification, although this seemed to be biased towards lower-level certificates. In contrast, 94% of those referred for surgery had received mainstream education and 78% had achieved academic qualifications, with the majority of the sample achieving at least 'O'-level standard. The surgical group are generally more able as measured by IQ (see Table 1), and this must certainly contribute to the differences in academic achievement between the two groups. Furthermore, the assessment unit sample tended to have an earlier age of onset such that it was more likely that seizures would actually influence their school career. However, it must be noted that the 71% of the surgery sample also experienced seizures while receiving secondary education.

Available evidence suggests that children with severe seizure disorders constitute an at-risk group regarding educational achievement (Thompson, 1987; Aldenkamp et al., 1987). Many reasons have been given, including hidden cognitive disability, absence from school due to 'illness' or hospital appointments, behaviour problems and effects of medication. Several subjects in the assessment centre sample had learning difficulties as demonstrated by their neuropsychological test performance. In addition, language difficulties were evident (Davey, personal communication). But in the majority of cases these learning difficulties had been undetected during their schoolyears. Early detection of such problems seems vital so that appropriate interventions can be undertaken (Wehrli, 1987). Furthermore, many individuals reported experiencing very unhappy schooldays, with bullying by classmates and blanket prohibition of some subjects, particularly sports, which may well have been unwarranted. Treatment of this sort can result in low self-esteem, reducing a child's confidence and motivation for learning. In the UK there is now material for teachers that can be used with entire classes and may improve the general understanding of epilepsy (Dowds, McCluggage and Nelson, 1983; Corbidge, 1987).

Moreover, for those adults in the assessment centre sample it may still be possible to improve their chances of work by undertaking further education or vocational training. We have found that some further educational courses run by other organizations, even those designed for people with disabilities, may sometimes have very unjust rules leading to the exclusion of people with epilepsy. One particular area of misunderstanding is the belief that people with epilepsy should not work with computers. There is a widespread misconception that visual display units will inevitably cause more seizures (Harding, 1986). Except in rare cases, new information technology offers increased opportunities for those with epilepsy to work in a safe environment, utilizing their full potential.

Expectations and attitudes of individuals with epilepsy may be another contributory factor leading to low employment prospects. Several patients, particularly in the assessment centre sample, had very unrealistic expectations, given the severity of their seizure disorder; for example, many expressed a wish to enter employment which involved driving. Appropriate career guidance during schoolyears is essential to make career choices more realistic. Other patients were waiting for their epilepsy to be cured so that they could undertake their chosen careers, when, in reality, the likelihood of full control of their attacks was extremely small. The need for accuracy and honesty in discussion of prognosis of seizure control between patient and physician cannot be overemphasized.

Psychological adjustment can also influence job-seeking skills. Low self-esteem, dependency and helplessness which can arise from frequent job rejections may result in a person becoming apathetic. Unemployment in all groups is found to engender such feelings; the longer this state continues, the more difficult people find it to motivate themselves (Hayes and Nutman, 1981). Other workers with groups less disabled in terms of seizure frequency than our two samples have also drawn attention to the importance of focusing on coping skills of the individual. Mittan (1986) felt that, in order to ensure success, vocational rehabilitation programmes must provide patients with endurance skills to cope with fears and job stress. There are patients in both our samples who believed that they had to prove themselves at work to be in some respect better than their colleagues. Such a belief would result in considerable stress which in itself might influence seizure control adversely (Temkin and Davis, 1984).

Other patients had very negative attitudes about employers and blamed all their problems of getting work on other people's lack of understanding about epilepsy. All job seekers, particularly those with disabilities, need to be aware of their own strengths and to be able to convey this information to prospective employers. There is some evidence that employers are not always negative in their attitude but rather lack appropriate information about epilepsy. Therefore, job applicants with epilepsy need to have a good understanding of their seizure disorder and be able to explain it in the right way to prospective employers, and correct misinformation.

However, the ability to do well in job interviews is not something that people are born with. It is a skill that needs to be learnt. Increasing awareness of these factors has led to the setting up of job clubs around the country which provide guidance on interview techniques. Some educational and vocational training programmes have been devised specifically for individuals with epilepsy but these are not widespread. A horticultural project supervised by the Epilepsy Association of Scotland with funding from the European Social Fund is an example of one such initiative.

Nevertheless, it would be wrong to give the impression that prejudice against epilepsy is not a problem in the job market. It does occur and people with epilepsy need to be prepared to cope with disappointment and frequent rejection. Job applicants with epilepsy are frequently presented with a dilemma when completing application forms. Many feel that they will be rejected automatically if they acknowledge their epilepsy. Floyd and Espir (1986) have advocated complete separation of medical information, which should only be considered after other recruitment procedures have been completed. These and other suggestions for a code of good practice for the employment of people with epilepsy have been outlined by Craig and Oxley (1988).

One employment opportunity available to people with uncontrolled seizures is setting up their own business. Naturally this is more feasible where an individual has a particular skill which is potentially marketable, the necessary intellectual resources or access to appropriate business input. Government grants can be obtained in the UK, at least in the short term. Indeed, two individuals in the surgical evaluation sample were self-employed and felt that this allowed them to arrange their working hours around their seizures.

There will always be a group of individuals with severe epilepsy and probably additional handicaps who will require sheltered employment. Few in our sample were in any sort of sheltered work scheme. Sheltered employment is available in special workshops and in sheltered placements where a disabled worker is employed alongside 'able-bodied' colleagues in an ordinary work environment. Sheltered workshop places are severely limited in the UK and usually concentrate on manufacturing and assembly work, requiring manual dexterity and speed which may place some of the young adults in our assessment unit sample at a disadvantage. Sheltered placements (which would be more appropriately called supported placements) are an alternative favoured both by government because they are cheaper to maintain, and by many disabled people because they avoid segregation.

For many individuals, even sheltered employment was not available. Alternatives to work which offer meaningful, structured daily activity are limited. A few of our assessment unit group attended training centres; the majority were attending centres for the mentally handicapped. Two attended centres for the physically disabled but these centres tended to cater for a very wide range of disabilities, often having a significant elderly population. Neither facility necessarily caters for the needs of people with epilepsy. Those in our groups with no structured daily activity were relatively young. Although it could be said that many non-disabled young people are without work, we would argue that people with additional difficulties may be less able than others to structure their own time and can benefit both medically and socially from some form of directed daily activity.

Social and Leisure Activities

Survey results   In the earlier report of our survey, this was the area in which the assessment centre sample expressed most dissatisfaction. A slightly lower percentage of this extended group expressed similar dissatisfaction. However, 67% still reported that they were unhappy about this aspect of their lives. On the other hand, only 22% of the patients referred for surgical evaluation expressed significant dissatisfaction; a finding that is comparable to the other groups given in Table 2. A supplementary question about the number of friends that each subject had was included as in our earlier report. Sixty-three per cent of the assessment centre sample admitted to having no personal friends and this contrasted with only 9% of the surgical sample. The striking difference between our two study groups requires further investigation. The following is an illustrative case example.

Social isolation: A case example   Mr S. was 35 years old when he was admitted to the Assessment Centre. Epilepsy was diagnosed at the age of 6 years. He had complex partial seizures which began with a vocalization followed by a few minutes of automatisms. These had always been difficult to control and occurred on approximately a monthly basis. Prior to admission, seizure frequency had increased. He had attended ordinary schools and is reported to have been the target of bullying and restrictions on activities, particularly sport and extracurricula activities. His family also restricted his activities and also family outings because he felt they were embarrassed about his attacks. He obtained no qualifications, and on leaving school he undertook a few jobs of an unskilled nature which he lost because of his seizures. At the time of admission he had had no structured daily activity, paid or otherwise, for the past 11 years. He spent his time at home doing gardening, decorating and more usually watching television. Relationship difficulties with his stepfather resulted in him moving to live with his grandparents, who were in their 80s.

An assessment revealed Mr S. to be an individual of average ability; in certain areas, particularly spatial and perceptual skills, his ability was well above average. He was a fairly anxious, moderately depressed individual. Socially he was assessed to have the skills necessary to form and maintain friendships. He believed that his rejection at school by his peers had strongly affected his ability to make social relationships throughout his life. Physically, he was an attractive man, and during his months at the assessment centre his confidence improved and he developed a number of friendships. On leaving he had a number of plans to seek work and undertake various leisure activities which might provide him with an environment to increase his social contacts. However, 18 months post-discharge, there seemed little improvement from his preadmission social situation.

Discussion   Other investigators have commented upon the restricted social life of patients with epilepsy and also that of their families. It has not, however, been given as much attention as other social difficulties such as employment and education. Intellectually intact children with epilepsy have been reported to have significantly fewer friends (Hermann, 1982), and in a survey of children with disabilities, Sillanpää (1987) found that children with epilepsy had no leisure-time activities outside the home and fewer friends and companions than healthy children or those with diabetes and asthma. Goodyear (1988) has commented on the social withdrawal syndrome that can occur in association with epilepsy. Mittan and colleagues, in a survey of adults with less severe epilepsy than either of our samples, reported that more than 50% spent nearly all their time at home (Mittan and Locke, 1982; Mittan, 1986).

Social participation and the ability to form friendships is vitally important, and the social isolation reported in our assessment centre referrals should be a matter of great concern. There are many reasons why this may have arisen. Seizures, being by their very nature unpredictable, can certainly contribute to the development of anxiety, making people fearful of going out because of possible injury or embarrassment (Dowds, McCluggage and Nelson, 1983). Mittan (1986) reported that one-fifth of their sample were frightened about going out socially. In our case study, fear certainly contributed to the restricted social life of Mr S., and may have affected his family in the same way. High levels of anxiety have been reported in patients with epilepsy (Arnston et al., 1986), and undoubtedly the unpredictable nature of the disorder is one important factor. It is likely, therefore, that people with epilepsy need to have psychological coping skills over and above those of the general population.

Anxiety may not only prevent individuals making social contact but can also interfere with social behaviour. A very anxious person may appear awkward in social situations. Psychological techniques that help to reduce anxiety may be helpful (Butcher and de Clive Lowe, 1985), as can group work which focuses upon understanding epilepsy and confidence in talking with other people. Experience may be obtained from self-help groups but, although there are over 80 such groups in the UK, very few patients in our samples were members of such groups. Many did not know of their existence, while others believed they were too often composed of older people and focused too much upon epilepsy.

We do not believe that anxiety resulting from poor seizure control is the only reason for restricted social life. Indeed, one individual in the surgical sample who blamed his seizures for his social isolation had a temporal lobectomy which resulted in complete control of his attacks as assessed 18 months post operatively. This loss of his seizures was not accompanied by any significant improvement in his social situation.

For some individuals, limited social contact stems from lack of opportunity. This may be due to unnecessary restrictions set by families and also patients themselves. Blanket bans on going to discotheques and pubs are positively harmful. Sporting activities offer another social environment for young people. Many of our samples had been dissuaded from participating in sports. We are increasingly a health-conscious society and if young people with epilepsy are denied such opportunities they may become not only a very lonely group but also a less healthy one. Encouragingly, however, we have recently had admissions to the assessment centre who were members of sports clubs and, despite uncontrolled attacks, participated in a variety of activities, including judo, badminton, swimming and yoga. The important role of physical activities in providing fitness and social outlets is increasingly being recognized and is strongly advocated in some assessment packages for people with epilepsy (Achterberg and Nelson, personal communication).

Geographical isolation certainly contributes to social difficulties in some of our patients. The inability to drive and poor public transport can isolate young people from their peer groups. One factor that probably contributed to the better social lives of our surgical referral group was that many lived within the London area where there is comprehensive public transport.

Several of our group displayed very good social skills when exposed to the social environment of the assessment centre. This is illustrated in the case example of Mr S. During his assessment period he made many friends and was a popular member of the group. Prior to discharge, many plans were made to enhance his social situation when he returned home. Unfortunately, as indicated, these plans did not materialize.

Merely providing opportunity for social contacts does not, however, always remedy social isolation. Some subjects were observed to display limited social skills when given a suitable social environment. As children, many had had restrictions placed on their social activities by families because of anxiety about safety, and often there was a history of rejection by schoolmates. Due to this lack of opportunity in their early years many had not learned how to form friendships. Overprotection has been considered by some authors to be psychologically more damaging than lack of protection can be physically hazardous (Dell, 1986; Scambler, 1987). Appropriate education about a child's epilepsy for the family and classmates may thus help to improve the social development of the child with problematic epilepsy. As most people learn how to behave socially from family and friends, effective interventions have been devised, including those based on structured groups which focus on social skills involving role play and modelling (Shepherd, 1983). More recent work suggests that success is more likely to occur when social skills training is undertaken in more natural contexts (Gaylord-Ross, Stremel-Campbell and Storey, 1986). Ideally, where social difficulties exist, interventions of this sort should be used as early as possible, and some success has been reported with children with epilepsy (Verdyn, 1987).

It has to be acknowledged that there were individuals in the assessment centre group who had evidence of significant brain damage and dysfunction. This is known to influence not only intellectual but also social development. Where hidden difficulties exist, such as subtle receptive language problems, these can greatly interfere with a person's social presentation, particularly when such deficits go unrecognized or are misunderstood. Even for this group, appropriate teaching can result in improved social skills.

In certain cases, medication may influence social opportunities. Some patients were found on admission to have high levels of medication such that they were very tired, needing to go to bed early and having little energy for social activities at the weekend. Careful monitoring of medication with the use of monotherapy can help to improve the situation.

The need to improve public attitudes towards epilepsy has been apparent for a long time. Changing the attitudes is not something that will happen quickly, but increased awareness, e.g. in sports and leisure centres and places of entertainment, will inevitably improve the situation for people with uncontrolled seizures. Social clubs for disabled groups exist and these are generally run by voluntary organizations. We would argue that, where possible, it is preferable for individuals to socialize within normal environments. Befriending schemes currently being developed with people with mental handicap would seem a valuable approach to adopt with our assessment sample (Walsh, 1985).

Family Life

Survey results   Nine per cent of the assessment centre sample were married or living with a partner at the time of admission. A further 7% had a steady relationship, 5% were divorced and 2% were widowed. The majority (78%), however, were not in a relationship and 50% of these reported never having had a relationship. In contrast, 45% of the surgical evaluation sample were married or cohabiting. No individuals were divorced or widowed.

The SPQ enquired whether individuals either had a problem with their relationship, e.g. not being able to confide in their partner, or if they did not have a relationship, how satisfied they were with this situation. Forty-nine per cent of the assessment centre sample reported dissatisfaction in the area of relationships and for all of these it was because they did not have a partner. Twenty-eight per cent of the surgical evaluation sample reported dissatisfaction with their relationships, and for the majority it was for the same reason. However, three patients who had a partner reported significant problems, mostly of a sexual nature. Nine per cent of patients in the assessment centre sample had children at the time of admission and one woman was pregnant. Six of the group reported difficulties with their children, and for five of these it was due to lack of contact. In each case the children were no longer living with them. A larger proportion of the surgical evaluation sample had children (26%) and only one reported significant difficulties, and this concerned the behaviour of her teenage daughter.

Further questions on the SPQ enquired about relationships with any adults or relatives with whom the respondent is living. This question was more often applicable to the assessment centre sample, who were still living with their parents. Few reported major difficulties.

Discussion A low incidence of marriage and relationship in the assessment centre sample was perhaps not unexpected. Evidence already exists that people with epilepsy, particularly when the disorder is severe or there are additional handicaps, are less likely to marry and have children (Lechtenberg, 1984; Hoare, 1988). Many factors may underlie this finding. One reason that has been given little attention is the more basic problem of forming friendships as outlined in the previous section. Difficulties of this sort must be relevant. A further reason cited in the literature for this reduced desire to seek a sexually satisfying relationship is lack of sex drive. This has been attributed to hormonal factors, possibly as a side-effect of certain antiepileptic medications (Fenwick, 1988). Research in this area is limited, and the possibility that environmental factors may also influence libido or even hormonal levels cannot be ruled out.

Our survey would suggest that for adults with epilepsy still living within the parental home, relationship difficulties were few. Discussions with family members of this sample, however, suggested that such problems are likely to be underestimated by our patient group. Little research on the impact of intractable epilepsy on family relationships has been undertaken. The majority of this work has concerned children with epilepsy, and existing evidence suggests that having a child with epilepsy can place considerable psychological strain on family members (Goodyear, 1988). If difficulties of this sort exist in childhood, then it seems likely that problems may be intensified when a person with epilepsy becomes adult. Further research work in this area is necessary.

Finances

Thirty-four per cent of the assessment centre sample and 22% of the surgical referrals reported significant dissatisfaction with their finances. These figures are not markedly different from those of the other groups given in Table 2. This finding may be surprising given that the majority of our assessment centre sample were not employed. Many of this sample, however, were still living with their parents, who might be experiencing economic difficulties because of the need to provide financial support. Indeed, in a survey by Sillanpää (1987), 27% of families of children with epilepsy reported unsatisfactory or poor financial circumstances. Increased difficulties would be expected when the child with epilepsy becomes an adult. Furthermore, as the parents get older and retire, then economic hardships may increase. For some of our families, one parent, and in some cases both parents, had given up work to look after their son or daughter with epilepsy, and relied upon state benefits.

Housing

The assessment centre and surgical evaluation samples reported 27% and 6% dissatisfaction respectively with their accommodation. This makes it a low area of concern for both groups in comparison with other areas.

Table 4 gives the living situation of our two samples. The majority of the assessment centre sample were living at home and 54% were assessed to be highly dependent for basic needs on their family. Needs catered for included clothing care, cooking, paying bills and house repairs. This contrasts with the surgical referral sample, where only a minority were assessed to be dependent on their family for basic needs.

There are many reasons why individuals remain within the parental home, and the differences observed between our two samples suggests that it cannot be solely due to frequent seizures. Naturally, financial resources must contribute to this situation. The majority of our assessment centre sample were unemployed. The high cost of housing, whether to buy or to rent, means that many young adults are generally forced to stay at home for longer periods of time. Although local authority housing is one alternative, the demand greatly exceeds the supply, and frustration with living in the parental home does not often enhance eligibility. This lack of opportunity to live independently may further increase social isolation, reducing the likelihood of relationships and marriage.

In contrast, many of the surgical evaluation sample had moved away from their parental homes because they had formed new relationships and had their own families. In the assessment centre sample it could be argued once more that difficulties in making friends denies individuals the opportunity to form relationships, and there is therefore no drive to leave the family home, as parents are their only friends. Dependency on parents for basic needs may be fairly acceptable in a child with epilepsy, but this becomes a problem without an obvious solution as the individual and the parents get older. We can cite several cases where a crisis has arisen because one or both parents have died, leaving a very dependent person in their 40s or 50s who, while having the cognitive resources to cope with looking after themselves, has never been expected to undertake such tasks. We would argue that to avoid such situations there is a need early in adulthood to teach independent living skills and to encourage normal movement from the parental home while keeping regular contact with the family.

There is an impetus in the UK for people with even severe disabilities to be cared for in the community rather than in institutions. Unfortunately, the resources do not keep up with the demand (Fiedler, 1988). Housing associations (voluntary organizations funded from government or other sources) offer certain groups the opportunity to move away from the parental home with varying levels of support. But often such sheltered housing can be difficult to obtain if an individual has uncontrolled epilepsy. Indeed, certain supported

Table 4. Housing

	Assessment centre (%)	Surgical evaluation (%)
Parental home		
High dependency	54	19
Low dependency	12	31
Own home	13	47
Own home		
Support external services	7	0
Sheltered housing	14	3

housing schemes give as an exclusion criterion, along with alcoholism and drug addiction, 'uncontrolled grand mal epilepsy'. This is unfair discrimination and contrary to assessment on the basis of individual needs. Professionals working in the field of epilepsy should actively educate those who are responsible for providing housing of all kinds. In addition, work can be done with the care staff in sheltered housing schemes so that they feel comfortable in coping with seizures and come to recognize them as not being a medical emergency. There are a few housing projects in the UK which demonstrate that even people with poorly controlled seizures can learn to achieve a high level of independence. These include the St Katherine's Housing Trust in Croydon and the Stonham Housing Association in Buckinghamshire, where people with epilepsy live together in small units. It could be argued that grouping disabled people in this way constitutes a form of segregation. However, the evidence suggests that these schemes work very well, particularly as movement into fully independent housing is encouraged for those with the necessary skills.

Multiple Problems

Table 5 gives the total number of problem areas experienced by the different groups. The majority of our assessment centre sample have multiple problems with more than one-third experiencing more than three problems. In contrast, only a minority (13%) of the surgical evaluation group experienced a comparable number of problems. Indeed, this figure is in keeping with that reported by epilepsy outpatients and less than that reported for the social work referrals. Surprisingly, less than 20% of our assessment centre sample had received any professional social work input, other than a brief assessment required for admission purposes.

Thus our assessment centre sample are a group with multiple problems. In national terms they are a relatively small group and as such their wide-ranging needs can be overlooked. This is particularly the case because their problems

Table 5. Number of problem areas in the different samples

Problem areas	Epilepsy assessment patients	Surgical evaluation	Epilepsy outpatients	Social work referrals	GP attenders (Inner London)
None	3	41	39	3	42
One	20	28	22	25	23
Two	17	9	17	28	14
Three	16	9	9	20	11
More than three	36	13	13	25	10

are often seen as stemming from the seizures and thus the solution to their difficulties is seen only in terms of improved seizure control. In many cases this is a medical impossibility. Failure to identify their needs at an appropriate time, often due to an overconcentration on the purely medical aspects of the condition, will often lead to a slow but inexorable descent down the dependency spiral. With the passage of time, this process becomes harder and harder to reverse.

Conclusion

This survey shows that people with epilepsy admitted to an assessment centre have a high level of social problems. These are greater than those of another group with frequent seizures, namely neurosurgical referrals, and other groups who are thought to have a high level of social problems, such as social work referrals. It seems likely that these additional problems contributed to their referral to the assessment centre. We have looked at reasons that may underlie reported difficulties and have mentioned some of the interventions that exist which may help to reduce the problems experienced. These interventions can be undertaken irrespective of seizure control. Ideally, the wider implications of complicated epilepsy should be realized in childhood. Careful evaluation and targeted interventions may reduce future problems. Unfortunately, patients and families are often waiting for a new drug or an operation that will result in seizure relief. These are often not forthcoming, and as the child with epilepsy and the parents grow older, the problems of dependency become more intractable.

Further research work into the psychological and social needs of people with problematic epilepsy is necessary. It is probable that as a group they are not fully utilizing existing resources. Furthermore, unless we examine this group in detail we cannot plan effectively for future needs. The existence of the dependency spiral is obvious from our results; the solutions will be more difficult to identify.

But whatever future research may reveal, it is clear that existing services for people with disabilities, including epilepsy, remain fragmented and lack coherence. Many government departments, including Health, Education, Employment and Social Services, are involved, as well as local authorities and voluntary bodies to an ever-increasing extent. Every person severely disabled by epilepsy will meet many professionals and most will experience the frustrations of inadequate interprofessional communication and a lack of continuity of care, even a lack of a common purpose. A government working party which reviewed services for people with epilepsy in the UK (Department of Health and Social Security, 1986) recommended the setting up of epilepsy clinics, specifically for patients with severe epilepsy. The clinics, as advocated, should cater not only for medical needs but also for other psychological and social problems, utilizing a multidisciplinary team of professionals as appropriate. Partly because of lack of special funding, only a few such clinics are in operation, but the nature of their services suggests that the quality of care for people with epilepsy should improve (Richens, 1988). It is suggested that more difficult cases could be referred to residential centres such as the Chalfont Centre. It is perhaps from these clinics and assessment centres that enhanced co-operation may arise. Without improved co-ordination of services, precious resources will continue to be wasted, and patients and their families suffer unnecessarily.

Opportunities for people with intractable epilepsy need to be created to enable them to fulfil their potential for independent living, for work and for forming friendships. It is not enough to say that people with problematic epilepsy will have a high level of problems.

References

Aldenkamp AP, Alpherts WCJ, Meinhardi H, Stores G. Education and epilepsy. Netherlands: Swets and Zeitlinger, 1987.
Arnston P, Droge D, Norton R, Murray E. The perceived psychosocial consequences of having epilepsy. In: Whitman S, Hermann BP (eds) Psychopathology in epilepsy: Social dimensions. New York: Oxford University Press, 1986: 143–61.
Beardshaw V. Last on the list: Community services for people with a physical disability. London: Kings Fund Institute, 1988.
Beran RG, Flanagan PS. Psychosocial sequelae of epilepsy. The role of associated cerebral pathology. Epilepsia 1987; 28: 107–10.
Butcher P, de Clive-Lowe S. Strategies for living: Teaching psychological self-help as adult education. Br J Med Psychol 1985; 58: 207–16.
Corbidge P. Teacher training—attitudes towards epilepsy. In: Oxley J, Stores G (eds) Epilepsy and education. London: Medical Tribune Group, 1987: 31–4.
Corney RH, Clare AW. The construction and development of a self-report questionnaire to identify social problems. Psychol Med 1985; 15: 637–49.
Craig A, Oxley J. Social aspects of epilepsy. In: Laidlaw J, Richens A, Oxley J (eds) A textbook of epilepsy. 3rd ed. Edinburgh: Churchill Livingstone, 1988: 566–609.
Craig AG, Oxley J, Dowds C. Children and young people with epilepsy: An educational package for teachers. Chalfont St. Peter: National Society for Epilepsy, 1985.

Dell JL. Social dimensions of epilepsy: Stigma and response. In: Whitman S, Hermann BP (eds) Psychopathology in epilepsy: Social dimensions. New York: Oxford University Press, 1986: 185–210.

Department of Health and Social Security. Report of the Working Group on Services for People with Epilepsy. London: HMSO, 1986.

Dodrill CB. Correlates of generalised tonic–clonic seizures with intellectual, neuropsychological, emotional and social functioning. Epilepsia 1986; 27: 399–411.

Dowds N, McCluggage J, Nelson J. A survey of the socio-medical aspects of epilepsy in a general practice population in Northern Ireland. Leeds: British Epilepsy Association, 1983.

Edwards F, Espir M, Oxley J (eds). Epilepsy and employment: A medical symposium on current problems and best practices. Royal Society of Medicine International Congress and Symposium, Series 86. London: Royal Society of Medicine, 1986.

Fenwick P. Sexual behaviour: The epileptic and his family. In: Hoare P (ed.) Epilepsy and the family. Manchester: Sanofi UK Limited, 1988: 29–38.

Fenwick P, Fenwick E (eds). Epilepsy and the law—a medical symposium on the current law. Royal Society of Medicine International Congress and Symposium, Series 81. London: Royal Society of Medicine, 1985.

Fielder B. Living options lottery. London: Prince of Wales Advisory Group, 1988.

Floyd M, Espir MLE. Assessment of medical fitness for employment: the case for a code of practice. Lancet 1986; ii: 207–9.

Gaylord-Ross R, Stremel-Campbell K, Storey K. Social skills training in natural contexts. In: Horner RH, Meyer LH, Bud Fredericks HH (eds). Education of learners with severe handicaps. Exemplary service strategies. Baltimore: Paul H. Brooks Publishing Co., 1986: 161–87.

Godwin-Austen RB, Espir MLE (eds). Driving and epilepsy—and other causes of impaired consciousness. Royal Society of Medicine International Congress and Symposium, Series 60. London: Royal Society of Medicine, 1983.

Goodyear I. The influence of epilepsy on family functioning. In: Hoare P (ed.) Epilepsy and the family. Manchester: Sanofi UK Limited, 1988: 11–18.

Harding G. Photosensitive epilepsy and employment. In: Edwards F, Espir M, Oxley J (eds). Epilepsy and employment: A medical symposium on current problems and best practices. Royal Society of Medicine International Congress and Symposium, Series 86. London: Royal Society of Medicine, 1986: 75–87.

Hayes J, Nutman P. Understand the unemployed. Bungay: Chaucer Press, 1981.

Hermann BP. Neuropsychological functioning and psychopathology in children with epilepsy. Epilepsia 1982; 23: 545–54.

Hoare P (ed.). Epilepsy and the family. Manchester: Sanofi UK Limited, 1988.

Lechtenberg R. Epilepsy and the family. Cambridge, Massachusetts: Harvard University Press, 1984.

McClelland DL. Epilepsy and employment. J Soc Occup Med 1987; 37: 94–9.

Mittan RJ. Fear of seizures. In: Whitman S, Hermann BP (eds) Psychopathology in epilepsy: Social dimensions. New York: Oxford University Press, 1986: 90–121.

Mittan R, Locke G. Fear of seizures: Epilepsy's forgotten symptom. Urban Health 1982; 11: 30–2.

Oxley J, Stores G (eds). Epilepsy and education. London: Medical Tribune Group, 1987.

Richens A. Epilepsy clinics: A specialist service for families. In: Hoard P (ed.) Epilepsy and the family. Manchester: Sanofi UK Limited, 1988: 39–43.

Rodin E. Factors which influence prognosis in epilepsy. In: Hopkins A (ed.) Epilepsy. London: Chapman Hall, 1987: 339–71.

Scambler G. Sociological aspects. In: Hopkins A (ed.) Epilepsy. London: Chapman Hall, 1987: 497–609.

Shepherd GL. Interpersonal relationships. In: Watts FN, Bennett DH (eds) Theory and practice of psychiatric rehabilitation. Chichester: John Wiley & Sons, 1983: 267–88.

Sillanpää M. Social adjustment and functioning of chronically ill and impaired children and adolescents. Acta Paediatr Scand 1987; suppl. 340.

Temkin NR, Davis GR. Stress as a risk factor for seizures among adults with epilepsy. Epilepsia 1984; 25: 450–6.

Thompson PJ. Educational attainment in children and young persons with epilepsy. In: Oxley J, Stores G (eds) Epilepsy and education. London: Medical Tribune Group, 1987: 15–24.

Thompson PJ, Oxley JR. Socioeconomic accompaniments of severe epilepsy. Epilepsia 1988; 29 (suppl. 1): S9–S18.

Verdyn C. Social skills training and the promotion of self-esteem. In: Oxley J, Stores G (eds) Epilepsy and education. London: Medical Tribune Group, 1987: 43–6.

Walsh J. Setting up a friendship scheme. Mental Handicap 1985; 13: 58–9, 110–16.

Wehrli A. Function deficits and remedial techniques. In: Aldenkamp AP, Alpherts WCJ, Meinardi H, Stores G (eds) Education and epilepsy. Netherlands: Swets and Zeitlinger, 1987: 110–17.

10
Some Behavioural Consequences of Epileptic Seizures

M.R. Trimble
Institute of Neurology, London, UK

Introduction

Although the relationship between epilepsy and disturbances of cognitive function, in particular associations between certain seizure types and some patterns of cognitive impairment, is now becoming accepted (see Chapter 8), associations of seizures and behaviour problems continue to be an area of controversy. This is in spite of a long history attesting to a clear relationship between psychopathology and epilepsy which may properly be said to have crystallized in the nineteenth century, particularly with the contributions of the French authors who developed concepts such as 'larval epilepsy', describing cases in which automatic activity or acute behavioural disturbance was seen in epileptic patients without necessarily including loss of consciousness. Morel (1860), who introduced the term 'larval epilepsy', drew attention to the paroxysmal nature of the clinical features of these states and also noted certain personality characteristics of chronic epileptic patients. The latter ideas, over time, led to the concept of the epileptic personality, and attempts to further clarify the interictal psychiatric states of epileptic patients.

The divisions of historical thinking since the nineteenth century were outlined by Guerrant et al. (1962) into four epochs, as shown in Table 1. The first, referred to as the period of epileptic deterioration, reflected ideas towards the end of the last century which assumed that because patients had epilepsy this was enough for deterioration of their personality and behaviour to occur. These ideas stemmed directly from the degeneracy theory of mental disorder,

Table 1. Changing ideas of the relationship between epilepsy and psychopathology. After Guerrant et al. (1962)

Period of epileptic deterioration	(–1900)
Period of the epileptic character	(1900–1930)
Period of normality	(1930–)
Period of psychomotor peculiarity	(1930–)

prevalent in continental Europe at that time, in which it was considered that psychopathology, including epilepsy, was the result of a progressive heredity degenerative condition which would pass from one generation to another, ultimately leading to the decline of the progeny and to imbecility.

The period of the epileptic character, referring to concepts which were prevalent earlier in this century, led to a marked change of thinking. The epilepsy itself, and associated behaviour or personality change, were seen as secondary to an underlying third principle, namely patients' constitution, and their 'personality'. A major exponent of this line of thought was Pierce-Clark (1929). It was claimed that it was possible to discern certain patterns of developmental personality traits which could be identified in patients prior to the onset of seizures, implying an 'epileptic constitution'. This era became bound up with Freudian psychodynamics such that epilepsy and a number of other conditions were thought to reflect upon infantile motives and inadequate development of an individual's affects and instincts, leading to the later development of symptoms. This was the era of psychosomatic medicine, in which various disease personalities were identified. In the case of epilepsy this led to the delineation of the epileptic character, and to so-called epileptic equivalents. These were behaviour disorders which resembled epilepsy in their paroxysmal and explosive nature, but which were not associated with overt seizures.

The mid-part of this century saw a change in views, and ideas that patients with epilepsy were somehow susceptible to the development of specific psychopathologies were abandoned. It was considered that patients with epilepsy were essentially normal people, and any changes of personality or psychopathology that developed were secondary to head injuries, to the long-term prescription of anticonvulsant drugs, or to the consequences of psychosocial stigmatization. This was most forcibly stated by Lennox (1944), and is still a view which is vehemently held by many today. The alternative view, which to some extent is a return to the nineteenth century views in the sense that it is more deterministic in nature, is that not all patients with epilepsy are liable to develop psychopathology, but it is those with chronic temporal lobe abnormalities, in particular those who have limbic epilepsy, who are most susceptible. This 'period of psychomotor peculiarity' was summed up by Gibbs and Stamps (1958) as follows: 'the patient's emotional reactions to his seizures, to his family and to his social situation are less important determinants of psychiatric disorder than the site and type of the epileptic discharge'.

Association with Seizure Type

The discovery that bilateral lesions of the temple lobes in animals could lead to marked behaviour changes, referred to as the Kluver–Bucy syndrome, substantiated the view that disorder in certain regions of the brain could be associated with relatively clearly defined behaviour patterns. The principle had earlier been established with the acknowledgement of frontal lobe syndromes. The idea that there may therefore be a recognizable temporal lobe syndrome, and thus distinctive behavioural characteristics of patients with temporal lobe epilepsy, gained ground. Indeed, much of the controversy in this field relates to the specificity of temporal lobe abnormalities in relationship to psychopathology, many people accepting that patients with epilepsy suffer from more psychopathology than would be expected in the normal population, but attributing this to secondary factors such as anticonvulsant drugs or social stigmatization. Unfortunately, resolving this issue has been difficult, partly on account of the lack of adequate epidemiological surveys, but further because many patients with epilepsy arising from the temporal lobes have a number of differing characteristics from patients with generalized seizures, for example often displaying more than one seizure type, or taking more anticonvulsant medications. Pond and Bidwell (1959), in a general practice survey, noted that nearly 30% of epileptic patients had 'psychological difficulties', 7% having been in a psychiatric hospital before or during the survey year. A temporal lobe group had a higher rate of hospitalization to psychiatric hospitals and a higher rate of severe personality change and psychosis. Gudmundsson (1966), in a survey of the population of Iceland, was able to compare the prevalence rates for psychiatric illness in epilepsy with those without epilepsy. In the epilepsy population some 8% were psychotic, this again being greater in the temporal lobe sample. In a similar extensive survey, Zielinski (1974) provided further information on non-selected epileptic patients in a community population of Poland. Fifty-eight per cent showed some 'mental abnormality' and approximately 3% had psychotic symptoms. In that survey, psychopathology was again over-represented in those with temporal lobe epilepsy.

Edeh and Toone (1987) completed a general practice survey in which they compared the incidence of psychopathology in patients with generalized epilepsy, and compared this with focal epilepsy. The latter were divided into those with a temporal lobe focus, and those with a non-temporal lobe focus. The incidence of psychopathology was higher in the non-focal group, but did not differ between the temporal and non-temporal subgroups. Almost half of their sample were rated as psychiatric cases.

Another way to approach the problem has been to give personality rating scales such as the Minnesota Multi-Phasic Personality Inventory (MMPI). Hermann and Whitman (1984) carried out a meta-analysis on a large number of epileptic patients who had been studied with this rating scale, and compared their profiles with those of patients with non-neurological but chronic medical conditions, and neurological disorders other than epilepsy. Patients with epilepsy showed significantly higher rates of severe psychopathology than the neurological controls, who in turn showed a higher rate than the chronic medically ill controls. They suggested that if psychopathology was associated with epilepsy, it was more likely to be more severe. The same group (Hermann et al., 1982) made a significant contribution to the temporal lobe epilepsy debate by comparing patients with temporal lobe epilepsy with those with generalized epilepsy on the MMPI, but separated out a temporal lobe group that had an aura of fear to contrast with those who had different auras. The fear group displayed pathological elevations on several MMPI scales, especially depression and psychosis. Since ictal fear is known to relate to activity from medial temporal structures, especially the peri-amygdaloid region, these data suggest that it is medial temporal lesions, in particular limbic system lesions, that are more likely to be associated with the susceptibility to develop severe pathology. Similar data have been noted for both personality change (Nielsen and Kristensen, 1981) and psychosis (Kristensen and Sindrup, 1978).

The Geschwind Syndrome

The concept that a personality change secondary to a chronic temporal lobe focus was clinically readily identifiable was most strongly supported by Geschwind and colleagues (Waxman and Geschwind, 1975). They particularly emphasized hyposexuality, religiosity and hypergraphia—a tendency towards extensive and compulsive writing. This hypergraphia is characteristically meticulous, containing moral or religious overtones, and there is preoccupation with detail and often a compulsive quality to that which is written. Words or sentences may be repetitive, as may the themes. Variants include the hiring of public stenographers to record events or outpourings, or extensive drawings or paintings. The religiosity may take the form of sudden religious conversions, or of an increasing preoccupation with religious behaviour, compulsive Bible reading and church attendances. Patients may develop philosophical notions about the nature of their epilepsy, and how they have 'been chosen' to suffer from epilepsy.

Much of the controversy about this syndrome relates less to its occurrence than to its frequency. It is clear that it is not universal, but clinically the finding of some features of this syndrome is commoner than its critics assume. Aspects of the syndrome are easily missed unless specifically asked for. For example, it is not customary to ask patients if they keep extensive diaries, write books, or

Behavioural Consequences

are over-concerned with philosophical matters. Further, the syndrome fluctuates in its intensity, and is often not counterproductive to the patient's life in society. Bear (1986) discusses three different aspects of behaviour which comprise this interictal behaviour syndrome. The first relates to alteration of physiological drives, including sexuality, aggression and fear. The second group he summarizes as 'nascent intellectual interests', showing preoccupation with religious, moral, cosmological or philosophical themes. The third group are termed 'dispositions' in association with interpersonal relationships. Under this heading he includes preoccupation with details (obsessiveness), circumstantiality, and a tendency to prolong and deepen social encounters, sometimes referred to as viscosity. He contrasts, as did Geschwind, these aspects of the behaviour of patients with temporal lobe epilepsy with the Kluver–Bucy syndrome of temporal lobe destruction, where aggression is diminished, sexual behaviour is increased and social cohesion is diminished.

Aggression and Epilepsy

This association is also one of considerable controversy and recrimination. A major problem has been the difficulty of recording and quantifying aggressive behaviour, particularly as most of it is interpersonal and situational in nature. There have been few recorded cases of ictal aggression using such techniques as ambulatory monitoring or video telemetry, but this is not surprising because of the environmental precipitants associated with the aggressive act, which are rarely found in the highly structured setting of the EEG laboratory. Nevertheless, ictal aggression is occasionally observed and does have forensic relevance in that the violent episodes may lead to harming another (Fenwick, 1986).

During automatisms, aggressive behaviour is sometimes seen, but it is poorly directed and often provoked by inadequate handling of the confused patient. Increased aggressive behaviour as a personality trait has been noted in several studies, but reviews of the literature (Kligman and Goldberg, 1975) note major methodological criticisms associated with most of them. Serafetinides (1965), in a study of 100 patients operated on for temporal lobectomy, noted that a history of explicit aggressive outbursts was associated with an early onset of seizures, with left-sided resections, and with epigastric autonomic and complex automatisms. Following operation, aggression improved but only in those in whom the epilepsy was improved. Although in animal models the association between aggressive behaviour and some limbic system structures, particularly the amygdala and its associated hypothalamic nuclei, has been clearly established, the relationship of any particular seizure type to the release of aggression in human studies has still to be further clarified.

Depressive Illness

The relationship between depression and epilepsy has been reviewed by Robertson, Trimble and Townsend (1987). Although some authors (Flor Henry, 1969) have suggested direct associations between seizure type (temporal lobe seizures), seizure frequency (infrequently expressed), and site of the focus (non-dominant hemisphere) and affective disorder, these studies have stemmed from highly selected populations, and the psychopathology essentially refers to the more severe forms of affective disorder, especially manic depressive (bipolar) illness. The studies of depression in epileptic patients tend to emphasize an association between anticonvulsant medications, particularly polytherapy with barbiturates, and the subsequent psychopathology, rather than clear associations with seizures or epilepsy per se. Nonetheless, individual case histories are described lending support to Flor Henry's view that the non-dominant hemisphere is in some way interlinked with some forms of affective disturbance in epilepsy, and a subgroup of patients appears to exist with a tendency to recurrent affective disorder who have a clinical diagnosis of complex partial seizures (Robertson, Trimble and Townsend, 1987).

Psychosis

That there is an association between psychosis and epilepsy cannot be doubted by anybody who deals with a large number of epileptic patients. The sudden onset of an acute psychosis in association with a flurry of seizures, namely ictally-associated psychosis, is not infrequently encountered in neurological practice. This clinical pattern is often interlinked with seizure characteristics, occurring following a flurry of major tonic–clonic seizures, and followed by a lucid interval of 24–48 h before the onset of the psychosis. Patients with temporal lobe epilepsy are more likely to have a psychosis with relatively clear consciousness, as opposed to those with a generalized seizure disorder, who are more likely to show confusion.

Complex partial and absence seizure status epilepticus, while rare, provide other examples of associations between seizures and psychosis. In both, consciousness is clouded and the patient shows overt confusion, with difficulty in manipulating cognitive tasks, which, with complex partial seizure status, may be subtle. Such episodes can continue for many days, the patient presenting psychopathological phenomena which sometimes resemble schizophrenia in the absence of epilepsy.

The schizophrenia-like psychosis of epilepsy, rather like the personality disorders, has occasioned considerable controversy. Slater and Beard (1963) reported on 69 cases and they noted the similarity to schizophrenia in the absence of epilepsy. Delusions of religion and delusions of persecution were often reported, but hebephrenic deterioration and catatonic phenomena were rare. Certain features distinguish the schizophrenia-like psychosis of epilepsy from schizophrenia, and they are the absence of a premorbid schizoid personality type, the absence of a family history of psychopathology, and the maintenance of affective responses without deterioration of the personality. Slater and Beard, and several others following them (for review see Trimble (1988)), found associations between temporal lobe lesions and the schizophrenia-like psychosis of epilepsy, implying either that there was underlying structural damage in the temporal lobes which led both to the seizures and, at a later date in time, to the psychosis, or that there was something special about the seizures of temporal lobe epilepsy which led on to the development of psychosis. The latter view was strongly supported by Flor Henry (1969), who noted associations between seizure frequency and the psychotic presentations, implying that infrequently released seizures were associated with the condition. Unlike the case with affective disorders, particularly of a less severe variety, links between anticonvulsant medications and psychoses have not been established by those who have studied this, except for some idiosyncratic cases. Amongst the latter must be included the forced normalization concept of Landolt (1958). Essentially, some patients are reported in whom cessation of seizures, either spontaneously or with anticonvulsant medications, is associated with an abrupt or a gradual onset of a psychotic condition during which time the electroencephalogram tends to 'normalize'. These states have particularly been noted with atypical absence seizures in adolescents or adults, especially following the use of succinimide drugs. Although they are not common, their presentation, with this reciprocal link between seizures and psychotic symptoms, clearly establishes some biological associations between psychosis and epilepsy, which to some extent mirror the alternative, namely the resolution of psychotic states in some patients with artificially induced convulsions during electroconvulsive therapy.

A further important consideration of the link between epilepsy and psychosis was the association of dominant hemisphere lesions with schizophrenia-like presentations suggested initially by Flor Henry (1969). This association has been found by several other workers since (for review see Trimble (1988)), and it has been suggested that one explanation of this link is that temporal lobe epilepsy, in some patients, particularly with lesions in limbic system structures, represents a model for the development of psychotic symptoms in the absence of epilepsy. The dominant hemisphere relates only to certain schizophrenic symptoms, in particular some 'positive' phenomena, notably Schneiderian first-rank symptoms (Trimble, 1988). The fact that many such symptoms relate to alteration of symbolic language, and thought disorder, is consistent with our knowledge that the dominant hemisphere modulates language processes, and it is not unreasonable to suggest that disruption in this hemisphere at certain times of life, as may occur in patients with longstanding temporal lobe lesions which later flower into temporal lobe seizures, may cause disturbed developments of these precious human faculties.

Conclusions

Patients with epilepsy develop psychiatric problems, and to ignore this leads to a restriction of the clinical services that should be made available to patients with epilepsy, and to a limitation on the help that can often be provided for them. It is not suggested that all patients with epilepsy develop psychiatric problems, but it is suggested that a significant minority do so, and that in some cases the psychopathology can be severe. There are many reasons for this, and direct associations with the process of epilepsy, or with seizures, have yet to be clarified for many psychopathological states. The persistent stigmatization that patients receive, the saddened and restricted social lives, with the attendant loneliness which pervades the lives of many patients with epilepsy, is surely a provoking factor for many problems. Further, the long-term use of anticonvulsant drugs, particularly polytherapy and barbiturate use, can be associated with psychopathology, especially of an affective disorder, dysphoria, irritability and instability of mood. Nonetheless, for some conditions discussed here, in particular the more severe psychoses and possibly some personality characteristics as defined by the Geschwind syndrome, there may be more direct biological associations with the underlying epileptic process. Further exploration of these, and identification of subgroups of patients who may, with longstanding and continuous seizure disorders, go on to develop such psychopathologies, is of importance clinically, but also has many theoretical implications. Not the least is the possibility of prevention.

References

Bear DM. Behavioural changes in temporal lobe epilepsy: conflict, confusion, challenge. In: Trimble MR, Bolwig TG (eds) Aspects of epilepsy and psychiatry. Chichester: John Wiley & Sons, 1986: 19–29.

Edeh J, Toone B. Relationship between inter-ictal psychopathology and type of epilepsy. Br J Psychiatry 1987; 151: 95–101.

Fenwick P. Aggression and epilepsy. In: Trimble MR, Bolwig TG (eds) Aspects of epilepsy and psychiatry. Chichester: John Wiley & Sons, 1986: 31–57.

Flor Henry, P. Psychosis and TLE: a controlled investigation. Epilepsia 1969; 10: 363–95.

Gibbs FA, Stamps FW. Epilepsy handbook. Springfield, Illinois: Charles C. Thomas, 1958.

Gudmundsson G. Epilepsy in Iceland. Acta Neurol Scand 1966; 43 (suppl. 25): 1–124.

Guerrant J, Anderson C, Fischer A, Weinstein MR, Jarros RM, Deskins A. Personality and epilepsy. Springfield: Thomas, 1962.

Hermann BP, Whitman S. Behavioural and personality correlates of epilepsy. Psychol Bull 1984; 95: 451–93.

Hermann BP, Dickmen S, Schwartz MS, Carnes WE. Interictal psychopathology in patients with ictal fear: A quantitative investigation. Neurology 1982; 32: 7–11.

Kligman D, Goldberg DA. Temporal lobe epilepsy and aggression. J Nerv Ment Dis 1975; 160: 324–41.

Kristensen O, Sindrup EH. Psychomotor epilepsy and psychosis. Acta Neurol Scand 1978; 57: 361–70.
Landolt H. Serial electroencephalographic investigations during psychotic episodes in epileptic patients and during schizophrenic attacks. In: Lorenz de Haas AM (ed) Lectures on epilepsy. Amsterdam: Elsevier, 1958: 91–133.
Lennox WG. Epilepsy. In: Hunt (ed.) Handbook of epilepsy and behaviour problems. New York: Ronald Press, 1944.
Morel BA. Traité des maladies mentales. Paris: 1860.
Nielsen H, Kristensen O. Personality correlates of sphenoidal EEG foci in temporal lobe epilepsy. Acta Neurol Scand 1981; 64: 289–300.
Pierce-Clark L. A psychological interpretation of essential epilepsy. Brain 1929; 43: 38–49.
Pond D, Bidwell BH. A survey of epilepsy in fourteen general practices. Epilepsia 1959; 1: 285–99.
Robertson MM, Trimble MR, Townsend HRA. Phenomenology of depression in epilepsy. Epilepsia 1987; 28: 364–72.
Serafetinides EA. Aggressiveness in temporal lobe epilepsies and its relation to cerebral dysfunction and environmental factors. Epilepsia 1965; 6: 33–42.
Slater E, Beard AW. The schizophrenia-like psychoses of epilepsy. Br J Psychiatry 1963; 109: 95–100.
Trimble MR. Biological psychiatry. Chichester: John Wiley & Sons, 1988.
Waxman SG, Geschwind N. The interictal behaviour syndrome of temporal lobe epilepsy. Arch Gen Psychiatry 1975; 32: 1580–6.
Zielinski JJ. Epidemiology and medical–social problems of epilepsy in Warsaw. Warsaw: Warsaw Psychoneurological Institute, 1974.

11

Strategies of Antiepileptic Drug Treatment in Patients with Chronic Epilepsy

John S. Duncan
National Hospital for Nervous Diseases, London, UK

Introduction

One in 200 people endure chronic epilepsy. Despite the advent of new and powerful antiepileptic drugs (AEDs), many of these patients are likely to remain intractable and present a challenge to the clinical neurologist. The views in this chapter reflect the experience at the epilepsy clinics of the National Hospital for Nervous Diseases and the Chalfont Centre for Epilepsy, and the results of studies undertaken with Drs S.D. Shorvon and M.R. Trimble at these centres.

First, there is a suggested strategy for the treatment of naïve and chronic patients with AEDs. There follows a discussion of the withdrawal of individual AEDs from the polytherapy regimens of patients with chronic epilepsy, with particular reference to the rates of reduction of the individual drugs. Finally, practical issues relating to the withdrawal of individual AEDs are considered.

AED Prescribing Strategy

About 70–80% of patients may expect to become seizure-free with optimal AED therapy. Approximately 80% will be best controlled with a single drug, and 10–15% with a combination of two agents. Poor compliance, drug interactions and long-term toxicity are all more likely to occur if more than one drug is prescribed (Reynolds and Shorvon, 1981; Schmidt, 1982; Thompson and Trimble, 1982). The goal of therapy should be complete seizure control with a single drug taken once or twice a day, without side-effects. Careful recording of seizures and side-effects is essential if rational management decisions are to be made.

Although the maximally tolerated dose of each drug used should be explored if control is difficult to attain, a balance needs to be struck between side-effects and control of seizures, and drugs that do not contribute to seizure control should be discontinued. In all cases in which treatment appears to be ineffective, the diagnosis of epilepsy and compliance with therapy should be reviewed. Consideration should also be given to the presence of a progressive cerebral disorder, such as a tumour or metabolic defect, and the patient investigated accordingly. There follows a suggested stepwise treatment strategy for naïve patients with epilepsy.

(1) A patient should be commenced on a small dose of one of the first-line AEDs for their type of seizure, and dose increments made if seizures continue and side-effects do not occur, with increments being guided by the measurement of serum drug concentrations. Zealous adherence to quoted therapeutic ranges of serum AED concentrations is inappropriate. These data should always be subordinate to the clinical picture of whether the patient continues to have seizures and/or dose-related side-effects from AEDs, or not. When employed as a guide to dosing, measurement of serum concentrations of phenytoin are particularly useful. Assay of concentrations of carbamazepine and phenobarbitone are moderately helpful, and valproate levels are of little utility.

(2) If seizures continue despite a maximally tolerated dose of a first-line AED, reconsider the diagnosis of epilepsy and its putative aetiology and check compliance with tablet counts and measurement of the serum drug concentration.

(3) Another first-line drug should then be commenced, and built up to an optimal dose, and the initial agent should then be withdrawn. The ideal rate of drug withdrawal in this situation is controversial; phenytoin and sodium valproate probably may be safely withdrawn over a few days, but carbamazepine, barbiturate and benzodiazepine withdrawal should probably be over a period of weeks (Duncan, Shorvon and Trimble, 1987; Duncan, 1988).

(4) The dose of the second drug, taken alone, should then be adjusted to optimum, as was the initial agent.

(5) If seizures continue despite a maximally tolerated dose of all the individual first-line drugs, the next step is to try a combination of two first-line drugs for that seizure type (e.g. ethosuximide and sodium valproate for generalized absences or phenytoin and carbamazepine for partial seizures). The chances of duotherapy controlling seizures when monotherapy has been unsuccessful is of the order of 10–15% (Shorvon and

Reynolds, 1977; Reynolds and Shorvon, 1981; Schmidt, 1982; Mattson et al., 1985).

(6) Should a combination of two first-line agents be unhelpful, the drug which appears to have the most effect, and least side-effects, should be continued, and the other AEDs replaced with a second-line drug, or clobazam (see Chapter 14).

(7) If the second-line drug is effective, withdrawal of the initial agent should be considered. Prescription of an unhelpful second-line drug should not be continued.

(8) Consider the use of a novel AED. As a general rule, the use of such drugs should only be as part of a formal organized trial, with very accurate documentation of seizures and side-effects. Drug trials are demanding for patients and should not be entered into lightly.

(9) The above scheme will generally take a number of months or even years to work through. If satisfactory control cannot be obtained with drugs, and the patient has partial seizures, consideration should be given to evaluating the possibility of surgical treatment of their epilepsy. Such evaluation should be carried out in a specialized unit. The most commonly performed operation is a temporal lobectomy, and amongst the minority of patients that are suitable for surgery, 50–60% become seizure-free and a further 25% have a marked improvement in seizure control (Falconer and Taylor, 1968; Jensen, 1975; Duncan and Sagar, 1987; Polkey, 1988) (Chapter 16).

AED Treatment in Patients with Chronic Epilepsy

The minority of patients who suffer intractable, chronic epilepsy should be treated with a single, or at most two, AEDs that have been shown to have some efficacy, at doses that do not given rise to intolerable side-effects. This is a difficult area, and referral to a specialist is appropriate. The general principles are as follows:

(1) Review seizure history. Classify current seizure types on clinical and EEG grounds. Is there evidence for pseudoseizures? Is there an identifiable aetiology?

(2) Check serum concentrations of AEDs and question compliance.

(3) Review past and present AED treatment for efficacy and side-effects. Has the patient had a good trial with a maximally tolerated dose of all the major AEDs?

(4) Select the AED that is most likely to be efficacious and with the least side-effects. This information needs to be determined from a detailed drug and seizure history. Adjust the dose of this drug to the optimum. The drug to

be retained will usually be selected on the grounds that it has not been used to its full potential, and/or that it appears to have had a definite beneficial effect. In rare cases, e.g. patients with primary generalized epilepsy, there is a clear indication to use a particular agent. Other AEDs may then be withdrawn if their prescription has not aided seizure control, and they may be giving rise to adverse effects.

(5) Attempt to reduce and discontinue the other AEDs, recognizing that seizures may worsen at this time. Frequently, however, reduction of the number of AEDs results in the patient feeling better and improved seizure control (Shorvon and Reynolds, 1979; Thompson and Trimble, 1982; Theodore and Porter, 1983; Callaghan, O'Dwyer and Keating, 1984; Albright and Bruni, 1985).

(6) If seizures remain uncontrolled, consider other first-line drugs and second-line agents, and surgical treatment, as above.

The Optimum Rates at Which to Withdraw AEDs

Once a decision to withdraw a particular AED from a regimen of polytherapy has been made, and the doses of remaining AEDs have been optimized, the next question to address is the rate at which the drug should be tailed off. There has been a very wide range of rates of drug reduction employed in studies of polytherapy reduction (Jeavons, Clark and Maheshwari, 1977; Milano Collaborative Group for Studies on Epilepsy, 1977; Callaghan et al., 1978; Shorvon and Reynolds, 1979; Schobben, 1979; Maheshwari and Padmini, 1981; Gannaway and Mawer, 1981; Thompson and Trimble, 1982; Covanis, Gupta and Jeavons, 1982; Fischbacher, 1982; Bennett, Dunlop and Ziring, 1983; Schmidt, 1983; Theodore and Porter, 1983; Roman et al., 1983; Alvarez and Hazlett, 1983; Callaghan, O'Dwyer and Keating, 1984; Albright and Bruni, 1985; Schmidt and Richter, 1986), ranging from 7 days to 12 months, reflecting a lack of consensus amongst physicians. This impression was confirmed by a survey of the practice of consultant neurologists in the UK and Eire (Duncan and Shorvon, 1987). This survey employed a set of case histories, with questions relating to the rate of reduction of individual AEDs. The time taken to withdraw 1400 mg of carbamazepine, for example, varied from 12 days to 170 weeks.

There are several arguments in favour of making rapid AED reductions rather than slow changes, provided that the former does not carry an increased risk of an exacerbation of seizures. These arguments may be summarized as:

(1) It is possible to supervise patients closely over a short period of time.
(2) The strategy is more likely to be followed through.
(3) The effect of the drug change on seizures, medication side-effects and concomitant AED levels may be rapidly determined.

(4) Potentially beneficial drug treatments can be explored quickly, and the patient established on optimal therapy as soon as is possible.

We have recently undertaken a prospective, double-blind study of the withdrawal of phenytoin, carbamazepine and sodium valproate, at two different rates, from the polytherapy of patients with chronic, intractable epilepsy (Duncan, Shorvon and Trimble, 1987; Duncan, 1988). Phenytoin was withdrawn in 50 mg decrements every 2 or 5 days, carbamazepine was discontinued at 200 mg every 2 or 5 days, and sodium valproate at 200 mg every 2 or 4 days. Among the practical implications from this study, it was concluded that:

(1) The rapid reduction of phenytoin and valproate appeared to be generally problem-free in these patients with active epilepsy, who were under close supervision. The optimal rates of carbamazepine reduction remain uncertain; withdrawal of this drug was often associated with an increase in seizures, and its discontinuation should be approached with caution, even if its use does not appear to have helped seizure control. If further studies show that slower carbamazepine reduction is associated with a lower incidence of difficulties than was found in the current study, then rapid withdrawal of that agent would be inappropriate in routine clinical practice.
(2) Whilst the acute effects of drug changes may be rapidly determined, the longer-term consequences need more prolonged observation, particularly if seizures occur only infrequently.
(3) If a marked increase in seizures occurs on reduction and withdrawal of an AED, and serum concentrations of concomitant drugs have not fallen, the increase in seizures is likely to continue until the withdrawn drug is recommenced. In the event of a serious increase in seizures, diazepam should be given and the withdrawn drug reintroduced. This action would be expected to restore the seizure frequency to the baseline level immediately.
(4) In cases of failed AED withdrawal, the withdrawn drug may be recommenced at the dose that was being taken prior to the increase in seizures, and then increased further as necessary. In the case of reintroduction of phenytoin or phenobarbitone, a loading dose might be necessary.
(5) The optimal dose of the restarted drug should be reviewed. It may be that a higher dose than that which was being given at the baseline will improve seizure control. On the other hand, a lower dose may be equally efficacious.
(6) If a drug change does result in an increase in seizures, this can be managed safely, and the clinician and the patient can be reasonably confident that, with appropriate treatment, there will be no long-lasting deterioration of control of the seizure disorder.

Further studies are necessary to confirm these findings and to determine the optimal rates of removal of carbamazepine, when it is desired to discontinue that agent.

Conclusion

Patients whose epilepsy is chronic and intractable are the most difficult to treat. Careful attention may improve these patients' lot, with improved control of seizures and reduction of the toxic effects of antiepileptic drug therapy, so that they are more able to cope satisfactorily with life's demands.

Acknowledgements

These studies were supported by Ciba–Geigy Pharmaceuticals and the Brain Research Trust. I am grateful to Drs S.D. Shorvon and M.R. Trimble for encouragement and support.

References

Albright P, Bruni J. Reduction of polypharmacy in epileptic patients. Arch Neurol 1985; 42: 797–9.
Alvarez N, Hazlett J. Seizure management with minimal medications in institutionalized mentally retarded epileptics: A prospective study. First report after 4½ years of follow-up. Clin Electroencephalogr 1983; 14: 164–73.
Bennett HS, Dunlop T, Ziring P. Reduction of polypharmacy for epilepsy in an institution for the retarded. Dev Med Child Neurol 1983; 25: 735–7.
Callaghan N, O'Dwyer R, Keating J. Unnecessary polypharmacy in patients with frequent seizures. Acta Neurol Scand 1984; 69: 15–9.
Callaghan N, O'Callaghan M, Duggan B, Feely M. Carbamazepine as a single drug in the treatment of epilepsy. J Neurol Neurosurg Psychiatry 1978; 41: 907–10.
Covanis A, Gupta AK, Jeavons PM. Sodium valproate: monotherapy and polytherapy. Epilepsia 1982; 23: 693–720.
Duncan JS. The withdrawal of individual antiepileptic drugs from patients taking polytherapy. Oxford University, DM thesis, 1988.
Duncan JS, Sagar HJ. Seizure characteristics, pathology, and outcome after temporal lobectomy. Neurology 1987; 37: 405–9.
Duncan JS, Shorvon SD. Rates of antiepileptic drug reduction in active epilepsy—current practice. Epilepsy Res 1987; 1: 357–64.
Duncan JS, Shorvon SD, Trimble MR. Antiepileptic drug reduction in active epilepsy. Neurology 1987; 37 (suppl. 1): 352.
Falconer MA, Taylor DC. Surgical treatment of drug-resistant epilepsy due to mesial temporal sclerosis. Arch Neurol 1968; 19: 353–61.
Fischbacher E. Effect of reduction of anticonvulsants on wellbeing. Br Med J 1982; 285: 423–4.
Gannaway DJ, Mawer CE. Transfer from multiple to single antiepileptic drug therapy. Lancet 1981; i: 217.
Jeavons PM, Clark JE, Maheshwari MC. Treatment of generalized epilepsies of childhood and adolescence with sodium valproate ('Epilim'). Dev Med Child Neurol 1977; 19: 9–25.

Jensen I. Temporal lobe surgery around the world. Acta Neurol Scand 1975; 52: 354–73.
Maheshwari MC, Padmini R. Role of carbamazepine in reducing polypharmacy in epilepsy. Acta Neurol Scand 1981; 64; 22–8.
Mattson RH, Cramer JA, Collins JF et al. Comparison of carbamazepine, phenobarbital, phenytoin and primidone in partial and secondarily generalized tonic–clonic seizures. N Engl J Med 1985; 313: 145–52.
Milano Collaborative Group for Studies on Epilepsy. Long term intensive monitoring in the difficult patient. Preliminary results of 16 months of observations—usefulness and limitations. In: Gardner-Thorpe C, Janz D, Meinardi H, Pippenger CE (eds) Antiepileptic drug monitoring. Tunbridge Wells: Pitman, 1977: 197–213.
Polkey CE. Neurosurgery. In: Laidlaw J, Richens A, Oxley J (eds). A textbook of epilepsy. 3rd ed. Edinburgh: Churchill Livingstone, 1988: 484–510.
Reynolds EH, Shorvon SD. Monotherapy or polytherapy for epilepsy? Epilepsia 1981; 22: 1–10.
Roman EJ, Lambert JB, Buchanan N, Barrah N. Rationalization of therapy in severe epilepsy. Aust NZ J Med 1983; 13: 601–4.
Schmidt D. Two antiepileptic drugs for intractable epilepsy with complex partial seizures. J Neurol Neurosurg Psychiatry 1982; 45: 1119–24.
Schmidt D. Reduction of two drug therapy in intractable epilepsy. Epilepsia 1983; 24: 368–76.
Schmidt D, Richter K. Alternative single anticonvulsant drug therapy for refractory epilepsy. Arch Neurol 1986; 19: 85–7.
Schobben AFAM. Pharmacokinetics and therapeutics in epilepsy. Nijmegan: Stichting Studentenpers, 1979: 251–8.
Shorvon SD, Reynolds EH. Unnecessary polypharmacy for epilepsy. Br Med J 1977; 1: 1635–7.
Shorvon SD, Reynolds EH. Reduction in polypharmacy for epilepsy. Br Med J 1979; 2: 1023–5.
Theodore WH, Porter RJ. Removal of sedative–hypnotic antiepileptics from the regimens of patients with intractable epilepsy. Ann Neurol 1983; 13: 320–4.
Thompson PJ, Trimble MR. Anticonvulsant drugs and cognitive functions. Epilepsia 1982; 23: 531–44.

12
Management of Chronic Epilepsy in Children

Kevin Farrell
University of British Columbia, and British Columbia's Childrens Hospital, Vancouver, British Columbia

Introduction

It has been suggested that in some patients epilepsy is an active process where each seizure may predispose the patient to further seizures (Reynolds, 1988). This implies that failure to control seizures during the early phase of the disorder may play a role in the development of seizures which persist despite antiepileptic therapy. Because the majority of patients with epilepsy develop seizures during childhood, effective early treatment of seizures in children may play an important role in the prevention of chronic epilepsy.

Establishment of a precise diagnosis is fundamental to the optimal management of a child with chronic epilepsy. Thus, the seizure type, the epileptic syndrome and the aetiology may influence significantly the choice of treatment and prognosis. Recognition and management of associated neurological and emotional problems is equally important. In this context, unemployment and lack of social skills are perceived by many adults with chronic epilepsy to be a greater handicap than the seizures themselves (Thompson and Oxley, Chapter 9). Factors other than organic brain dysfunction and poor control of seizures may contribute to these problems. Thus, low self-esteem and emotional dependence are often observed in patients with chronic epilepsy and may relate to failure of both physicians and families to address and prevent these problems during childhood. In addition, the use of excessive doses and numbers of medications, particularly phenobarbitone and the benzodiazepines, may limit

---

Chronic Epilepsy, Its Prognosis and Management
Edited by M.R. Trimble. © 1989 John Wiley & Sons Ltd

the child's opportunity to learn and interact with other children. Clearly, failure to consider the impact of these factors during childhood may contribute significantly to the morbidity associated with chronic epilepsy in adults.

Establishing the Diagnosis

Establishing an accurate diagnosis is critical to the management of the child with chronic epilepsy. This involves determination of whether or not the episodes are in fact seizures, classification of seizure types, identification of a recognized epilepsy syndrome, and determination of the aetiology.

Non-epileptic Events

Recurrent, paroxysmal episodes in children are often due to causes other than epilepsy (Rothner, 1989). The diagnosis of many of these entities is based solely on the description of the event. A careful history is the most effective method of establishing the diagnosis, and investigations are rarely helpful. However, in some instances, intensive video–EEG monitoring may be useful in excluding a diagnosis of epilepsy, particularly when the events are due to psychological factors.

Pseudoseizures and Munchausen's syndrome by proxy are disorders which may simulate epilepsy and are often difficult to diagnose and treat. In a study of patients between 10 and 20 years of age with intractable seizures, pseudoseizures were documented by video–EEG telemetry in 21% (Holmes et al., 1980). Epileptic seizures were documented also in the majority of these patients, emphasizing the difficulty in establishing a clinical diagnosis. Most pseudoseizures in children resemble tonic–clonic or complex partial seizures. Incontinence is rare and postictal confusion is often conspicuously absent. Finally, the episodes are often exacerbated by periods of stress, and are rarely influenced by changes in medication (Holmes et al., 1980). Documentation of the episodes by video–EEG telemetry will usually establish the diagnosis. However, it is also important to investigate any underlying psychological factors, and involvement of a psychologist or psychiatrist is usually necessary in the management of these children.

Fictitious epilepsy is the commonest manifestation of 'Munchausen syndrome by proxy' (Meadow, 1984) and may be difficult to distinguish from true epilepsy. The episodes are usually reported by the parent (nearly always the mother) as clonic seizures which occur most often at night. The children are usually under 5 years of age but this disorder has even been described in adults. The average duration of the disorder prior to diagnosis is 4 years, which reflects the difficulty in making the diagnosis. Many mothers demand to stay all of the time with the child in hospital and appear to thrive on the social contact with the ward staff. Despite the fact that they involve themselves in many ward activities, they rarely appear to have other close friends outside the hospital.

Seizure Type

Determination of seizure type(s) is of major importance in the management of chronic epilepsy. Thus, certain seizure types respond only to specific medications and may be exacerbated by others. Ethosuximide and valproic acid are usually effective for control of absence seizures, while carbamazepine may in fact increase the frequency of this seizure type (Shields and Saslow, 1983). Classification of the seizure type can normally be achieved by careful clinical history and interictal EEG recording. Inaccurate classification of seizure type may be an important cause of poor seizure control. Thus, in a series of adults with intractable seizures, intensive video–EEG monitoring demonstrated unrecognized seizure types in 20% and resulted in a diagnostic reclassification in 48% (Sutula et al., 1981).

Typical absence seizures are often controlled by valproic acid, ethosuximide or clonazepam. However, because of the neurotoxic side-effects of clonazepam, this drug is used most often as a second-line therapy. Acetazolamide, nitrazepam, clobazam, methsuximide and primidone may also be effective in the treatment of patients with resistant absence seizures (Henriksen, 1986). The first-line drugs for prevention of tonic–clonic seizures are carbamazepine, phenytoin and valproic acid. Phenobarbitone is effective in the treatment of tonic–clonic seizures, but the neurotoxicity associated with this drug usually precludes its use as a first-line medication in children, except as prophylaxis against febrile seizures. Valproic acid is often the most effective drug in patients in whom the tonic–clonic seizures are associated with generalized spike and wave activity on the EEG and in those with primary generalized epilepsy.

In children, partial seizures are best treated initially with carbamazepine because of its relative lack of toxicity. Phenytoin, valproic acid, phenobarbitone and primidone are effective also in prevention of this seizure type. If single-drug therapy is ineffective, the addition of clobazam, valproic acid or acetazolamide may be effective (Heller, Ring and Reynolds, 1988; Oles et al., 1989).

Myoclonic, tonic, atonic and atypical absence seizures are often difficult to control. These seizure types often occur in combination and are difficult to quantify in terms of seizure frequency and duration. This has limited the evaluation of antiepileptic medications in these seizure types. Valproic acid and the benzodiazepines are the most effective medications. Of the benzodiazepines, clobazam has an advantage over clonazepam and nitrazepam in that it is associated with less neurotoxicity (Farrell, 1986). Development of tolerance is a major problem with clobazam therapy and occurs most commonly within 4 months of the start of this medication (Farrell, 1986). Tolerance may occur less frequently in patients treated with smaller doses and may respond to an increase in clobazam dosage or to a brief 'drug holiday'. These seizure types appear to be more vulnerable to exacerbation by certain antiepileptic drugs, including carbamazepine, phenytoin, clonazepam and chlormethiazole (Bittencourt and Richens, 1981; Levy and Fenichel, 1965; Shields and Saslow, 1983).

The prognosis of many seizure types is determined more accurately when viewed in the context of the epileptic syndrome or associated neurological findings. Thus, the prognosis for remission of absence seizures and for development of tonic–clonic seizures differs between childhood absence epilepsy (pyknolepsy) and juvenile absence seizures (Berkovic et al., 1987). Similarly, the prognosis of partial and myoclonic seizures is influenced by whether the patient has one of the benign epileptic syndromes associated with these seizure types.

Epileptic Syndromes

A number of epileptic syndromes have been described in children based on certain criteria, including seizure type(s), age of onset, diurnal frequency, associated neurological abnormalities and ictal and interictal EEG features (Roger et al., 1985). These are described more comprehensively by Pellock in Chapter 6. Many children with chronic seizures do not fit clearly into a specific epileptic syndrome. However, in a child with chronic seizures, identification of a recognized epileptic syndrome may be helpful in decisions concerning the most appropriate investigations and the most effective medications, and in prediction of outcome.

The benign partial epilepsies may be associated with centro-temporal spikes, occipital paroxysms or affective symptoms (Dalla Bernardina, 1985a). These syndromes are characterized by absence of an underlying brain lesion, normal neurological development, and a family history of epilepsy in a high percentage of patients. The prognosis for recovery from epilepsy is excellent and does not appear to be influenced by the degree of seizure control. The rationale for obtaining good seizure control in these patients is to alleviate symptoms rather than to influence prognosis. Thus, it may be reasonable to accept less than perfect seizure control in this group of children in situations where medication side-effects are present. A similar conservative approach to treatment is advocated for benign, febrile convulsions, which are associated with normal development and a very low incidence of afebrile seizures in later life.

Classification of the epileptic syndromes associated with secondary generalized epilepsy, which affect a large number of children with chronic epilepsy, is less satisfactory. Many children possess some, but not all, of the features of a specific syndrome, and analysis of other factors may be more helpful in these patients.

Infantile spasms (IS) are often resistant to antiepileptic therapy. Corticotrophin (ACTH), corticosteroids, benzodiazepines, valproic acid and intravenous immunoglobulin G (IVIG) have been demonstrated to be effective in the treatment of IS. Corticosteroids and ACTH are the most commonly used drugs and there is no strong evidence that one drug is better than the other (Hrachovy et al., 1983). There is considerable variation in the dosages used, the type of ACTH and the duration of therapy. The most common dosage is 20–40 IU daily, although higher dosages (up to 180 IU daily) have been used (Aicardi, 1986a). Natural ACTH is considered to have fewer side-effects than synthetic ACTH (Riikonen, 1984).

Benzodiazepines and valproic acid have been shown to be effective in the treatment of IS. Because of the side-effects associated with steroid therapy, these antiepileptic drugs are preferred by some for the treatment of symptomatic IS (Aicardi, 1986a). Nitrazepam may be more effective than clonazepam (Hanson and Menkes, 1972). Valproic acid monotherapy at dosages of 40–100 mg kg day^{-1} was effective in controlling IS in 20 of 22 patients after 6 months (Siemes et al., 1988). Hypotonia was a side-effect observed in nearly all patients, and thrombocytopenic purpura, occurring after a viral infection and responding to a reduction in dosage, was observed in 7 of the 22 children. Recent studies suggest that IVIG may also be helpful in the treatment of IS (Ariizumi et al., 1987). This therapy has the advantage of being administered at monthly intervals and is associated with few side-effects.

Control of seizures in the Lennox–Gastaut syndrome is difficult to achieve. Valproic acid and the benzodiazepines are the most effective drugs. Clobazam, a 1,5-benzodiazepine, should be tried before clonazepam or nitrazepam, because of the higher incidence of cognitive side-effects associated with the latter drugs. Corticosteroids or ACTH are often effective in Lennox–Gastaut syndrome but, in most patients, the antiepileptic effects persist only for a brief period. In children who do not respond to the above medications, ethosuximide, acetazolamide, imipramine and methsuximide may occasionally be effective for prevention of myoclonic, tonic, atonic or atypical absence seizures. The ketogenic diet may also be effective in this type of epilepsy but most parents have difficulty maintaining the child on the diet over prolonged periods. Carbamazepine or phenytoin may control tonic–clonic seizures when these occur in children with Lennox–Gastaut syndrome, but these drugs occasionally exacerbate the other seizure types. Because medications are often ineffective or their antiepileptic action is transient, it is very important to withdraw drugs which may not be active.

Classification of the myoclonic epilepsies is complicated by the frequent occurrence of other seizure types and the overlap with other epileptic syndromes. Thus, exact classification of an individual patient is often difficult. However, identification of a specific myoclonic syndrome may be of prognostic value. Patients with severe myoclonic epilepsy of infancy (SMEI) present in the first year of life with unilateral or generalized clonic seizures, often associated with fever, and myoclonic seizures appear within the next 3 years (Dravet, Bureau and Roger, 1985b). The EEG is often normal initially but later shows fast, generalized spike–waves. The seizures are difficult to control and the prognosis is poor. Despite normal development in the first 2 years of life, these patients become progressively retarded and often ataxic. In contrast, benign myoclonic epilepsy in infants has a more favourable prognosis. This syndrome is characterized by onset of myoclonic seizures in the first 2 years of life (Dravet, Bureau and Roger, 1985a). There are no other seizure types and the child's development is normal. Unlike with SMEI, the seizures are easily controlled by antiepileptic medication. Although few patients develop mental retardation, educational and behavioural difficulties are common (Aicardi and Gomes, 1989). Myoclonic seizures are a frequent clinical feature in certain neurodegenerative disorders, especially when associated with progressive neurological deterioration (Aicardi, 1986b).

Aetiology

In the majority of children with chronic seizures, an aetiology cannot be established. This may relate to the fact that the predisposition to seizures is multifactorial (e.g. constitutional factors, specific brain lesions, systemic factors modulating the excitability of the brain) (Aicardi, 1986b). Structural lesions of the brain are less likely to be demonstrated in children who develop a chronic seizure disorder over the age of 4 years. This relates in part to the high incidence of genetically influenced epilepsies in this age group. Nevertheless, even in the primary generalized epilepsies, slight abnormalities of neural architecture are often observed (Meencke and Janz, 1984).

The history and neurological examination often suggest the underlying aetiology and determine the extent of investigations. Perinatal and postnatal causes of epilepsy are often apparent from the history. Similarly, the presence of dysmorphic features or other congenital abnormalities on examination suggests an underlying cerebral dysgenesis. Careful examination of the skin for neurocutaneous lesions is particularly important and should include examination with a Wood's lamp. The investigation of children with chronic seizures is influenced also by the epileptic syndrome. Thus, a structural abnormality is demonstrated rarely in children with pyknoleptic absence epilepsy or one of the benign, partial epilepsies. Conversely, an underlying structural abnormality is demonstrated often in children with infantile spasms, Lennox–Gastaut syndrome and epilepsy associated with progressive neurological deterioration.

Developmental abnormalities of the brain are an important cause of chronic seizures in children. In a retrospective review of 68 children with neuronal migration abnormalities diagnosed by CT scan, 36 had seizures (Buckley et al., 1989). MRI is a more sensitive diagnostic method of demonstrating small migration abnormalities (Smith et al., 1988).

Tumours are a rare cause of chronic epilepsy in children. Thus, it has been demonstrated that only 0.2–0.3% of children with seizures have a brain tumour (Aicardi, 1986b). However, 25–50% of hemispheric tumours in children present with seizures (Gjerris, 1976; Millichap et al., 1962), which may be the only clinical manifestation of a tumour for many years (Page, Lombroso and Matson, 1969). Most epileptogenic tumours are benign gliomas, usually situated in the central, temporal or parietal areas. Partial seizures are the most common seizure type in children with tumours and this diagnosis should be considered in children with chronic partial seizures when there is no other obvious cause, particularly if the child is of normal intelligence and has a normal neurological examination (Blume et al., 1982). Persistent focal delta activity on serial EEGs also suggests the possibility of a cerebral tumour (Blume, Girvin and Kaufmann, 1982). Olfactory symptoms are classically associated with an underlying brain tumour, although the relationship may be less strong than was considered previously (Howe and Gibson, 1982). The syndrome of gelastic seizures, precocious puberty, behaviour disorder and mental retardation is often associated with a tumour located in the floor of the third ventricle (Berkovic et al., 1988).

The initial CT scan, particularly if performed soon after the onset of the seizures, may be normal in patients in whom seizures are the initial manifestation of a tumour (Aicardi, 1986b). Small tumours of the temporal lobe in particular may be especially difficult to detect. The use of CT with contrast enhancement or MRI may help to demonstrate small tumours. The CT head scan may reveal cerebral lesions which are incidental to the epilepsy, and careful evaluation should precede any decision to deal with the lesion surgically on the basis that it is related to the seizures (Aicardi, 1986b).

The possibility of an underlying metabolic or degenerative disease should be considered in children with unexplained, secondary, generalized epilepsy or with seizures associated with progressive neurological deterioration. Underlying metabolic disorders are a rare cause of intractable seizures. However, they have important genetic implications and some may be amenable to treatment. Thus, pyridoxine dependency should be considered in any child with intractable seizures with onset in the first 18 months of life (Goutieres and Aicardi, 1985). Similarly, biotinidase deficiency, which may present with seizures and ataxia, is a treatable form of seizures in infancy (Wolf et al., 1983). Neuronal ceroid-lipofuscinosis may present with Lennox–Gastaut syndrome and visual failure may be a late feature (Santavuori, 1988). Myoclonic epilepsy associated with progressive neurological dysfunction, in particular, should raise the suspicion of a neurometabolic disease (Aicardi, 1986b).

Medical Therapy

Treatment of seizures with a single drug is the preferred method. Polytherapy is often associated with pharmacokinetic interactions, which may result in a higher incidence of side-effects and poorer control of seizures. Phenobarbitone, carbamazepine and phenytoin induce hepatic microsomal metabolism of several antiepileptic drugs, resulting in lower serum concentrations. This effect may account in part for the improved seizure control which has been described in patients changed from polytherapy to monotherapy. Variability in protein binding may make serum drug concentrations difficult to interpret in patients on polytherapy. For example, valproic acid increases the free fraction of phenytoin by displacing the phenytoin from its binding sites (Gugler and von Unruh, 1980). This may result in phenytoin toxicity at serum total phenytoin concentrations within the accepted therapeutic range. Finally, metabolites of certain antiepileptic drugs possess pharmacological properties. Induction of a specific metabolic pathway may increase the serum concentration of an active metabolite and result in adverse side-effects. Such a mechanism may be responsible for the increased incidence of hepatic failure observed in children on valproic acid polytherapy.

The therapeutic range of an antiepileptic medication is usually established prior to its general release and frequently is based on limited data. Seizure control may be obtained only at concentrations well above the upper end of the therapeutic range. Thus, it is particularly important in patients with chronic epilepsy to use the highest tolerated dose of a medication before concluding that the seizures are refractory to that medication. If a drug is ineffective, the first step should be to replace it with a different drug. This has been shown to be effective in the management of tonic–clonic and partial seizures, which were refractory to maximum tolerated doses of other monotherapy (Schmidt and Richter, 1986).

The role of polytherapy in the management of chronic seizures is controversial. Improved seizure control may be achieved by converting patients from polytherapy to monotherapy (Shorvon and Reynolds, 1977). This may relate to increased serum drug concentrations or to a reduction in drowsiness. Reduction of polytherapy in children has been demonstrated to result in a marked improvement in performance (Trimble and Cull, 1988). Reduction in polytherapy is more likely to be successful when there is only one seizure type (Albright and Bruni, 1985). Drugs with a sedative effect should be withdrawn first, and it has been suggested that withdrawal be gradual over a minimum of 12 months (Schmidt and Richter, 1986). Withdrawal may be difficult, especially when barbiturates or benzodiazepines are involved, and prevention of polytherapy is the most effective method of dealing with this problem.

Despite the problems associated with polytherapy, there is a reason for adding a second drug in patients who do not respond to single-drug therapy at maximum tolerated doses. The addition of a second drug with a different mechanism of action to the first may be a more effective strategy. However, even the use of a second-line antiepileptic drug may be effective, and this should be considered in those patients who are not surgical candidates

(Dasheiff, McNamara and Dickinson, 1986). The addition of primidone or valproic acid to carbamazepine has been associated with improved seizure control (Callaghan and Goggin, Chapter 13). The addition of clobazam has been shown to be effective also in both adults (Callaghan and Goggin, Chapter 13) and children (Farrell, 1986). Similarly, there is evidence that valproate and ethosuximide, used in combination, may be effective for control of absence seizures which were refractory to either drug alone (Rowan et al., 1983). The benefit of this combination may relate to a synergistic action between the two drugs.

Failure of the combination of two drugs to control the seizures should prompt a careful reassessment of the patient, with particular attention to factors which may exacerbate seizure control rather than the addition of a third drug. Seizure-inducing factors play an important role in refractory seizures, particularly in children. Thus, it has been demonstrated that treatment of emotional stress, fatigue and water retention resulted in complete seizure control in 14% and a greater than 50% reduction in seizure frequency in 20% of 150 children and adolescents with refractory seizures (Aird, 1988).

Failure of the patient to take the medication as prescribed is a common cause of apparent drug resistance. This may be due to poor compliance, particularly in the adolescent. If poor compliance is suspected, serial measurements of serum drug concentrations, at the same time each day, together with pill counts when the child attends the clinic, are useful methods by which to establish this diagnosis. In the adolescent, poor compliance may indicate a problem in adjustment to the diagnosis, in which case measures should be taken to address the psychosocial problems which may underlie the poor compliance. Discussion of the importance of complete seizure control prior to application for a driving licence may provide an incentive for the adolescent. Another important cause of poor compliance is failure of the patient or parents to understand the physician's instructions. Providing the patient with written instructions or having another professional review the medication protocol with the parent may help to reduce this cause.

Surgical Management

It is clear that certain patients have seizures that are refractory to all medical therapy. Resection of the epileptic focus, corpus callosotomy and hemispherectomy may be effective in preventing further seizures or in reducing the seizure frequency. In most instances, these operations are not performed until late adolescence or early adult life. Thus, most of the child's growth and development may take place in a setting of uncontrolled seizures, excessive medication and decreased social interaction. This may limit employment and social opportunities, even if seizure control is achieved following surgery. Thus, there is an increasing trend towards selection of patients for surgery at a much earlier age. Most adults with chronic epilepsy have had poor seizure control from the time of diagnosis (Reynolds, 1988). However, in many children, complex partial seizures remit spontaneously in later childhood (Porro et al., 1988). Our limited knowledge of the natural history of certain partial seizure disorders in children is a factor which limits our ability to select patients for surgery early in the course of their disorder.

In selection of patients for surgical resection of the epileptic focus, the area of brain from which the seizures arise must be demonstrated clearly, removal of the brain tissue should not result in neurological handicap, and the seizures must be intractable to medical therapy. Identification of the seizure focus involves serial interictal EEG recording and video–EEG monitoring (see Chapter 4). Neuropsychological assessment and neuroradiological studies may demonstrate a focal abnormality. Localization is more reliable if several different modalities point to the one area.

In patients with epilepsy associated with Sturge–Weber disease or hemiplegia, hemispherectomy may be of value (Ogunmekan, Hwang and Hoffman, 1989; Tinuper et al., 1988). In patients with Sturge–Weber disease, surgery at an earlier age has been especially beneficial (Ogunmekan, Hwang and Hoffman, 1989). Corpus callosotomy may be effective in the management of patients with secondary generalized epilepsy who have drop attacks, particularly if there is a focal abnormality on the EEG (Wyllie, 1988).

Psychosocial Management

In many instances, the impact of epilepsy on an individual relates to factors other than seizures. Thus, adults with chronic epilepsy often perceive unemployment and lack of social skills as greater problems than the seizures themselves (Thompson and Oxley, Chapter 9). Although seizures and brain dysfunction contribute to these difficulties, there are other influences which may be amenable to therapy in childhood. Patients with refractory epilepsy often have extremely limited social skills and form few friendships (Thompson and Oxley, 1988). Children with epilepsy have a lower self-esteem and a higher incidence of psychiatric disturbance than other children (Vining, 1989). This, of course, may relate to an underlying brain dysfunction. However, overprotection by the parent, fear of having a seizure in public, and the attitude of the public towards epilepsy clearly are important factors. Management of these problems in childhood may be important for the development of the patient's full potential as an adult.

The attitude of parents is critical in determining how the child adapts to the diagnosis of epilepsy. Lerman and Kivity (1986) observed a striking difference in the incidence of emotional problems, behaviour difficulties, social maladjustment and scholastic underachievement in children with benign rolandic epilepsy, when the parents had been told that the child had a poor prognosis.

Much of the emotional dependence and social inadequacy may relate to a tendency of parents to overprotect the child, which, in turn, decreases opportunities for social interaction. Thus, the child may not be permitted to take the necessary social and emotional risks which are necessary to develop independent living skills. Parent education is critical in the management of this issue. In addition, introduction of the parents to parents of similarly affected children may modify patterns of parental behaviour.

Several other factors may influence the behaviour of parents of children with chronic epilepsy. Thus, the absence of a specific aetiological diagnosis may make it difficult for some parents to accept the problem. Categorization of the epileptic syndrome may help to reassure the parent, even in the absence of a specific aetiological diagnosis. The lack of control over their child's epilepsy is another factor which may impair the parent's ability to cope. Teaching parents how to administer certain medications, e.g. rectal diazepam or sublingual lorazepam, may not only prevent admission to hospital but may also provide the parents with a certain degree of control over the situation. Parents of children with intractable seizures must also contend with frequent changes in different antiepileptic drug regimens. In such situations, they appear to deal better with the situation if an overall plan of therapy is outlined.

During the teenage years, it is important to address both social and employment issues. Adolescents with tonic–clonic seizures appear to have more difficulty coping if the seizures have not occurred in public (Hodgman et al., 1979). In addition, those who are normal neurologically appear to have the greatest difficulty in coping. This suggests that the fear of being recognized to have epilepsy may be the most difficult problem to deal with. Education and involvement in a social skills group in the early teenage years may be beneficial in the management of these problems.

Unemployment and underemployment are common in adults with epilepsy. The most appropriate time to address this problem is prior to completion of secondary school. Poor seizure control is only one of the factors which contribute to this problem. Patients with epilepsy may have unrealistic employment goals. Neuropsychological and vocational assessments performed towards the end of the formal schooling process may determine the most appropriate employment opportunities. Psychological factors, e.g. poor motivation, lack of self-esteem, and feelings of dependency, may also play an important role in job interviews and how subsequent employment stresses are dealt with. Identification of these difficulties in the early teenage years and provision of appropriate counselling may ameliorate the problem.

References

Aicardi J. Treatment of infantile spasms. In Schmidt D, Morselli PT (eds) Intractable epilepsy. New York: Raven Press, 1986a: 147–56.
Aicardi J. Epilepsy in children. International Review of Child Neurology Series. New York: Raven Press, 1986b.

Aicardi J. Clinical approach to the management of intractable epilepsy. Dev Med Child Neurol 1988; 30: 429–40.
Aicardi J, Gomes AL. The myoclonic epilepsies of childhood. Cleve Clin J Med 1989; 56: S34–9.
Aird RB. The importance of seizure-inducing factors in the control of refractory forms of epilepsy. Epilepsia 1988; 24: 567–83.
Albright P, Bruni J. Reduction of polypharmacy in epileptic patients. Arch Neurol 1985; 42: 797–9.
Ariizumi M, Baba K, Hibio S, Shiihara H, Michihiro N, Ogawa K, Okubo O. Immunoglobulin therapy in the West syndrome. Brain Dev 1987; 9: 422–5.
Berkovic SF, Andermann F, Andermann E, Gloor P. Concepts of absence epilepsies: Discrete syndromes or biological continuum? Neurology 1987; 37: 993–1000.
Berkovic SF, Andermann F, Melanson D, Ethier RE, Feindel W, Gloor P. Hypothalamic hamartomas and ictal laughter: Evolution of a characteristic epileptic syndrome and diagnostic value of magnetic resonance imaging. Ann Neurol 1988; 23: 429–39.
Bittencourt PRM, Richens A. Anticonvulsant-induced status epilepticus in Lennox–Gastaut syndrome. Epilepsia 1981; 22: 129–34.
Blume WT, Girvin JP, Kaufmann, JCE. Childhood brain tumors presenting as chronic uncontrolled focal seizure disorder. Ann Neurol 1982; 12: 538–41.
Buckley AR, Flodmark O, Roland EH, Hill A. Neuronal migration abnormalities can still be diagnosed by computed tomography. Pediatr Neurosci 1989; in press.
Callaghan N, Goggin T. Adjunctive therapy in resistant epilepsy. Epilepsia 1988; 29: S29–S34.
Dalla Bernardina B, Chiamenti C, Capovilla G, Colamaria V. Benign partial epilepsies in childhood. In: Roger J, Dravet C, Bureau M, Dreifuss FE, Wolf P (eds) Epileptic syndromes in infancy, childhood and adolescence. London: John Libbey, 1985a: 137–49.
Dalla Bernardina B, Chiamenti C, Capovilla G, Trevisan E, Tassinari CA. Benign partial epilepsy with affective symptoms (Benign psychomotor epilepsy). In: Roger J, Dravet C, Bureau M, Dreifuss FE, Wolf P (eds) Epileptic syndromes in infancy, childhood and adolescence. London: John Libbey, 1985b: 171–5.
Dasheiff RM, McNamara D, Dickinson LV. Efficacy of second-line antiepileptic drugs in the treatment of patients with mentally refractive complex partial seizures. Epilepsia 1986; 27: 124–7.
Dravet C, Bureau M, Roger J. Benign myoclonic epilepsy in infants. In: Roger J, Dravet C, Bureau M, Dreifuss FE, Wolf P (eds) Epileptic syndromes in infancy, childhood and adolescence. London: John Libbey, 1985a: 51–7.
Dravet C, Bureau M, Roger J. Severe myoclonic epilepsy in infants. In: Roger J, Dravet C, Bureau M, Dreifuss FE, Wolf P (eds) Epileptic syndromes in infancy, childhood and adolescence. London: John Libbey, 1985b: 58–67.
Farrell K. Benzodiazepines in the treatment of children with epilepsy. Epilepsia 1986; 27 (suppl. 1): S45–51.
Gastaut H. Benign epilepsy of childhood with occipital paroxysms. In: Roger J, Dravet C, Bureau M, Dreifuss FE, Wolf P (eds) Epileptic syndromes in infancy, childhood and adolescence. London: John Libbey, 1985: 159–70.
Gastaut H, Low MD. Antiepileptic properties of clobazam, a 1,5-benzodiazepine, in man. Epilepsia 1979; 20: 437–46.
Gjerris F. Clinical aspects and long term prognosis of intracranial tumours in infancy and childhood. Dev Med Child Neurol 1976; 18: 145–59.
Goutieres F, Aicardi J. Atypical presentations of pyridoxine-dependent seizures: a treatable cause of intractable epilepsy in infants. Ann Neurol 1985; 17: 117–20.

Gugler R, Von Unruh GE. Clinical pharamcokinetics of valproic acid. Clin Pharmacokinet 1980; 5: 67–83.
Hanson PA, Menkes JH. A new anticonvulsant in the management of minor motor seizures. Dev Med Child Neurol 1972; 14: 3–14.
Heller AJ, Ring HA, Reynolds EH. Factors relating to dramatic response to clobazam therapy in refractory epilepsy. Epilepsy Res 1988; 2: 276–80.
Henriksen O. Absence seizures: Multiple-drug therapy. In: Schmidt D, Morselli PL (eds) Intractable epilepsy. New York: Raven Press, 1986: 187–93.
Hodgman C, McAnarney R, Myers G et al. Emotional complications of adolescent grand mal epilepsy. J Pediatr 1979; 95: 309–12.
Holmes GL, Sackellares JC, McKiernan J, Ragland M, Dreifuss FE. Evaluation of childhood pseudoseizures using EEG telemetry and videotape monitoring. J Pediatr 1980; 97: 554–8.
Howe JG, Gibson JD. Uncinate seizures and tumors, a myth reexamined. Ann Neurol 1982; 12: 227.
Hrachovy RA, Frost JD, Kellaway P, Sion TE. Double-blind study of ACTH vs prednisone therapy in infantile spasms. J Pediatr 1983; 103: 641–5.
Janz D. Neurological morbidity of severe epilepsy. Epilepsia 1988; 29: S1–6.
Leppik IE, Sherwin AL. Anticonvulsant activity of phenobarbital and phenytoin in combination. J Pharmacol Exp Ther 1977; 200: 750–5.
Lerman P. Benign partial epilepsy with centro-temporal spikes. In: Roger J, Dravet C, Bureau M, Dreifuss FE, Wolf P (eds). Epileptic syndromes in infancy, childhood and adolescence. London, Paris: John Libbey, 1985: 150–8.
Lerman P, Kivity S. Benign focal epilepsy of childhood. Arch Neurol 1975; 32: 261–4.
Lerman P, Kivity S. The benign focal epilepsies of childhood. In: Pedley TA, Meldrum BS (eds) Recent advances in epilepsy. vol. 3. New York: Churchill Livingstone, 1986: 137–56.
Levy LL, Fenichel GM. Diphenylhydantoin activated seizures. Neurology 1965; 15: 716–22.
Meadow R. Fictitious epilepsy. Lancet 1984; ii: 25–8.
Meencke HJ, Janz D. Neuropathological findings in primary generalized epilepsy: A study of eight cases. Epilepsia 1984; 25: 8–21.
Millichap JG, Bickford RG, Miller RH, Backus RE. The electroencephalogram in children with intracranial tumors and seizures. Neurology 1962; 12: 329–36.
Ogunmekan AO, Hwang PA, Hoffman HJ. Sturge–Weber–Dimitri disease: Role of hemispherectomy in prognosis. Can J Neurol Sci 1989; 16: 78–80.
Oles KS, Penry JK, Cole DLW, Howard G. Use of acetazolamide as an adjunct to carbamazepine in refractory partial seizures. Epilepsia 1989; 30: 74–8.
Page LK, Lombroso CT, Matson DD. Childhood epilepsy with late detection of cerebral glioma. J Neurosurg 1969; 31: 253–61.
Porro G, Matricardi M, Guidetti V, Benedetti P. Prognosis of partial epilepsy. Arch Dis Child 1988; 63: 1192–7.
Reynolds EH. The prevention of chronic epilepsy. Epilepsia 1988; 29: S25–8.
Riikonen R. Infantile spasms: Modern practical aspects. Acta Paediatr Scand 1984; 73: 1.
Roger J, Dravet C, Bureau M, Dreifuss FE, Wolf P (eds). Epileptic syndromes in infancy, childhood and adolescence. London: John Libbey, 1985.
Rothner AD. Not everything that shakes is epilepsy: The differential diagnosis of paroxysmal nonepileptiform disorders. Cleve Clin J Med 1989; 56: 206–13.
Rowan AJ, Meijer JWA, De Beer-Pawlikowski N, Van der Geest P, Meinardi H. Valproate–ethosuximide combination therapy for refractory absence seizures. Arch Neurol 1983; 40: 797–802.

Santavuori P. Neuronal ceroid-lipofuscinoses in childhood. Brain Dev 1988; 10: 80–3.
Schmidt D, Richter K. Alternative single antiepileptic drug therapy for refractory epilepsy. Ann Neurol 1986: 85–7.
Shields WD, Saslow E. Myoclonic, atonic, and absence seizures following institution of carbamazepine therapy in children. Neurology 1983; 33: 1487–9.
Shorvon SD, Reynolds EH. Unnecessary polypharmacy for epilepsy. Br Med J 1977; 1: 1635–7.
Siemes H, Spohr HL, Michael TH, Nau H. Therapy of infantile spasms with volproate: Results of a prospective study. Epilepsia 1988; 29: 553–9.
Smith AS, Weinstein MA, Quencer RM, Murof LR, Stonesifer KJ, Li FC, Wener L, Soloman MA, Cruse RP, Rosenberg LH, Berke JP. Association of heterotopic gray matter with seizures: MR imaging. Radiology 1988; 168: 195–8.
Sutula TP, Sackellares JC, Miller JQ, Dreifuss FE. Efficacy of prolonged hospitalization and intensive monitoring in refractory epilepsy. Neurology 1981; 31: 243–7.
Thompson PJ, Oxley J. Socioeconomic accompaniments of severe epilepsy. Epilepsia 1988; 29: S9–18.
Tinuper P, Andermann F, Villemure JG, Rasmussen TB, Quesney LF. Functional hemispherectomy for treatment of epilepsy associated with hemiplegia: Rationale, indications, results, and comparison with callosotomy. Ann Neurol 1988; 24: 27–34.
Trimble MR, Cull C. Children of school age: The influence of antiepileptic drugs on behaviour and intellect. Epilepsia 1988; 29 (suppl. 3): S15–19.
Vining EPG. Psychosocial issues for children with epilepsy. Cleve Clin J Med 1989; 56: S214–20.
Wolf B, Grier RE, Allen RJ, Goodman SI, Kien CL. Parker WD, Howell DM, Hurst DL. Phenotypic variation in biotinidase deficiency. J Pediatr 1983; 103: 233–7.
Wyllie, E. Corpus callosotomy for intractable generalized epilepsy. J Paediatr 1988; 113: 255–61.

13
Adjunctive Therapy in Resistant Epilepsy

Noel Callaghan and Tim Goggin
Cork Regional Hospital and University College, Cork, Ireland

There are conflicting views about the prognosis for seizure control in epilepsy. Based on patients attending special clinics, with a strong representation of chronic patients, it has been suggested that the overall prognosis is poor and only 20–30% of patients will enter a remission (Rodin, 1968; Strobos, 1959). Studies in newly diagnosed patients followed from diagnosis show that up to 82% of patients enter a remission (Elwes et al., 1984; Reynolds, Elwes and Shorvon, 1983). Two community-based studies (Annegers, Hauser and Elveback, 1979; Goodridge and Shorvon, 1983) also suggest an overall good prognosis, with remission achieved in 69% and 70% of patients respectively. However, monotherapy does not result in satisfactory control in all patients. In a recent comparative study of phenytoin, carbamazepine and valproate as monotherapy in newly diagnosed and previously untreated patients, Callaghan et al. (1985) found that 22% of patients with generalized seizures and 24% of patients with partial seizures did not respond to treatment. Reynolds, Elwes and Shorvon (1983) have suggested that chronic refractory epilepsy develops in 25% of patients.

Thus, most patients will achieve satisfactory seizure control with monotherapy, and only when this has failed will other forms of treatment need to be considered. There are two alternatives for patients who do not respond to monotherapy: surgery or adjunctive treatment prescribed as polypharmacy. In patients who are not suitable candidates for surgery, the use of adjunctive treatment may have to be considered, but it is very important that patients not suitable for surgery be given optimum treatment with monotherapy before being considered for polypharmacy. Callaghan et al. (1985) have shown that of

41 patients who failed to respond to the first drug prescribed as monotherapy, only 6 (15%) were eventually prescribed polypharmacy, when a trial was carried out with a second and then a third drug given as monotherapy. Schmidt (1983, 1984) has shown that chronic partial seizures can be controlled with high-dose monotherapy, and suggests that the limit of efficacy is primarily imposed by toxicity.

Additive Treatment—Carbamazepine Used in Combination with Sodium Valproate or Primidone

A number of prospective studies have been carried out to assess the response to polypharmacy in patients who have failed to respond to one drug. Most of these studies have involved patients with chronic partial seizures. It has been shown that the addition of carbamazepine (Cereghino et al., 1974), primidone (Livingston and Petersen, 1956) or phenobarbitone (Merritt and Brenner, 1942) to the existing anticonvulsant drug did not result in complete seizure control in any patient. Schmidt (1982), in a more recent study, showed that a reduction of >75% in seizure frequency occurred in only 4 patients (13%) when a second drug was added to therapy in patients who failed to respond to optimal treatment with monotherapy, and in this study no patient became seizure-free. A better outcome was obtained by Kutt et al. (1977), who stated that when carbamazepine was added to therapy in 20 patients with intractable epilepsy, 12 (60%) had 50% reduction in seizure frequency. Shorvon and Reynolds (1977) carried out a retrospective study in 50 patients with chronic epilepsy, on two antiepileptic drugs, and found that a reduction of 50% or more in seizure frequency occurred in 36% of their patients.

A study was carried out at the Cork Regional Hospital in order to determine the response to polypharmacy in patients whose seizures failed to respond to monotherapy with carbamazepine at the maximum dose that they could tolerate. Thirty-one patients were included in the study, and were allocated to treatment with carbamazepine–valproate (15 patients) and carbamazepine–primidone (16 patients). The distribution of patients by age, sex and seizure type is given in Table 1, together with duration of epilepsy and duration of treatment. The response to treatment was classified as follows: excellent control, seizure-free for a minimum of 6 months; good control, >50% reduced seizure frequency; and poor control, <50% reduced seizure frequency, or no response.

The response to treatment for the separate drug combinations is illustrated in Figure 1. Overall, 1 patient (3%) had an excellent response, 14 patients (45%) a good response, and 16 patients (52%) a poor response. Side-effects occurred in 9 patients (29%); these were ataxia and nystagmus, severe drowsiness, aggressive behaviour, hyperactivity, rash, diplopia, depression, megaloblastic anaemia and neutropenia. Side-effects occurred in 4 patients on

Table 1. Demographic data for patients prescribed carbamazepine–valproate or carbamazepine–primidone

Number (N)	Sex M	Sex F	Seizure type G (N)	Seizure type CP (N)	Seizure type SP (N)	Seizure type P+2″G (N)	Age (years) (Mean ± SD)	Duration of epilepsy (years) (Mean ± SD)	Duration of treatment (years) (Mean ± SD)
Carbamazepine–Valproate 15	12	3	5	2	1	7	28 ± 8.9	14.2 ± 9.1	10.8 ± 4.8
Carbamazepine–Primidone 16	8	8	7	1	1	7	27 ± 8.2	15.8 ± 7.3	14.6 ± 6.5

G = Generalized tonic or tonic–clonic or myoclonic.
CP = Complex partial.
SP = Simple partial.
P + 2″G = Complex or simple partial seizures with secondary generalization.

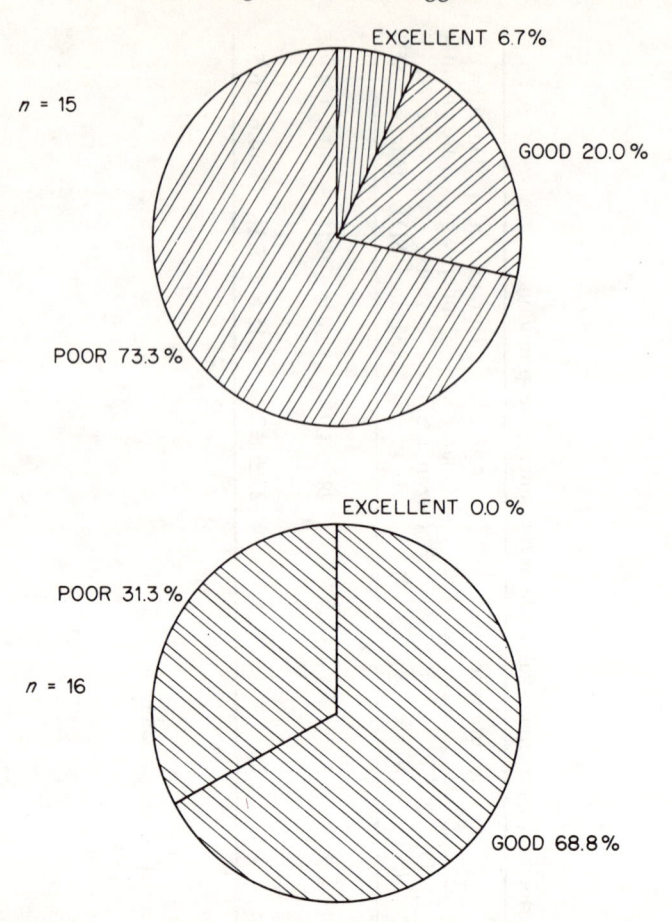

Figure 1. Response to treatment for separate drug combinations. Upper figure: carbamazepine–valproate; lower figure: carbamazepine–primidone

carbamazepine–valproate and in 5 patients taking carbamazepine–primidone (Callaghan and Goggin, 1988).

Clobazam as Adjunctive Treatment

Clobazam has been shown to have anticonvulsant activity (Barzaghi, 1973; Gastaut, 1981). It has been found to be most useful in the treatment of drug-resistant epilepsy, and both open and double-blind studies have shown that this drug is useful for this purpose (Martin, 1981; Critchley et al., 1981; Allen et al., 1983). Clobazam has also been found to be of benefit when prescribed on an intermittent basis in patients with catamenial epilepsy (Feely, Calvert and Gibson, 1982; Feely and Gibson, 1984). In one of these studies, clobazam was

Table 2. Patients' treatment prior to clobazam

Drug	No. of patients
Monotherapy	
Carbamazepine	7
Phenytoin	2
Sodium valproate	1
Polypharmacy	
Carbamazepine + Phenytoin[b]	4
Carbamazepine + Phenobarbital[a]	5
Carbamazepine + Valproate[b]	5
Carbamazepine + Primidone[b]	3
Carbamazepine + Nitrazepam[a]	2
Phenytoin + Phenobarbital[a]	2
Carbamazepine + Primidone + Valproate[a]	2
	33

[a] Polypharmacy when referred to seizure clinic.
[b] Monotherapy initially.

superior to placebo in 14 of 18 patients when given intermittently over a 10-day period, prior to the expected day of menstruation. Clobazam completely suppressed seizures in most patients and toxic effects were of low frequency and severity. The antiepileptic effect of clobazam has been demonstrated in animal models (Gent and Haigh, 1983), and it is felt that intermittent therapy avoided the onset of tolerance.

The effect of clobazam as adjunctive therapy in drug-resistant epilepsy was investigated in an open prospective study (Callaghan and Goggin, 1984). A total of 33 patients were studied; 10 patients were taking monotherapy prior to the prescription of clobazam, and 23 patients polypharmacy. The treatment that each patient was taking prior to the study is given in Table 2. Response to clobazam was classified as follows: excellent control, complete freedom from seizures; good control, >50% reduction in seizure frequency; and poor control, <50% reduction in seizure frequency.

The response to treatment of patients with generalized and partial seizures is summarized in Figures 2 and 3 respectively. The improvement that occurred at 6 months for both types of seizure was not maintained at 12 months, when control deteriorated in 38% of patients with generalized seizures, and 16% of patients with partial seizures who, initially, improved. A further 9% of patients with generalized seizures, and 8% of patients with partial seizures, deteriorated over a period that ranged from 15 to 18 months. Six per cent of patients maintained excellent control for the duration of the study, and 33% continued to maintain a >50% reduction in seizure frequency at the end of the study.

The drug was tolerated with minimal side-effects. Thirty per cent of patients

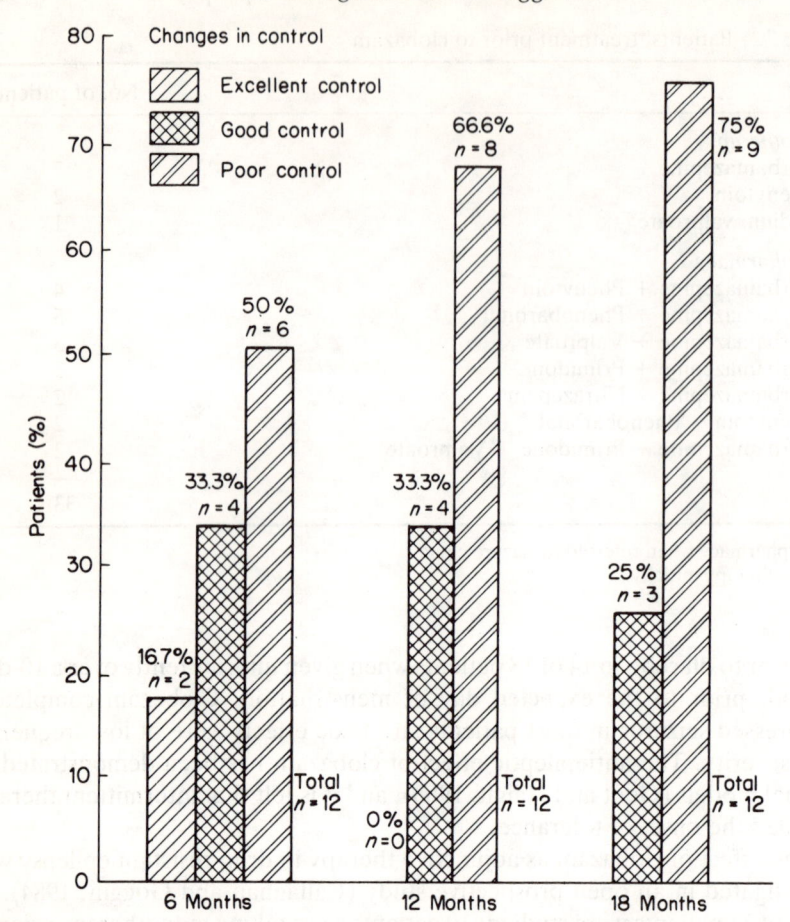

Figure 2. Response of patients with generalized seizures to clobazam

developed some side-effects—one patient suffered headache, two dry mouth, one apprehension, one lightheadedness and one sweating. All these effects were classified as mild or moderate. The drowsiness which occurred in four patients was dose-related, and severe drowsiness occurred in two patients when a dose in excess of 40 mg/day was prescribed.

The dose of clobazam used was related to seizure control, and this and seizure type are summarized in Table 3. Similar summaries of the serum levels of clobazam and N-desmethylclobazam are given in Tables 4 and 5. When a comparison was made between excellent and good or poor control, a significant difference was observed in the dose of clobazam used, and in the levels both of clobazam and its N-desmethyl metabolite. (Students t-test, comparison of means.) Excellent control was achieved at the lowest dose with the lowest

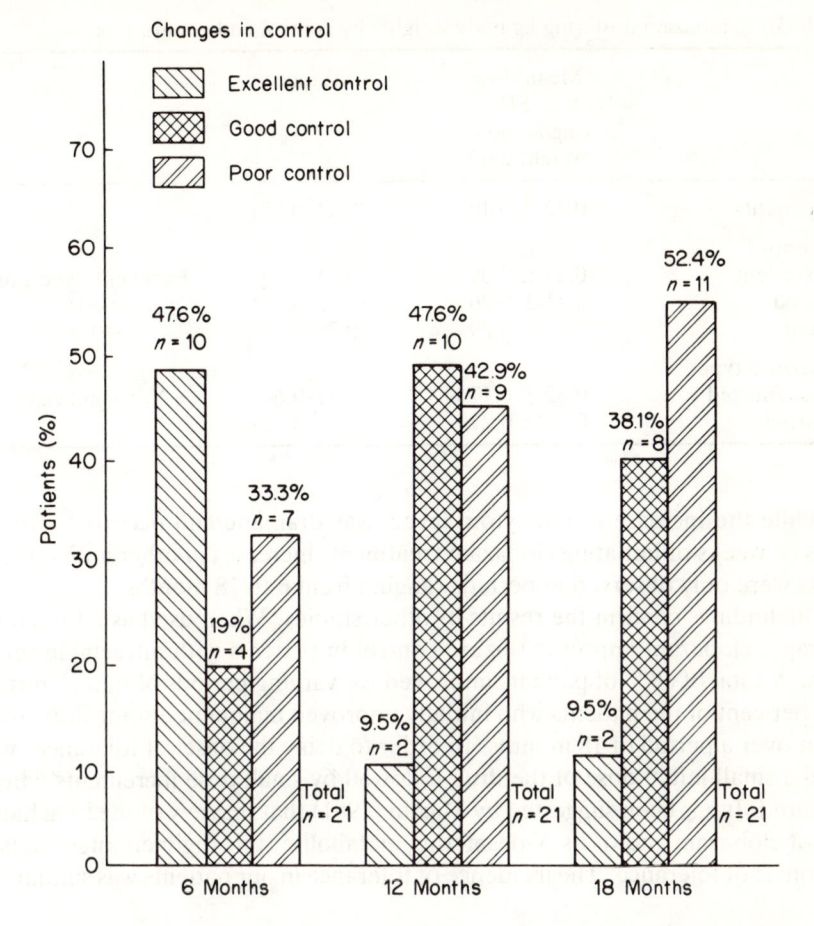

Figure 3. Response of patients with partial seizures to clobazam

levels of clobazam and *N*-desmethylclobazam. As seizure control diminished, an increase in the ratio of levels of clobazam to *N*-desmethylclobazam was observed. When comparisons of dose, levels and ratio were made between generalized and partial seizures in patients who achieved either excellent or good control, no significant differences were observed.

Drug interactions were assessed over each of the 6 months follow-up periods, comparing with baseline levels, based on three estimations in the 3 months prior to clobazam treatment. Patients whose baseline anticonvulsant medication was altered in any way were excluded from this analysis. Significant increases were observed in the levels of phenytoin, carbamazepine, sodium valproate and phenobarbitone. A decrease in the levels of primidone was observed.

Table 3. Clobazam dose (mg/kg body weight) by control and seizure type

	Mean dose ± SD (mg/kg body weight/day)	Range	
All patients	0.33 ± 0.19	(0.11–0.97)	
By control			
Excellent	0.23 ± 0.09	(0.11–0.39)	Excellent<good or
Good	0.41 ± 0.20	(0.15–0.73)	poor
Poor	0.51 ± 0.20	(0.29–0.97)	$P<0.005$
By seizure type			
Generalized	0.32 ± 0.17	(0.11–0.60)	Not significant
Partial	0.38 ± 0.21	(0.15–0.73)	

While the increase in phenytoin levels was dramatic and occurred within days or weeks of initiating clobazam treatment, increases in other anticonvulsants were only observed in periods ranging from 6 to 18 months.

The findings confirm the results of other studies. When used as adjunctive therapy, clobazam improves seizure control in patients with intractable seizures. A total of 60% of patients improved for varying periods of time. Thirty-five per cent of the patients who initially improved maintained some improvement over a period of 18 months. In order to delay the onset of tolerance, we used a small initial dose of the drug followed by small dose increments when required. It has been suggested by Martin (1981) that, in view of the long half-life of clobazam and of its N-desmethyl metabolite, this regimen might delay the onset of tolerance. The incidence of tolerance in our patients was similar to

Table 4. Clobazam levels

Serum level	Mean ± SD (ng/ml)	Range	No. of estimates
By control			
Excellent	77.2 ± 70.2	(24.8–289.9)	56
Good	162.6 ± 121.4	(27.2–782.6)	86
Poor	195.6 ± 108.1	(25.6–523.1)	62
By seizure type			
Generalized	123.1 ± 108.5	(26.4–782.6)	100
Partial	132.8 ± 89.3	(24.8–386.3)	42

Excellent control<good or poor control. $P<0.001$.
(To convert ng/ml to nmol/l, multiply by 3.33.)

Table 5. N-Desmethylclobazam levels and ratio to clobazam

Serum level	Mean ± SD (ng/ml)	Range	Ratio of clobazam to N-desmethyl-clobazam
By control			
Excellent	1061.7 ± 282.5	(309.9–2137.7)	0.07
Good	1747.3 ± 1047.7	(131.9–5900.0)	0.09
Poor	1890.7 ± 836.9	(549.4–4131.6)	0.11
By seizure type			
Generalized	1450.8 ± 898.0	(190.9–5900.0)	0.08
Partial	1524.5 ± 907.6	(131.9–4461.0)	0.09

Excellent control<good or poor control.
$P<0.005$.
(To convert ng/ml to nmol/l, multiply by 3.50.)

that described by Gastaut (1981) and Martin (1981). However, control was maintained in all patients who improved for a minimum period of 6 months, and in some patients for periods of 12–18 months. Our findings therefore suggest that a low-dose regimen may delay the onset of tolerance. Once tolerance developed, further dose increases, associated with increases in the blood levels of clobazam and its N-desmethyl metabolite, did not improve seizure control.

It has been shown (Martin, 1981) that as seizure control improved, it was possible to reduce the dose of other anticonvulsant drugs, and to discontinue some drugs. Our attempt to rationalize polypharmacy by discontinuing some anticonvulsant drugs proved disappointing. It was only possible to reduce polypharmacy from a three-drug combination to a two-drug combination in five patients, and to reduce the dose of anticonvulsant drugs in four other patients, three taking carbamazepine and one taking primidone. Although Gastaut (1981) found that better responses occurred in patients with partial complex seizures, we could not find any difference between the response of patients with partial complex attacks and simple partial seizures.

Interactions of clobazam with other anticonvulsants occurred, resulting in increased blood levels of phenytoin, carbamazepine, sodium valproate and phenobarbitone. In two patients, toxic levels of phenytoin were associated with ataxia. There was no evidence that these interactions alone resulted in improved seizure control. All patients but one had therapeutic levels of other anticonvulsants before clobazam was added, and seizure control did not improve in all patients with increased levels of other anticonvulsant drugs.

The value to the clinician of routine monitoring of clobazam and N-desmethylclobazam levels is limited. Interesting patterns developed with regard to the relationship of serum levels to control, but since tolerance developed in many patients and only 6% of patients maintained excellent control for a period greater than 18 months, changes in the pattern with time allow for no definitive 'optimal range' of serum levels for this drug in chronic usage. It is interesting, however, that where low doses in the range 0.11–0.39 mg kg^{-1} day^{-1}, resulting in serum levels of clobazam in the range 20–150 ng ml^{-1} and N-desmethylclobazam levels in the range 300–2100 ng ml^{-1}, were ineffective, further upward dose adjustments with increased serum levels were not helpful.

Drug Combinations for Intractable Seizures

When patients fail to respond to monotherapy, polypharmacy may have to be considered for some patients, in particular for patients whose lifestyle is compromised as a result of frequent seizures. On the basis of the evidence available at the present time, it is difficult to establish guidelines for the treatment of patients who fail to respond to monotherapy, and who are not suitable for surgery. In the absence of a placebo-controlled trial, it is difficult to establish if the reduction in seizure frequency is due to the effect of the additional drug or the natural history of the disease. Two drug combinations may increase seizure frequency. This may, in part, be related to changes in plasma concentrations due to drug interactions. It has been shown in one study (Hansen, Siersboek-Nielsen and Skovsted, 1971) that a reduction in phenytoin levels can occur in some patients when carbamazepine is used in combination with phenytoin. Feely (1977) studied the effect of phenytoin on carbamazepine levels in 14 patients, and demonstrated a drop in these levels when phenytoin was added to carbamazepine monotherapy in 9 of the 14 patients. An increase in seizure frequency has been documented to coincide with the decrease in the plasma level of one drug when carbamazepine and phenytoin are used in combination (Schmidt, 1981), the reduction in plasma level usually involving phenytoin. In addition, it has been shown that improved seizure control can be achieved in some patients following a reduction in polypharmacy (Shorvon and Reynolds, 1977; Callaghan, O'Dwyer and Keating, 1984; Schmidt, 1983).

In this chapter, the effects on seizure control of three different drug combinations have been discussed, carbamazepine in combination with valproate or primidone and clobazam as adjunctive treatment. Overall, the response was better with clobazam, in particular for generalized seizures, with 47% of patients being completely controlled for a period of 6 months. Only one patient achieved complete control of seizures using the other drug combinations. The improvement which occurred in patients taking clobazam as adjunctive treatment was achieved with side-effects which were of less severity than the side-effects which occurred with the other drug combinations. However, the initial improvement was not maintained in all patients; tolerance occurred in some patients to clobazam.

While in the absence of any control prospective studies it is difficult to suggest drug combinations which give the best chance of seizure control, we have shown that clobazam can be of benefit as adjunctive treatment in drug-resistant epilepsy. Although tolerance will occur in some patients, others may derive a long-term benefit from treatment. We have also demonstrated that carbamazepine in combination with primidone or sodium valproate improves seizure control in some patients, but only a small proportion of patients will obtain complete freedom from seizures. Therefore, clobazam as adjunctive treatment, or primidone combined with sodium valproate or carbamazepine, should be considered when polypharmacy is contemplated for the treatment of intractable seizures.

Summary

Patients who fail to respond to monotherapy, who are not suitable for surgery, and who continue to have frequent seizures may have to be considered for an alternative drug regimen. A review of the literature indicates that complete seizure control with adjunctive treatment is rare, but improved seizure control can be obtained in up to 40% of patients. In a study of clobazam as adjunctive treatment, 60% ($N = 20$) of our patients responded to treatment initially, and 33% maintained an improvement over an 18-month period. In 31 patients who failed to respond to carbamazepine as monotherapy, primidone ($N = 16$) or valproate ($N = 15$) were prescribed as adjunctive treatment. One patient obtained complete freedom from seizures and 14 (45%) had a > 50% reduction in seizure frequency. Suggested indications for the use of adjunctive treatment in epilepsy are discussed.

References

Allen JW, Oxley J, Robertson MM, Trimble MR, Richens A, Jawad SSM. Clobazam as adjunctive therapy in drug resistant epilepsy. Br Med J 1983; 286: 1246–7.

Annegers JF, Hauser WA, Elveback LR. Remission of seizures and relapse in patients with epilepsy. Epilepsia 1979; 20: 729–37.

Barzaghi F. Pharmacological and toxicological properties of clobazam (1-phenyl-5-methyl-8-chloro-2,4-diketo-3H-1,5-benzodiazepine), a new psychotherapeutic agent. Arzneimittelforsch 1973; 23: 683–9.

Callaghan N, Goggin T. Clobazam as adjunctive treatment in drug resistant epilepsy—Report on an open prospective study, Ir Med J 1984; 77: 240–4.

Callaghan N, Goggin T. Adjunctive therapy in resistant epilepsy. Epilepsia 1988; 29 (suppl. 1): S29–35.

Callaghan N, O'Dwyer R, Keating J. Unnecessary polypharmacy in patients with frequent seizures. Acta Neurol Scand 1984; 69: 15–19.

Callaghan N, Kenny RA, O'Neill B, Crowley M, Goggin T. A prospective study between carbamazepine, phenytoin and sodium valproate as monotherapy in previously untreated and recently diagnosed patients with epilepsy. J Neurol Neurosurg Psychiatry 1985; 48: 639–44.

Cereghino JJ, Brock JT, Van Meter JC, Penry JK, Smith LD, White BG. Carbamazepine for epilepsy, a controlled prospective evaluation. Neurology (Minneap) 1974; 24: 401–10.

Critchley EMR, Vakil SD, Hayward HW et al. Double blind clinical trial of clobazam in refractory epilepsy. R Soc Med Int Cong Symp Ser 1981; 43: 159–63.

Elwes RDC, Johnson AL, Shorvon SD, Reynolds EH. The prognosis for seizure control in newly diagnosed epilepsy. N Engl J Med 1984; 311: 944–7.

Feely M. M.D. Thesis, National University of Ireland, 1977.

Feely M, Calvert R, Gibson J. Clobazam in catamenial epilepsy. A model for evaluating anticonvulsants. Lancet 1982; ii: 71–3.

Feely M, Gibson J. Intermittent clobazam for catamenial epilepsy: tolerance avoided. J Neurol Neurosurg Psychiatry 1984; 47: 1279–82.

Gastaut H. The effects of benzodiazepines on chronic epilepsy in man. R Soc Med Int Cong Symp Ser 1981; 43: 141–9.

Gastaut H, Low MD. Antiepileptic properties of clobazam, a 1,5-benzodiazepine in man. Epilepsia 1979; 20: 437–46.

Gent JP, Haigh JRM. Development of tolerance to the anticonvulsant effects of clobazam. Eur J Pharmacol 1983; 94: 155–8.

Goodridge DMG, Shorvon SD. Epilepsy in a population of 6,000. 1. Demography, diagnosis and classification, and the role of the hospital services. 2. Treatment and prognosis. Br Med J 1983; 287: 641–7.

Hansen JM, Siersboeck-Nielsen K, Skovsted L. Carbamazepine induced acceleration of diphenylhydantoin and warfarin metabolism in man. Clin Pharmacol Ther 1971; 12: 539–43.

Kutt H, Solomon G, Wasterlain C, Peterson H, Louis S, Carruthers R. Carbamazepine in difficult to control epileptic outpatients. Acta Neurol Scand 1977; 75 (suppl. 60): 27–32.

Livingston S, Petersen D. Primidone (Mysoline) in the treatment of epilepsy. N Engl J Med 1956; 254: 327–9.

Martin AA. The antiepileptic effect of clobazam: a longterm study in resistant epilepsy. R. Soc. Med Int Cong Symp Ser 1981; 43: 151–7.

Merritt HH, Brenner CH. Treatment of patients with epilepsy with sodium diphenylhydantoinate and phenobarbital combined. J Nerv Ment Dis 1942; 96: 245–50.

Reynolds EH, Elwes RDC, Shorvon SD. Why does epilepsy become intractable? Prevention of chronic epilepsy. Lancet 1983; ii: 952–4.

Reynolds EH, Shorvon SD. Monotherapy or polytherapy for epilepsy? Epilepsia 1974; 22: 1–10.

Rodin EA. The prognosis of patients with epilepsy. Springfield, IL: Charles C. Thomas. 1968.

Schmidt D. Behandlung der Epilepsien. Stuttgart: Thieme Verlag, 1981.

Schmidt D. Two antiepileptic drugs for intractable epilepsy with complex–partial seizures. J Neurol Neurosurg Psychiatry 1982; 45: 1119–24.

Schmidt D. Single drug therapy for intractable epilepsy. Neurology 1983; 229: 221–6.

Schmidt D. Prognosis of chronic epilepsy with complex partial seizures. J Neurol Neurosurg Psychiatry 1984; 47: 1274–8.

Shorvon SD, Reynolds EH. Unnecessary polypharmacy for epilepsy. Br Med J 1977; 1: 1635–7.

Strobos R. Prognosis in convulsive disorders. Arch Neurol 1959; 1: 216–21.

14

Clobazam for Chronic Epilepsy: Factors Relating to a Dramatic Response

A.J. Heller, H.A. Ring and E.H. Reynolds
King's College Hospital, London, UK

Introduction

There are many reports of the usefulness of clobazam as an adjunctive treatment in chronic epilepsy, although its longer term value is limited by the development of tolerance (Koeppen, 1985; Robertson, 1986; Schmidt et al., 1986). In Koeppen's (1985) review of the literature, 69% of patients experienced some reduction of seizures, although this was often short-lived. In Robertson's (1986) review, clobazam was associated with an overall reduction of seizure frequency of 65%, and 29% of patients had complete abolition of seizures, but neither figure takes into account duration of follow-up.

Amongst those patients responding to clobazam is a subgroup who clearly show a dramatic reduction or complete abolition of seizures. At present there is no apparent indication as to which patients will benefit in this striking way. We have retrospectively reviewed our experience with clobazam to search for clues to predict such benefit (Heller, Ring and Reynolds, 1988).

Patients and Methods

Forty-one patients with drug-resistant complex partial seizures were included in the study. Seven patients had complex partial seizures alone and 34 had complex partial seizures with secondary generalization. Mean seizure frequency prior to clobazam therapy was 14 per month (range 1–60). Thirteen patients had an identified aetiology for their epilepsy: 4 post-traumatic, 4 perinatal trauma, 3 postinfective, 1 kernicterus and 1 West's syndrome.

There were 26 males and 15 females. The mean age was 32.1 years (range 15–60). The mean duration of epilepsy was 23.1 years (range 5–52). All patients were on at least one other anticonvulsant with an optimum blood level; 11 patients were on two other drugs.

Clobazam was added openly initially in a dose of 10 mg at night and, depending on clinical progress, increased to a maximum of 40 mg daily in two divided doses. The mean dose was 21.5 mg (range 10–40 mg). Previous medication was unchanged and monitored regularly. The mean duration of follow-up was 14.7 months (range 6–36).

Results

Response to the addition of clobazam was assessed at 1 month, 6 months and 1 year. Patients were divided into three groups. Group I (dramatic response) showed a greater than 90% reduction in seizure frequency or complete cessation of seizures. Group II showed less than 90% reduction in seizure frequency. Group III showed no response to clobazam. Twenty-five patients (61%) exhibited a dramatic response to clobazam (group I) by 1 month of follow-up, and of these 16 (39%) were seizure-free. However, at 6 months of follow-up nearly half the dramatic responders had developed tolerance; by 1 year of follow-up only 9 patients (22%) had maintained a sustained dramatic response (Figure 1). Eight patients (19.5%) were free of all seizures at 6 months, and 4 (10%) at 1 year.

The patients in group I were further divided into those with a sustained response for 1 year (group Ia) and those in whom tolerance developed (group Ib).

Patients in groups Ia, Ib, II and III were compared for as many variables as possible to examine factors that might influence response to clobazam. These included age, duration of epilepsy, seizure type (i.e. partial ± secondary generalization) and frequency, aetiology of epilepsy, associated neurological and psychiatric handicaps, mental retardation, concurrent anticonvulsant medication and CT scan or EEG abnormality. The results are summarized in Table 1, and analysed using χ^2 test. The only factor for which there was a significant difference was mental retardation, which was more common in group III than in group Ia ($p < 0.05$). A known aetiology for the epilepsy was more common in group Ia but this did not reach statistical significance. Comparing the 9 patients with sustained dramatic response (group Ia) with the 16 patients who developed tolerance after an initial dramatic response (group Ib), it was notable that in the former group two-thirds ($N = 6$) had a known aetiology in contrast to one-quarter in the latter; and that only 1 patient in the former had mental retardation compared to 7 in the latter.

We then combined the patients in groups Ia and Ib (i.e. sustained and unsustained dramatic response) and compared them with the combined groups

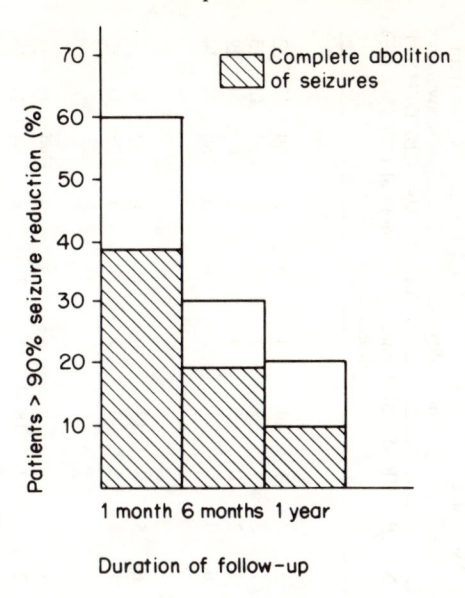

Figure 1. Development of tolerance to clobazam over 1 year

II and III, i.e. partial responders or non-responders (Table 1). There was no significant difference between the groups for any of the factors considered, although there were trends suggesting that partial seizures alone, a known aetiology and the absence of mental retardation were associated with a dramatic response.

Finally we compared the 9 patients who showed sustained response to clobazam (group Ia) with all the other patients (groups Ib, II and III) (Table 1). Sustained response was significantly associated with a known aetiology ($p < 0.05$) and with trends towards partial seizures alone and the absence of mental retardation.

Discussion

The overall response of our patients to clobazam is similar to that reported in previous studies. Thus we found that 61% of our patients showed a dramatic response at 1 month of follow-up, but that this figure had fallen to 32% at 6 months and 22% at 1 year of follow-up (Figure 1). The corresponding figures for complete cessation of seizures were 39% at 1 month, 19.5% at 6 months and 10% at 1 year (Figure 1).

None of the many studies of clobazam analysed which particular patients respond in a dramatic way. Our analysis suggests that three factors seem to be important—the presence of a known aetiology for the epilepsy, the absence of

Table 1. Response to the addition of clobazam

Group	N	Mean age (yrs)	Mean duration epilepsy (yrs)	Seizure type PS	Seizure type PS+2°	Pretreatment seizure frequency (attacks/month)	Aetiology Known	Aetiology Un-known	Associated handicap N	Associated handicap P	Associated handicap MR	EEG abnormality Focal	EEG abnormality Generalized	CT scan Normal	CT scan Ab-normal	Concurrent anticonvulsants CBZ (%)	Concurrent anticonvulsants DPH (%)	Concurrent anticonvulsants SVP (%)
Characteristics of all groups																		
Ia	9	40.9	26.5	3	6	14.1	6	3	5	2	1	4	4	5	2	89	22	22
Ib	16	31.4	25.5	3	13	16.7	4	12	1	3	7	9	6	10	4	94	13	13
II	9	30.3	16.8	1	8	10.6	2	7	1	2	0	5	4	7	1	67	44	22
III	7	23.3	11.8	0	7	11.8	1	6	0	0	5[a]	4	3	4	3	86	14	14
Dramatic responders versus partial and non-responders																		
I	25	35.2	25.9	6	19	15.7	10	15	6	5	8	13	10	15	6	92	16	16
II + III	16	27.2	16.2	1	15	11.1	3	13	1	2	5	9	7	11	4	75	31	12
Sustained dramatic responders versus rest of patients (Ib + II + III)																		
Ia	9	40.9	26.5	3	6	14.1	6[b]	3	5	2	1	4	4	5	2	89	22	22
Ib + II + III	32	29.3	20.7	4	28	13.8	7	25	2	5	12	18	13	21	8	84	23	13

[a] $p<0.5$ (group III versus group Ia). [b] $p<0.05$ (group Ia versus groups Ia + II + III).
PS = partial seizures; 2° = secondary generalization; N = neurological; P = psychiatric; MR = mental retardation; CBZ = carbamazepine; DPH = phenytoin; SVP = sodium valproate.

secondary generalization and the absence of mental retardation. Initially, 10 patients out of 13 with a known aetiology and 6 out of 7 with partial seizures alone responded dramatically to clobazam. Only 1 out of 9 patients with a sustained response was mentally retarded. Some studies have suggested that, overall, clobazam is more effective in partial than in generalized epilepsy (Allen et al., 1983; Wilson, Dellaportas and Clifford Rose, 1985).

The effectiveness of clobazam is clearly limited by the development of tolerance. In Robertson's review the incidence of tolerance ranged from 0 to 86%, with a mean of 36%. This is difficult to interpret because outcome will depend on the duration of follow-up, which varied from 7 days to 63 months in the studies reviewed. Figure 1 shows the evolution of tolerance in our series of patients. We found that out of 25 patients with initial dramatic response at 1 month of follow-up, 45% had developed tolerance at 6 months and 64% at 1 year. Comparing the patients who had a sustained response to those in whom tolerance developed, a known aetiology and absence of mental retardation again seemed to be important but the differences were not statistically significant.

Despite the high proportion of good responders who do relapse, it is apparent that clobazam can produce a sustained dramatic response in 22% of patients with intractable focal epilepsy. This is a remarkable achievement in such a drug-resistant population. We have found some evidence to suggest that selection of patients in whom marked benefit will occur may be possible, but further studies of this problem are needed. If the problem of tolerance to clobazam could be overcome, the potential value of this drug would be considerably increased.

Summary

Twenty-five out of 41 (61%) patients with drug-resistant complex partial seizures showed an initial dramatic response to clobazam. Sixteen of these responders developed tolerance to the effects of clobazam so that only 9 (22%) maintained a dramatic response for 1 year. Factors which appeared important in predicting a dramatic response to treatment were a known aetiology for the epilepsy, the occurrence of complex partial seizures alone (i.e. without secondary generalization) and the absence of mental retardation.

References

Allen J, Oxley J, Robertson M et al. Clobazam as adjunctive treatment in refractory epilepsy. Br Med J 1983; 286: 1246–7.
Heller AJ, Ring HA, Reynolds EH. Factors relating to dramatic response to clobazam therapy in refractory epilepsy. Epilepsy Res 1988; 2: 276–80.

Koeppen D. A review of clobazam studies in epilepsy. In: Hindmarch I, Stonier PD, Trimble MR (eds) Clobazam. Royal Society of Medicine International Congress and Symposium Series No. 74. London: Royal Society of Medicine, 1985: 207–15.

Robertson MM. Current status of the 1,4- and 1,5-benzodiazepines in the treatment of epilepsy: the place of clobazam. Epilepsia 1986; 27 (suppl. 1): S27–41.

Schmidt D, Rohde M, Wolf P, Roeder-Wanner U. Clobazam for refractory focal epilepsy. Arch Neurol 1986; 43: 824–6.

Wilson A, Dellaportas CI, Clifford Rose F. Low dose clobazam as adjunctive treatment in chronic epilepsy. In: Hindmarch I, Stonier PD, Trimble MR (eds). Clobazam. Royal Society of Medicine International Congress Symposium Series No. 74. London: Royal Society of Medicine, 1985: 173–8.

15
Strategies to Avoid the Development of Tolerance to Antiepileptic Benzodiazepine Effects

Dieter Schmidt, Sibylle Ried and Eberhard Rohrer
Ludwig-Maximilians University, Munich, West Germany

Oral benzodiazepines are among the most potent antiepileptic drugs for acute treatment of ongoing epileptic seizures or status epilepticus (Schmidt, 1989). The addition of clobazam is highly effective even in patients with intractable complex partial seizures, as shown in a recent controlled trial (Schmidt et al., 1985).

Inspired by the excellent antiepileptic effect even on intractable seizures, we tried to attenuate the development of tolerance in patients with epilepsy receiving clobazam as an add-on drug.

Experimental Evidence

Tolerance can be classified as metabolic or functional. Metabolic tolerance is caused by accelerated drug elimination and requires increased doses to maintain the original drug concentration in plasma and brain. In contrast, functional tolerance is caused by an adaptation of neurons and requires higher drug concentrations to maintain the original antiepileptic effect. The mechanism for tolerance to the antiepileptic effect of benzodiazepines has been suggested to involve reduced benzodiazepine receptor binding. This derives from studies in cultures of fetal mouse cortex cells in the presence of diazepam (Sher, 1983). Further, a subsensitivity of the dorsal raphé nucleus to iontophoretically applied GABA in rats treated with diazepam for 3 weeks has also been shown (Gallagher et al., 1984).

A possible involvement of 5-hydroxytryptamine has also been suggested (Jenner et al., 1975). A recently introduced animal model for epilepsy is the epileptic dog, where functional tolerance was shown to develop to diazepam and clonazepam. The antiepileptic effect declines over several weeks in spite of unchanged or even higher plasma drug concentrations (for review see Frey (1987)).

More recently, withdrawal effects have been shown when clorazepate, a prodrug for desmethyl diazepam, was discontinued after chronic exposure in epileptic dogs leading to fatal status epilepticus (Scherkl, Kurudi and Frey, 1989). Interestingly, withdrawal effects were observed in dogs which had not developed tolerance.

Following the initial observation that the development of tolerance to chronic diazepam administration in rodents is associated with the progressive development of GABAergic subsensitivity as discussed above, it has been shown that a single exposure to flumazenil, a benzodiazepine antagonist, reverses the GABA subsensitivity and reverses the tolerance to antiepileptic effects of chronic diazepam treatment in rats (Gonsalves and Gallagher, 1988). These experimental observations led us to investigate whether the use of flumazenil would reverse tolerance in patients, and furthermore whether intermittent exposure to clobazam, which may lead to a transient decrease in the number of benzodiazepine receptors occupied by the drug or its metabolites, may attenuate the development of tolerance.

Use of Flumazenil, a Benzodiazepine Receptor Antagonist

Flumazenil has been shown experimentally to reverse tolerance to antiepileptic effects of diazepam in rodents, and experiments in primates have indicated that periodic exposure to flumazenil decreases the physical dependence produced by chronic diazepam exposure (Gallagher et al., 1986; Gonsalves and Gallagher, 1988). In addition to its antagonistic nature, flumazenil may have slight antiepileptic effects, and this is currently being tested in a clinical trial. A major concern is the potential precipitation of withdrawal seizures in epileptic patients chronically exposed to benzodiazepines when flumazenil is given. We therefore undertook a controlled trial of the acute effects of the intravenous injection of flumazenil in several patients.

Case 1

A 48-year-old female patient with refractory complex partial seizures and occasional secondary generalization became seizure-free for 4 weeks after the addition of clobazam to her medication of carbamazepine and primidone. After 6 weeks the frequency of seizures returned to the level prior to the

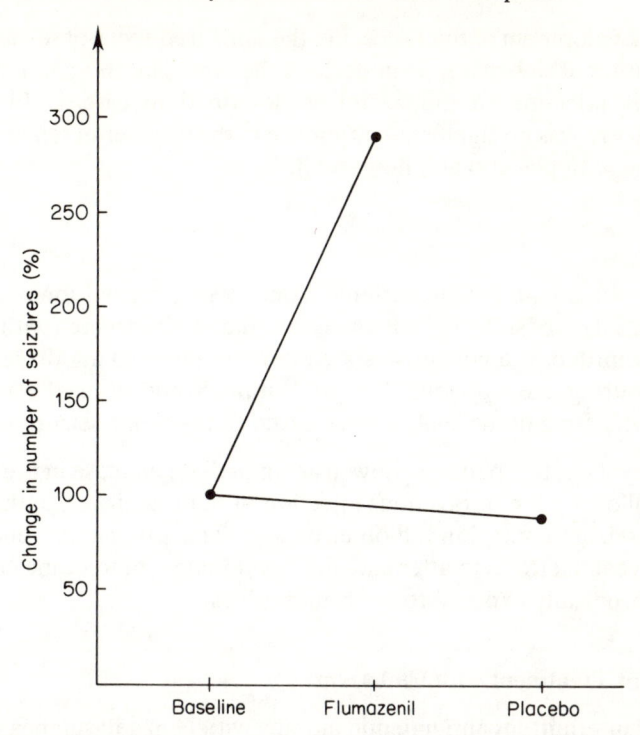

Figure 1. Marked increase in the number of seizures following the intravenous injection of flumazenil (0.15 mg kg^{-1}) in case 1. Three separate injections of flumazenil resulted in a 289% increase in the number of seizures compared to the 24 h prior to injection taken as baseline (5.3 versus 20.7 seizures). Four separate injections of physiological saline served as controls (10.3 versus 9.3 seizures)

administration of clobazam. In an attempt to reverse tolerance, we undertook a placebo-controlled trial of intravenous injection of 10 mg flumazenil (Anexate). Counting and averaging the number of seizures within 24 h before (baseline) and after application of physiological saline (placebo, four trials) and flumazenil (Anexate, three trials), we compared the percentage change in the number of seizures (Figure 1). There was no significant difference in the frequency of seizures between baseline and placebo, but, compared with baseline, the patient had, after application of flumazenil, nearly three times more seizures, 45% of the seizures occurring within 30 min following the intravenous injection of flumazenil.

Case 2

A 30-year-old male patient with intractable complex partial seizures became seizure-free for some weeks after clobazam had been added to carbamazepine.

After the development of tolerance, i.e. the same frequency of seizures prior to the application of clobazam, we undertook the same placebo-controlled trial of intravenous injection of flumazenil as described in case 1. In this case, however, there was no significant difference in the number of seizures comparing baseline with placebo and flumazenil.

Case 3

A 69-year-old female patient suffered from six generalized tonic–clonic seizures within 3 days of suffering pneumococcal meningitis treated with penicillin. She was admitted in a comatose state after receiving 80 mg diazepam intravenously during the previous 3 days. Within 5 min after the intravenous injection of 0.5 mg flumazenil, a generalized tonic–clonic seizure occurred.

In summary then, two patients showed an immediate increase in the number of seizures following the intravenous injection of flumazenil, while there was no change in seizure control in the other patient. This preliminary finding introduces a caveat in efforts to attenuate the development of tolerance in epileptic patients chronically exposed to benzodiazepines.

Intermittent Treatment with Clobazam

The use of intermittent antiepileptic therapy with benzodiazepines is accepted in preventing the recurrence of febrile seizures (Tondi et al., 1987) and in the control of clusters or series of seizures. Several investigators have demonstrated a reduction in benzodiazepine receptor binding after long-term exposure. Such receptor changes have been suggested to contribute to the development of tolerance. To minimize receptor alterations, several patients with intractable seizures received alternate-day clonazepam treatment, resulting in improved seizure control (Sher, 1985). Furthermore, intermittent clobazam was given for catamenial epilepsy to avoid tolerance (Feely and Gibson, 1984). Clobazam was given in a dose of 20–30 mg day^{-1} for 10 days around menstruation in several menstrual cycles to thirteen women who earlier had responded well to clobazam. Tolerance did not develop when treatment was confined to 10 days in each month. An increase in seizures between periods of clobazam therapy was observed in three patients, leading to discontinuation in two of these patients; another drop-out was due to sedative side-effects (Feely and Gibson, 1984).

Increase of Dose After Development of Tolerance

A fairly widely held view holds that the tolerance can be reversed by increasing the dose of benzodiazepines. A recent study shows, however, that on only one of thirteen occasions did an increase in dose produce clinically relevant improvement (Haigh et al., 1988). In conclusion, then, increase of dose is not an effective measure to reverse tolerance.

Conclusions

Clobazam is a very effective add-on drug for partial intractable epilepsy on a short-term basis. The chronic use is hampered by the development of tolerance. Various strategies to reverse or attenuate tolerance are currently under scrutiny, which include administration of a benzodiazepine antagonist, intermittent treatment or increasing the dose. None of the proposed measures can be definitely assessed until more data are available.

References

Feely M, Gibson J. Intermittent clobazam for catamenial epilepsy: tolerance avoided. J Neurol Neurosurg Psychiatry 1984; 47: 1279–82.
Frey HH. Tolerance to antiepileptic drug effects. Experimental evidence and clinical significance. Pol J Pharmacol Pharm 1987; 39: 495–504.
Gallagher DW et al. Chronic benzodiazepine treatment decreases postsynaptic GABA sensitivity. Nature 1984; 308: 74–7.
Gallagher DW et al. Periodic benzodiazepine antagonist administration prevents benzodiazepine withdrawal symptoms in primates. Eur J Pharmacol 1986; 132, 31–8.
Gonsalves SF, Gallagher DW. Persistent reversal of tolerance to anticonvulsant effects and GABAergic subsensitivity by a single exposure to benzodiazepine antagonist during chronic benzodiazepine administration. J Pharmacol Exp Ther 1988; 244: 79–83.
Haigh JRM et al. Disappointing results of increasing benzodiazepine dose after the development of anticonvulsant tolerance. J Neurol Neurosurg Psychiatry 1988; 51: 1008–9.
Jenner P et al. Clonazepam-induced changes in 5-hydroxytryptamine (5-HT) metabolism in animals and man. J Pharm Pharmacol 1975; 27: 38.
Scherkl R, Kurudi D, Frey HH. Clorazepate in dogs: tolerance to the anticonvulsant effect and signs of physical dependence. Epilepsy Res 1989; in press.
Schmidt D. In: Diazepam antiepileptic drugs. 3rd ed 1989, in press.
Schmidt D et al. Clobazam for refractory epilepsy. A controlled trial. Arch Neurol 1986; 43: 824–6.
Sher PK. Reduced benzodiazepine receptor binding in cerebral cortical cultures chronically exposed to diazepam. Epilepsia 1983; 24: 313–20.
Sher PK. Alternate-day clonazepam treatment of intractable seizures. Arch Neurol 1985; 42: 787–8.
Tondi M et al. Intermittent therapy with clobazam for simple febrile convulsions. Dev Med Child Neurol 1987; 29: 830–5.

16
Surgical Treatment of Chronic Epilepsy

C.E. Polkey
Maudsley Hospital, London, UK

Introduction

There are difficulties in relating the experimental data on the pathophysiology of epilepsy with those on clinical neurophysiology and the surgical management of drug-resistant epilepsy. Some of these difficulties relate to species differences, others to the uncontrolled nature of the 'experiment' in human epilepsy, and yet others to the restrictions imposed by the need for practical safe surgery. It is valuable to review the theoretical basis for the surgical management of uncontrolled epilepsy even though historically the operations have been used empirically.

Cells in an epileptic focus in an experimental animal have similar intracellular physiology, whether it is a primary or a secondary focus (Morrell, 1970). It is the means of spread of their autonomous discharge which is of interest when considering the surgical treatment of epilepsy. A number of studies, especially those of Morrell, have shown that after a primary focus has been established in the cortex of an experimental animal then a secondary or 'mirror' focus will appear in the homologous area of the contralateral cortex. This secondary focus will go through three stages. First there is complete dependence upon the primary focus so that the secondary focus fires when the primary focus fires, and if the primary focus is excised then the secondary focus will disappear. In the second, intermediate, stage, the firing of the secondary focus is independent of the primary focus but it will disappear if the primary focus is removed. In the third stage, the secondary focus becomes completely independent of the primary focus and is unaffected by its removal. This process has been called secondary epileptogenesis (Morrell, 1960). The position of the animal on the phylogenetic scale influences the rapidity and the certainty of the development of secondary epileptogenesis (Wilder, King and Schmidt, 1968).

Patients with bilateral temporal EEG foci tend to have a longer duration of their epilepsy than those with unilateral foci (Hughes and Schlagendorf, 1961; Gupta, Dharampaul and Singh, 1973). There is anecdotal evidence from patients subjected to hemispherectomy and those with bilateral EEG changes from unilateral temporal lesions that EEG abnormalities contralateral to the structural lesion can regress after operation (Falconer and Kennedy, 1961; Wieser and Yasargil, 1982). Convincing evidence for human secondary epileptogenesis has been presented by Morrell (Morrell, Wada and Engel, 1987). Among patients undergoing temporal lobe surgery at the Montreal Neurological Institute, he found a small number who had clinical and electrographic evidence of bilateral foci. The majority, but not all, of the secondary foci regressed after surgical resection of the primary focus. In those patients where the foci persisted, the appropriately lateralized seizures also persisted.

The process of 'kindling', first described by Goddard (1967), is thought by Wada (1982) to play little part in the persistence of epilepsy after resective surgery.

Resective surgery may be effective for each of three reasons. First, it removes pathology, including the primary focus; second, it disconnects a focus from the rest of the brain when the removal of the primary focus is incomplete; third, it reduces the mass of neurons which behave abnormally. Functional operations tend to achieve only one or two of these aims, whereas resective operations are hybrid in nature and encompass all three. Chronic epilepsy is a dynamic process which has a continuing influence in some brains. Therefore the length of time for which this adverse influence operates may be important in determining the outcome of the surgery.

Selection for Surgery

The selection process is complex and related to the intended surgical procedure. In this limited review it is only possible to deal with the broad principles of the selection process.

In resective surgery the aim is to demonstrate that the seizures originate from one area whose removal will not have any unfavourable consequences. Such selection depends upon evidence from the clinical history and examination, and the results of brain imaging, neuropsychological assessment and neurophysiological studies.

Clinical History and Examination

The clinical history should elicit any incident in the past which could have given rise to brain injury sufficient to cause the epilepsy. Such incidents include trauma, including birth trauma, meningitis and encephalitis, febrile convulsions and so forth. The absence of any such incident may suggest clinically silent lesions such as hamartomas, low-grade gliomas and so on. The level of social and intellectual functioning gathered from the educational and social history and the presence of psychiatric disease may also be important.

The clinical history should also include an adequate description of the patient's seizures. A detailed description from the patient and an independent observer is important and should be in everyday language to avoid misunderstandings.

Clinical examination between fits is usually normal, except where there is gross neurological disease. Postictal examination may reveal transient focal neurological deficits.

Brain Imaging Studies

Recent improvements in methods of imaging have made the detection of gross structural lesions inevitable. In patients with focal epilepsy or focal EEG abnormalities, CT examinations on high-definition machines will reveal a lesion in 60–70% of cases (Kendall, 1988). The majority of such lesions produce a definite change in tissue density such as tumours or arteriovenous malformations (AVMs). The detection of scarring in the temporal lobe is more difficult but appropriate angling of the scanner gantry helps. Some centres use intrathecal contrast to detect these changes, and claim 94% accuracy (Wyler and Bolender, 1983).

MRI scanning has improved the detection of structural lesions in patients with negative CT examinations. The Los Angeles group demonstrated such lesions in 7 of 35 patients (Sperling et al., 1986). The detection of gliotic lesions, such as mesial temporal sclerosis (MTS), is more contentious. In the same study all 18 patients who had this lesion at operation had normal MRI scans. Other groups have shown atrophy in the medial temporal structures on MRI and confirmed it at operation (McLachan et al., 1985; Meencke, Schorner and Janz, 1987). Functional studies of the temporal lobes, both ictal and interictal, using PET and SPECT, although lacking definition, are useful as confirmatory evidence of lateralization (Engel et al., 1982; Bonte et al., 1983).

Neuropsychological Assessment

This is important both to detect focal brain dysfunction and to predict the results of surgery, especially temporal lobe surgery. Early workers showed that bilateral temporal lobe surgery, or the equivalent thereof, produced a severe global amnesia (Scoville and Milner, 1957). However, unilateral temporal lobe surgery may produce material-specific deficits (Milner, 1975).

The Wada test is an important tool for predicting the results of temporal lobe surgery (Wada, 1949; Powell, Polkey and Canavan, 1987; Jack et al., 1988).

Neurophysiological Assessment

This is the most complex and diverse of the preoperative assessments. Information can be obtained by both interictal and ictal recordings but there is evidence that interictal recordings, especially in temporal and frontal lobe epilepsy, may be either unhelpful or misleading. A recent survey of centres in the Western Hemisphere found that some 30% were using only extracranial recording for their preoperative assessment (Engel, 1987a). Invasive ictal recordings increase the number of candidates for surgery by 30% (Spencer, 1981). The methods used for intracranial recording are diverse. They include the placement of electrodes through the foramen ovale to record adjacent to the mesial temporal structures (Wieser, Elger and Stodieck, 1985), and the use of plastic mats and strips placed extradurally (Goldring and Gregorie, 1984) and subdurally (Hahn and Luders, 1987). Electrodes may also be implanted in deep brain structures using a diversity of electrode types and stereotactic methods, including the use of CT and MRI imaging to identify the targets (Talairach et al., 1974; Olivier et al., 1987; Flanigin and Smith, 1987).

Each patient is investigated in stages, including correlation with the results of other investigations, until a clear decision is possible as to whether operation is appropriate or not.

In patients where functional surgery is being offered, the selection process is less precise. The clinical, neuroradiological and neuropsychological assessments remain important. The neurophysiological investigations are less crisp because of the nature of the abnormalities in these patients. On very rare occasions a single deep focus has been identified by depth recordings and this area of brain destroyed stereotactically (Hood, Siegfried and Wieser, 1983). More commonly, there are diffuse bilateral abnormalities whose presence is noted, but they have little influence on the choice of procedure. Much neurophysiological and neuropsychological investigation in these cases is directed to noting changes related to the surgery and its outcome.

Results of Surgery

The variety of operations available for the treatment of epilepsy, and the different protocols used for the selection of patients, make detailed comparison between different centres impossible. Indeed, in some centres certain operations may be precluded by the selection procedure. Certain broad criteria can be used to judge the results of surgery. The following criteria seem to be appropriate in this respect:

(1) Freedom from, or significant control of, the seizures.
(2) Complications of the surgery, including intellectual and behavioural changes.

Table 1. Frequency of resective operations for epilepsy

Resection	Montreal Neurological Institute (1929–1980)[a]		Maudsley Hospital (1975–1988)	
	Number	%	Number	%
Temporal	1210	56	156	71
Frontal	402	18	23	11
Central	151	7	3	1
Parietal	141	6	12	6
Occipital	30	1	4	1
Multilobe including hemisphere	243	11	20	9
Total	2177		218	

[a] From Rasmussen (1987).

(3) Mortality, short-term and long-term.
(4) Social and behavioural improvements.

The results of operation can be assessed easily if sufficient careful follow-up data are available. At present there is no agreement about the minimum or optimum period of follow-up but most serious workers would require a minimum period of 2 years and an optimum period of at least 5 years. The data available from the follow-up of resective operations suggest that the longer the patient is followed the less likely they are to remain fit-free. However, the significance of this residual liability to epilepsy is hard to judge, partly due to the way in which the data are collected and presented. Analysis of the same data using actuarial methods of analysis (Elwes et al., 1984) might present a more realistic view of this residual risk.

Resective Surgery

Resective operations can be described in groups according to the anatomical area resected and the size of the resection. Certain operations are commoner than others; this may relate to the predilection of certain parts of the brain to specific pathologies and also to the liability of that part of the brain to epilepsy (see Table 1). There is a rough correlation between the clinical material and the susceptibility of cerebral areas to experimental epilepsy, involvement of the temporal areas being common, and that of the occipital lobe being rare. The resective operations will be described in five groups, namely: temporal, frontal, centro-parietal, occipital and major resections including hemispherectomy.

Temporal Lobe Resections

Because the temporal lobe contains a variety of structures, there is a diversity of operations to be described. Historically, temporal lobe surgery has proceeded from the early gyrectomies or topectomies, through more extensive lobectomies to include the deep structures, including 'en bloc' lobectomy to preserve the pathology and recent modifications to improve the result.

Currently there are three options for temporal lobe resection: neocortical removal with preservation of the deep structures, removal of both neocortical and deep structures, and removal of the deep structures alone or virtually so as in selective amygdalo-hippocampectomy.

Neocortical removal only This is currently practised by only a minority of surgeons. The earliest operations, based upon corticographic findings, were of this nature. The first case operated upon by Bailey was a success (Bailey, 1954) but this was not consistent and later it was seen that seizure relief was poor (Bailey, 1961). This technique has been revived by Coughlan and co-workers in Dublin, who use a standard block removal of temporal neocortex. Among 24 patients followed for at least 2 years after operation, 54% are fit-free and 33% improved. There are no details of morbidity or mortality but they are likely to be low. Effects on cognitive function are not given (Coughlan et al., 1987).

Removal of neocortical and deep structures These are the most frequently reported procedures and are subject to variation and modification in various centres. In most centres the surgeon removes, in an adult, between 4.5 cm and 6.5 cm of temporal neocortex as measured from the pole. An equivalent portion, usually 2–3 cm of hippocampus and a part of the amygdala, is removed either 'en bloc' (Falconer, 1971) or separately. Different operators have different ways of dealing with dominant and non-dominant resections; a good description is given by Olivier (Olivier, 1987).

There are two important variations. The first attempts to overcome the verbal memory deficit which may follow left temporal lobectomy. The neocortical removal is restricted to preserve the relevant verbal memory area after mapping it under local anaesthesia (Ojemann and Dodrill, 1985). The deep structures are also removed. Unfortunately, the effect of the restriction of the neocortical removal on the relief of epilepsy is not known.

The second variation has been introduced because, with some pathologies, especially hippocampal sclerosis, the extent of hippocampal involvement may vary. Where the pathology extends to the posterior margin of the hippocampal resection, the outcome of surgery may be poor (Babb and Jann-Brown, 1987). In those patients where chronic depth recordings have shown spikes in the midposterior hippocampus, the Yale group have restricted the neocortical removal to 4.5 cm from the pole. Having thus gained access to the temporal horn, the

Surgical Treatment

hippocampal removal is extended with good results and no extra complications (Spencer et al., 1984).

Seizure control is improved by these operations. The position up to 1973 was summarized by Jensen (1975a). Reports of 2282 cases of anterior temporal lobectomy from the literature were analysed and 885 cases had been adequately investigated and followed; the majority of these were from the Montreal Neurological Institute. Overall, 43.6% of these patients were free of seizures (range 29–62%) and the unimproved patients, those with less than a 75% reduction in their seizure frequency, averaged 33.8% (range 14–58%). Where several consecutive series were quoted from the same centre, there was always an improvement in the seizure relief in the later series. Engel (1987b) analysed data provided by participants in an international symposium on the surgical treatment of epilepsy. There were 2336 lobectomies, reported from 40 centres, and 55.5% of the patients were fit-free (range 26–80%) and 16.8% (range 6–29%) were unimproved. Perhaps these results are not surprising in view of the diverse methods of selection and the periods of time over which these patients were treated. The variation could be attributed to differences in the population presented to each surgeon and in the pathology in the resected specimens. The improvements in neurophysiological assessment and brain imaging must be responsible for some of the improvement seen when compared with Jensen's figures. The most plentiful data about the durability of resective surgery relates to temporal lobe resections.

It is the common experience that the longer the patients are followed up after operation, the fewer remain absolutely fit-free. Whether this represents a total failure of the operative treatment is a matter of philosophy. Patients who obtain significant relief from operation, say a greater than 75% reduction in their seizure frequency, seldom relapse to their preoperative seizure frequency. Among 90 consecutive lobectomies at the Maudsley Hospital, only one patient reverted to the preoperative seizure frequency after a substantial period of relief. Fits can recur after a seizure-free period of many years. Thirteen patients among these 90 had recurrent seizures after periods of freedom ranging from 2 to 10 years. In eleven patients the fits were generalized seizures, which in six of them were completely abolished by a restitution of one anticonvulsant drug. In this group of 90 patients there were 16% who failed to benefit from the operation and this was clear by the end of the first postoperative year. In Van Buren's series, if a patient had remained seizure-free for 5 years their chance of relapsing thereafter was about 10% (Van Buren et al., 1975). Similar data are available for 106 patients undergoing temporal lobectomy at UCLA (Engel, 1987b). They note, as we have, that in any particular year after operation, say the third year, up to 40% of patients may be fit-free but that these are not the same patients who will constitute the 40% who are fit-free the following or previous year. This has to be partly an artificial effect of grouping patients together and could perhaps be overcome by using actuarial methods of analysis.

The perioperative mortality from temporal lobe resection is low. In Jensen's review (Jensen, 1975a) the overall mortality was 1.1%; it has fallen to 0.39% (Van Buren, 1987) with no mortality in more recent series. The late mortality is another matter. Taylor and Marsh (1977) looked at the deaths in Murray Falconer's series; there were 37 deaths in 193 patients who were followed for at least 5 years. Twenty-three of these deaths occurred in circumstances which might be related to either epilepsy or suicide. The suicides tended to occur a decade earlier than the expected peak for suicide, and half the patients who died by suicide were fit-free. Jensen found a late mortality of 4.76%, two-thirds of whom died of suicide or in an epileptic attack (Jensen, 1975b). Although the death rate in these patients (47.6 out of 1000) is in excess of that expected for a similar Danish population (2.9 out of 1000), it is better than that quoted for a representative group of Danish epileptics (59.4 out of 1000) (Brink-Henriksen, Juul-Jensen and Lund, 1970).

The morbidity is equally low. Jensen (1975a) gives a rate of 1% for permanent hemiparesis, and the more recent figures (Van Buren, 1987) are about the same. It seems more likely with 'en bloc' resections. Other hazards such as a transient third nerve palsy and a complete homonymous hemianopia are equally rare. In all series the majority of patients have an upper quadrant-anopia. Focal fits in the immediate postoperative period are also uncommon and have no influence on the eventual outcome of operation.

The intellectual sequelae of temporal lobectomy are complex and important. They depend upon the pathology in the resected temporal lobe and the age of onset of the illness. Blakemore and Falconer (1967) described an auditory learning deficit after dominant temporal lobectomy, and other workers also began to describe material-specific deficits. The whole topic has been well reviewed by Milner (1975). A more recent investigation (Powell, Polkey and McMillan, 1985) has shown that changes in cognitive function across the operation are small. Whereas the intellectually more able and older patients, whose epilepsy tends to be of later onset, acquire material-specific deficits, the opposite group, in whom the pathology tends to be some form of hippocampal sclerosis, do not. This is thought to be because the insult occurs at an age when they still have some ability to reorganize cognitive function. Improvement in cognitive function after operation is also related to improvement in seizure control (Novelly et al., 1984).

Behavioural changes after temporal lobectomy are well documented and fall into two groups.

The first group consists of those patients with uncontrolled partial seizures who have an aggressive behaviour disorder; the proportion varies from series to series. In Falconer's series, few of the patients were of normal personalilty and behaviour and only 13% were normal before operation but 32% were normal afterwards (Taylor and Falconer, 1968). In another review of 100 patients, there were 27 who had troublesome aggressive behaviour before operation, 10 of whom improved (Falconer, 1973). Jensen (1976) reports 74 patients who were socially disadvantaged prior to operation, but 39% were in full-time employment afterwards. The effects of uncontrolled epilepsy on the behaviour and development of children and the beneficial results of surgery have been reviewed in a careful longitudinal study by the Oxford group (Ounstead, Lindsay and Richards, 1987).

The second group consists of patients who either have a recognizable psychosis before operation or acquire one afterwards. Psychosis supervening upon chronic epilepsy, usually a schizophreniform psychosis, occurs late in the illness. Serafetidines and Falconer (1962) described twelve such patients, in all of whom temporal lobectomy had no effect on the psychosis, as has been reported by others (Jensen and Larsen, 1979).

Operation can also produce psychoses, both a schizophreniform psychosis usually associated with left-sided lobectomy, and a depressive psychosis usually associated with right-sided lobectomy. Jensen and Larsen (1979) report the development of psychosis in 12% of their patients, and Taylor (1975) the appearance of a schizophreniform psychosis in 15% of Falconer's series. He also noted that this was more likely to be associated with 'alien tissue' pathology. The same investigators report depressive psychoses which may be resistant to treatment and lead to suicide. All of these aspects have been reviewed in detail by Taylor (1987).

Removal of deep structures alone   Niemeyer (1958) described a transventricular approach to enable removal of the deep structures alone. This selective amygdalo-hippocampectomy has been revived. The indications suggested by the Zurich group are a unilateral medio-basal focus demonstrated by foramen ovale telemetering or by chronic SEEG studies, or a structural lesion in or adjacent to the hippocampus or amygdala (Wieser, 1986). In addition, Olivier (1987) notes that this operation may be used in patients where there is significant memory on the side of operation.

There are two methods of performing this operation. Yasargil describes a microsurgical approach through the insular cortex after splitting the Sylvian fissure, and this is more difficult than the method described by Olivier, where a similar removal is made through an incision in the middle temporal gyrus about 1.5 cm from the temporal pole.

Wieser reports 80% seizure relief with selective amygdalo-hippocampectomy. This is a reflection of the high proportion of patients with benign tumours in their series, and in patients with mesial temporal sclerosis the seizure relief rate is 61%, which compares favourably with 'en bloc' lobectomy.

The Zurich series is virtually free of morbidity; this is not so in less skilled hands, but it is to be expected that the morbidity, with practice, will be similar to that for formal lobectomy. These patients do not have the quadrantanopia which is inevitable with lobectomy.

The intellectual consequences of the operation seem much less than those of formal lobectomy, even in cases with more risk of amnesia. Wieser, analysing in detail the effects on cognitive function in seventeen patients, found only one to have deteriorated, and we have had the same experience in a smaller series of fourteen patients. Wieser describes a beneficial effect on patients whose epilepsy is relieved, as we have also found.

The pathology in the specimens from temporal lobe resections determine the outcome, to some extent independently of the operative procedure. In both 'en bloc' resection and selective amygdalo-hippocampectomy, benign lesions such as indolent tumours have an 80% seizure relief rate, mesial temporal sclerosis (MTS) about 60% and non-specific pathology about 15%.

Frontal Lobe Resections

There are a number of well-recognized patterns for seizures originating in the frontal lobe, such as adversive attacks or supplementary motor area-type seizures. Nevertheless, the recognition of frontal lobe seizures may be difficult and they can take very bizarre forms (Williamson et al., 1985). Depth electrode studies have shown that the adversive movements of the head and eyes are a poor lateralizing feature (Robillard et al., 1983). When the causative lesion lies on the medial side of the hemisphere there may be no abnormality in scalp EEG recordings even when a fit occurs. The range of pathology encountered in frontal lobe resections is different from that seen in temporal lobes. Rasmussen (1975a), reporting 346 frontal resections over 45 years, notes that 97 (28%) had tumours, 5 (1.4%) arteriovenous malformations (AVMs) and 167 (48%) scarring, often caused by head trauma. When there is a clear abnormality, the size and position of the resection can be guided by that abnormality with corticographic control. The resection may be limited by corticographic findings or by the practical size of a frontal lobe resection, which should leave one gyrus anterior to the pre-central gyrus, and respect Broca's area in the dominant hemisphere.

The results of frontal resection are satisfactory. The largest series from the Montreal Neurological Institute reports 212 patients followed for 2–39 years. There were 22 patients (10%) who had been absolutely seizure-free, and a total of 76 patients had suffered less than one seizure per year of follow-up (35%), with a further 42 patients experiencing a significant reduction of seizures, so that a total of 118 patients (55%) had benefited from the surgery. There has been no mortality in the last 160 operations and no morbidity. There are minor intellectual sequelae to frontal lobe resections.

Centro-parietal and Occipital Resections

The number of patients submitted to surgery in the centro-parietal regions is low, because this is an eloquent area, and in the occipital area because focal epilepsy rarely affects this area. The focal motor and focal sensory seizures which emanate from the central and parietal areas are easy to identify. Occipital seizures may begin with visual auras. Again the Montreal Neurological Institute has the only substantial series of resections from these areas. Goldring (1987) reported cortical resections from the central areas after assessment of the seizure origin and identification of motor and sensory cortex using epidural mat electrodes. Rasmussen (1975b) reported 68 patients undergoing central resections in 40 years. Eighteen per cent were rendered absolutely fit-free, 45% were down to less than one fit per year of follow-up, and overall 59% were significantly improved. In parietal resections, of which there were 132 cases, the results were almost identical. Goldring reports the results of extra-temporal resections in 40 patients; 18 (45%) became fit-free, and a further 8 obtained a significant improvement, giving an overall success rate of 65%. In a number of these cases, unsuspected indolent gliomas were found. In Rasmussen's material, 266 patients underwent central or parietal resections; 103 patients had tumours (38.7%) and 110 (41.3%) some other pathology, leaving 45 (20%) with no specific pathology. Rasmussen describes 23 patients undergoing occipital resections and notes that 68% achieved a significant reduction in their epilepsy.

Resection in these areas has to be tailored, often by operation under local anaesthesia, to avoid worsening a pre-existing deficit or introducing one. In occipital operations there may be a high risk of producing a homonymous hemianopia.

Major Resections

Where the insult is large it may still be possible to resect up to one-third or half of the hemisphere, but the surgery and its complications are similar to those of more restricted operations. However, sometimes the insult or disease process is so widespread that resection of 80% or more of the hemisphere is needed. This major procedure, known as hemispherectomy, was first described by Krynauw (1950). Applied to patients with an infantile hemiplegia and drug-resistant seizures, who often had a behaviour disorder and were dementing, it was very successful, with an 80% seizure relief and an improvement in the behaviour. This was soon confirmed by others (Wilson, 1970). Within 10 years or so it became clear from numerous reports (Falconer and Wilson, 1969) that there was a serious morbidity and mortality in between one-third and one-quarter of patients from late complications associated with chronic or delayed bleeding. In Montreal it was noticed that such complications occurred in 35% of patients undergoing anatomically complete hemispherectomy but was virtually absent after lesser resections. They therefore modified their practice twice. Between 1968 and 1974 they carried out only subtotal hemispherectomies, sparing the least epileptogenic area, usually either the frontal or occipital pole. This reduced the late complications but also reduced the seizure relief, so that whereas 80% of patients were virtually fit-free after complete hemispherectomy, only 69% were so relieved by subtotal hemispherectomy. Since 1974 they have carried out a functionally complete hemispherectomy in which the central and temporal areas, including the deep temporal structures, are removed and the corpus callosum divided in the frontal and parietal regions. They have 80% of patients seizure-free and only one late delayed complication in fourteen cases followed for between 2 and 10 years (Rasmussen, 1987).

Adams (1983) modified the classical hemispherectomy technique to avoid the late complications. In a recent report he noted the freedom from late complications in ten patients operated upon using this technique (Beardsworth and Adams, 1988). There was total seizure relief in 70% of these patients, with improvement in behaviour and in some intellectual function similar to the results reported for classical hemispherectomy (Wilson, 1970).

Mention should be made at this point of the clinically distinct, but ill-understood, disease called 'Rasmussen's encephalitis'. It is characterized by the onset of unilateral focal motor seizures, usually in childhood or occasionally in adolescence, followed by a progressive hemiparesis within 2-4 years. The disease usually progresses rapidly but occasionally halts. In advanced cases there is a good response to hemispherectomy (Rasmussen, 1978).

Functional Surgery

This is less widely practised than resective surgery. There are three options: to make lesions in the appropriate part of the brain using stereotactic techniques to reach the target, various disconnection operations which divide fibre tracts deep in the brain to restrict the spread of epileptic activity, and brain stimulation.

Stereotactic Lesions

These procedures have a long history but only since the development of CT and MRI scanning has it been possible to locate lesions accurately and verify them in the living patient. Pallidal lesions to control seizures were reported by Spiegel as early as 1958 (Spiegel, Wycis and Baird, 1958). Subsequently, various subcortical targets were used, including the fields of Forel, thalamus and globus pallidus. These methods were used to treat the more difficult cases, usually with multiple targets and in small numbers, and tended to control rather than cure the fits. Most reviewers feel that these methods are of limited application (Ojemann and Ward, 1975; Flanigin, King and Gallagher, 1985; Spencer et al., 1987).

Lesions in the temporal structures have been more rewarding, possibly because the patient population is more uniform and it is also easier to compare with resective surgery. Narabayashi et al. (1963) noted that in patients where he was using amygdala lesions to treat aggression, if they also had resistant epilepsy then both tended to respond to the lesion. He described improvement both in children (Narabayashi and Shima, 1973) and in adults (Narabayashi, 1979). It was noted by Mundinger that the best results were seen in patients with unilateral foci (Mundinger et al., 1976). The Paris group noted that only 23% of patients were rendered fit-free by stereotactic lesions and considered that resective surgery was better when it was possible (Talairach et al., 1974). The Danish group reported the results of 45 amygdalotomies. Both bilateral amygdalotomies (18 patients) and unilateral amygdalotomies (27 patients) rendered 18% of these patients fit-free. Eight of the 12 patients who did badly with unilateral amygdalotomies subsequently underwent unilateral temporal lobectomy with a good result (Vaernet, 1972).

Disconnection Procedures

Section of the corpus callosum was first introduced in 1940 (Van Wagenen and Herren, 1940). It fell into disrepute because of the undesirable neuropsychological sequelae until it was subsequently shown that these could be ameliorated if the splenium was spared (Gordon, Bogen and Sperry, 1971). At the same time it was used for patients with unilateral cerebral disease (Luessenhop, Dela-Cruz and Fairchild, 1970). The Dartmouth group described a microsurgical technique which gave better results with fewer complications (Wilson, Reeves and Gazzaniga, 1982). The current indications for the use of callosotomy are complex and empirical. Certain points emerge. First, there is some but not complete desynchronization of the EEG after callosotomy. This can be seen at acute corticography during the operation and perhaps can be used as an indication of when the section is sufficient (Marino, 1985). A complete section is more effective than a partial section and perhaps carries less risk of complications if carried out in stages at least 2 months apart. Patients with known unilateral cerebral pathology do better than those without (Williamson, 1985). Akinetic seizures such as drop attacks do best and partial complex seizures are least affected by the operation. Precise figures are variable between the series but an overall reduction of 50% in seizure frequency occurs in 60% or more of patients (Spencer et al., 1987).

After anterior section there may be a period of mutism, incontinence and variable limb weakness lasting between a few days and weeks; these generally disappear. The neuropsychological sequelae of anterior, posterior and complete section are demonstrable and well documented but are not necessarily of great practical significance. In certain circumstances this is not so, especially after complete section, and patients of mixed dominance should have a carotid amytal test (Spencer et al., 1987).

Brief mention is made of temporal lobotomy, in which the deep white matter of the temporal lobe is divided unilaterally or bilaterally (Turner, 1963). In a recent summary of his work, which is methodologically difficult to understand, it appears that 25–30% of patients were rendered fit-free, but some had lesions in other parts of the brain (Turner, 1982).

The operation of multiple subpial transection described by Morrell should be mentioned (Morrell, Whisler and Bleck, 1989). Accepting the idea that epileptic discharges propagate horizontally whereas the impulses controlling voluntary movement propagate vertically, then if a series of vertical cuts are made in the motor cortex the epilepsy will be controlled and normal function unaffected. In 32 patients there has been no practical neurological deficit, although subtle changes could be detected on formal examination. In 20 patients followed for more than 5 years there has been complete seizure control in 55%. Seizures recurred in some patients with progressive pathology such as Rasmussen's disease but always away from the treated area.

Brain Stimulation

There are currently no effective methods of chronic brain stimulation for control of epilepsy. Cerebellar stimulation introduced by Cooper (1973) has been discredited in controlled trials (Wright, McLellan and Brice, 1985).

Summary

The surgical management of intractable epilepsy is complex and requires a multidisciplinary approach.

Resective surgery is more successful than functional surgery and will virtually cure the epilepsy in a substantial number of cases. The degree of success depends upon the site and nature of the resection and on the pathological lesion.

Functional surgery is less well documented than resective surgery and is applied to more heterogeneous and difficult populations; it has to be seen as controlling rather than curing epilepsy.

Both kinds of surgery have acceptable morbidity and mortality rates.

References

Adams CBT. Hemispherectomy—a modification. J Neurol Neurosurg Psychiatry 1983; 46: 617–19.
Babb TL, Jann-Brown W. Pathological findings in epilepsy. In: Engel J (ed.) Surgical treatment of the epilepsies. New York: Raven Press, 1987: 511–40.
Bailey P. Betrachtungen uber die chirugische Behandlung der psychomotorische Epilepsie. Zentral Neurochir 1954; 14: 195–206.
Bailey P. Surgical treatment of psychomotor epilepsy. Five year follow-up. South Med J 1961; 54: 299–301.

Beardsworth ED, Adams CBT. Modified hemispherectomy for epilepsy: Early results in 10 cases. Br J Neurosurg 1988; 2: 73–84.
Blakemore CB, Falconer MA. Long-term effects of anterior temporal lobectomy on certain cognitive functions. J Neurol Neurosurg Psychiatry 1967; 30: 364–7.
Bonte FJ, Devous MD, Stokely EM, Homan RW. Single photon tomographic determination of regional cerebral blood flow in epilepsy. Arch Neurol 1983; 40: 267–70.
Brink-Henriksen P, Juul-Jensen P, Lund M. The mortality of epileptics. In: Brackenridge RDS (ed.) Life assurance medicine. Proceedings of the 10th International Congress of Life Assurance Medicine. London: Pitman, 1970: 139–48.
Cooper I. Chronic stimulation of the paleo-cerebellum in man. 1973; Lancet i: 206.
Coughlan A, Farrell M, Harriman O, Moore B, Staunton H. Appendix II. Presurgical evaluation protocols. In: Engel J (ed.) Surgical treatment of the epilepsies. New York: Raven Press, 1987: 689.
Elwes RDC, Johnson AL, Shorvon SD, Reynolds EH. The prognosis for seizure control in newly diagnosed epilepsy. N Engl J Med 1984; 311: 944–7.
Engel J. Approaches to the localisation of the epileptogenic lesion. In: Engel J (ed.) Surgical treatment of the epilepsies. New York: Raven Press, 1987a: 75–100.
Engel J. Outcome with respect to epileptic seizures. In: Engel J (ed.) Surgical treatment of the epilepsies. New York, Raven Press, 1987b: 553–71.
Engel J, Jann-Brown W, Kuhl DE, Phelps ME, Maziotta JC, Crandall PH. Pathological findings underlying focal temporal lobe hypometabolism in partial epilepsy. Ann Neurol 1982; 12: 518–28.
Falconer MA. Anterior temporal lobectomy for epilepsy. In: Logue V (ed.) Operative surgery. vol. 14. Neurosurgery. London, Butterworths, 1971: 142–9.
Falconer MA. Reversibility by temporal lobe resection of the behavioural abnormalities of temporal lobe epilepsy. N Engl J Med 1973; 289: 451–5.
Falconer MA, Kennedy WA. Epilepsy due to small focal temporal lesions with bilateral independent spike-discharging foci. A study of seven cases relieved by operation. J Neurol, Neurosurg Psychiatry 1961; 24: 205–12.
Falconer MA, Wilson PJE. Complications related to delayed haemorrhage after hemispherectomy. J Neurosurg 1969; 30: 413–26.
Flanigin H, King D, Gallagher B. Surgical treatment of epilepsy. In: Pedley TA, Meldrum BS (eds) Recent advances in epilepsy. No 2. Edinburgh; Churchill-Livingstone, 1985: 515–59.
Flanigin HF, Smith JR. Depth electrode implantation at the Medical College of Georgia. In: Engel J (ed.) Surgical treatment of the epilepsies. New York, Raven Press, 1987: 609–12.
Goddard GV. Development of epileptic seizures through brain stimulation at low intensity. Nature 1967; 214: 1020–1.
Goldring S. Surgical management of epilepsy in children. In: Engel J (ed.) New York: Raven Press, 1987: 445–64.
Goldring S, Gregorie EM. Surgical management of epilepsy using epidural mats to localise the seizure focus. Review of 100 cases. J Neurosurg 1984; 60: 457–66.
Gordon HW, Bogen JE, Sperry RW. Absence of deconnexion syndrome in two patients with partial section of the neocommissure. Brain 1971; 94: 327–36.
Gupta PC, Dharampaul SN, Singh B. Secondary epileptogenic EEG focus in temporal lobe epilepsy. Epilepsia 1973; 14: 423–6.
Hahn JF, Luders H. Placement of subdural grid electrodes at the Cleveland Clinic. In: Engel J (ed.) Surgical treatment of the epilepsies. New York: Raven Press, 1987: 621–7.
Hood TW, Siegfried J, Wieser HG. The role of stereotactic amygdalotomy in the treatment of temporal lobe epilepsy associated with behavioral disorders. Appl Neurophysiol 1983; 46: 19–25.

Hughes JR, Schlagendorf RE. Electro-clinical correlation in temporal lobe epilepsy with emphasis on inter-areal analysis of the temporal lobe. Electroencephalogr Clin Neurophysiol 1961; 13: 333–9.

Jack CR, Nichols DA, Sharbrough FW, Marsh WR, Petersen RC. Selective posterior cerebral amytal test for evaluating memory function before surgery for temporal lobe seizure. Radiology 1988; 168: 787–93.

Jensen I. Temporal lobe surgery around the world. Results, complications, mortality. Acta Neurol Scand 1975a; 52: 354–73.

Jensen I. Temporal lobe epilepsy. Late mortality in patients treated with unilateral temporal lobe resections. Acta Neurol Scand 1975b; 52: 374–80.

Jensen I. Temporal lobe epilepsy: Social conditions and rehabilitation after surgery. Acta Neurol Scand 1976; 54: 22–44.

Jensen I, Larsen JK. Mental aspects of temporal lobe epilepsy. Follow-up of 74 patients after resection of a temporal lobe. J Neurol, Neurosurg Psychiatry 1979; 42: 256–65.

Kendall B. Neuroradiology. In: Laidlaw J, Richens A, Oxley J (eds) A textbook of epilepsy. Edinburgh: Churchill-Livingstone, 1988: 307–49.

Krynauw RA. Infantile hemiplegia treated by removing one cerebral hemisphere. J Neurol, Neurosurg Psychiatry 1950; 13: 243–67.

Luessenhop AJ, Dela-Cruz TC, Fairchild DM. Surgical disconnection of the cerebral hemispheres for intractable seizures. Results in infancy and childhood. JAMA 1970; 213: 1630–6.

Marino R. Surgery for epilepsy. Selective partial microsurgical callosotomy for intractable multiform seizures: Criteria for clinical selection and results. Appl Neurophysiol 1985; 48: 404–7.

McLachan RS, Nicholson RL, Black S, Carr T, Blume W. Nuclear magnetic resonance imaging, a new approach to the investigation of refractory temporal lobe epilepsy. Epilepsia 1985; 26: 555–62.

Meencke HJ, Schorner W, Janz D. Magnetic resonance tomography studies in patients with temporal lobe epilepsy. In: Wolf P, Dam M, Janz D, Dreifuss FE (eds) Advances in epileptology. vol 16. New York: Raven Press, 1987: 279–82.

Milner B. Psychological aspects of focal epilepsy and its management. Adv Neurol 1975; 8: 299–314.

Morrell F. Secondary epileptogenic lesions. Epilepsia, 1960; 1: 538–60.

Morrell F. Cellular pathophysiology of focal epilepsy. In: Niedermeyer E (ed.) Modern problems in pharmacopsychiatry. vol. 4. Epilepsy. Basel: Karger, 1970: 1–12.

Morrell F, Wada J, Engel J. Appendix III. Potential relevance of kindling and secondary epileptogenesis to the consideration of surgical treatment of epilepsy. In: Engel J (ed.) Surgical treatment of the epilepsies. New York: Raven Press, 1987: 701–7.

Morrell F, Whisler WW, Bleck TP. Multiple subpial transection: A new approach to the surgical treatment of focal epilepsy. J Neurosurg 1989; 70: 231–9.

Mundinger F, Becker P, Grolkner E, Bachschmid G. Late results of stereotactic surgery of epilepsy, predominantly temporal lobe type. Acta Neurochir 1976; suppl. 23: 177–82.

Narabayashi H. Long range results of medial amygdalotomy on epileptic traits in adult patients. In: Rasmussen T, Marino R (eds) Functional neurosurgery. New York: Raven Press, 1979: 243–52.

Narabayashi H, Shima F. Which is the better amygdalar target, the medial or lateral nuclei? (For behaviour problems and paroxysm in epileptics.) In: Laitinen LV, Livingstone KE (eds) Surgical approaches in psychiatry. Lancaster, UK: MTP, 1973: 129–34.

Narabayashi H, Nagao T, Sato Y, Yoshida M, Nagahato M. Stereotactic amygdalotomy for behaviour disorder. Arch Neurol 1963; 9: 1–16.

Niemeyer P. The transventricular amygdalo-hippocampectomy in temporal lobe epilepsy. In: Baldwin M, Bailey P (eds), Temporal lobe epilepsy. Springfield, Illinois: Charles C. Thomas, 1958: 461–82.
Novelly RA, Augustine EM, Mattson RH, Glaser GH, Williamson PD, Spencer DD, Spencer SS. Selective memory improvement and impairment in temporal lobectomy for epilepsy. Ann Neurol 1984; 15: 64–7.
Ojemann GA, Dodrill CB. Verbal memory deficits after left temporal lobectomy for epilepsy: Mechanism and intraoperative prediction. J Neurosurg 1985; 62: 101–7.
Ojemann GA, Ward AA. Stereotactic and other procedures for epilepsy. In: Purpura DP, Penry JK, Walter RD (eds) Neurosurgical management of the epilepsies. New York: Raven Press, 1975: 241–63.
Olivier A. Commentary: Cortical resections. In: Engel J (ed.) Surgical treatment of the epilepsies. New York: Raven Press, 1987: 405–16.
Olivier A, Marchand E, Peters T, Tyler J. Depth electrode implantation at the Montreal Neurological Institute and Hospital. In: Engel J (ed.) Surgical treatment of the epilepsies. New York: Raven Press, 1987: 595–601.
Ounstead C, Lindsay J, Richards P. Developmental aspects of focal epilepsies of childhood treated by neurosurgery. In: Temporal lobe epilepsy. A Biographical Study 1948–1986. Oxford: Blackwell Scientific Publications Ltd, 1987: 70–86.
Powell GE, Polkey CE, Canavan AGM. Lateralisation of memory function in epileptic patients by use of the sodium amytal (WADA) technique. J Neurol Neurosurg Psychiatry 1987; 50: 665–72.
Powell GE, Polkey CE, McMillan TM. The new Maudsley series of temporal lobectomy I: Short term cognitive effects. Br J Clin Psychol 1985; 24: 109–24.
Rasmussen T. Surgery of frontal lobe epilepsy. Adv Neurol 1975a; 8: 197–205.
Rasmussen T. Surgery for epilepsy arising in regions other than the temporal or frontal lobes. Adv Neurol 1975b; 8: 207–26.
Rasmussen T. Further observations on the syndrome of chronic encephalitis with epilepsy. Appl Neurophysiol 1978; 41: 1–12.
Rasmussen T. Cortical resection for multilobe epileptogenic lesions. In: Wieser HG, Elger CE (eds) Presurgical evaluation of epileptics. Berlin: Springer-Verlag, 1987: 344–51.
Robillard A, Saint Hilaire JM, Mercier M, Bouvier G. The localising and lateralising value of adversion in epileptic seizures. Neurology 1987; 33: 1421–2.
Scoville WB, Milner B. Loss of recent memory after bilateral hippocampal lesions. J Neurol, Neurosurg Psychiatry 1957; 20: 11–21.
Serafetidines EA, Falconer MA. The effects of temporal lobectomy in epileptic patients with psychosis. J Ment Sci 1962; 108: 584–93.
Spencer DD. Postscript: Should there be a surgical treatment of choice and if so how should it be determined? In: Engel J (ed.) Surgical treatment of the epilepsies. New York: Raven Press, 1987; 477–84.
Spencer DD, Spencer SS, Mattson RH, Williamson PD, Novelly RA. Access to the posterior medial temporal lobe structures in the surgical treatment of epilepsy. Neurosurgery 1984; 15: 667–71.
Spencer SS. Depth electroencephalography in selection of refractory epilepsy for surgery. Ann Neurol 1981; 9: 207–14.
Spencer SS, Gates JR, Reeves AR, Spencer DD, Maxwell RE, Roberts D. Corpus callosum section. In: Engel J (ed.) Surgical treatment of the epilepsies. New York: Raven Press, 1987: 425–44.
Sperling MR, Wilson G, Engel J, Babb TL, Phelps M, Bradley W. Magnetic resonance imaging in intractable partial epilepsy: Correlative studies. Ann Neurol 1986; 20: 57–62.

Spiegel EA, Wycis HT, Baird MW. Long-range effects of electropallido-ansotomy in extra-pyramidal and convulsive disorders. Neurology 1958; 8: 734–40.

Talairach J, Bancaud J, Szilka G, Bonis A, Geier S, Vedrenne C. Approche nouvelle de la neurochirugie de l'epilepsie. Methodologie stereotaxique et resultats therapeutiques. Neurochirugie 1974; suppl. 2:

Taylor DC. Factors influencing the occurrence of schizophrenia-like psychosis in patients with temporal lobe epilepsy. Psychol Med 1975; 5: 249–54.

Taylor DC. Psychiatric and social issues in measuring the input and outcome of epilepsy surgery. In: Engel J (ed.) Surgical treatment of the epilepsies. New York: Raven Press, 1987: 485–503.

Taylor DC, Falconer MA. Clinical, socio-economic and psychological changes after temporal lobectomy for epilepsy. Br J Psychiatry, 1968; 114: 1247–61.

Taylor DC, Marsh SM. Implications of long-term follow-up studies in epilepsy: With a note on the cause of death. In: Penry JK (ed.) Epilepsy, the Eighth International Symposium. New York: Raven Press, 1977: 27–34.

Turner EA. A new approach to unilateral and bilateral lobotomies for psychomotor epilepsy. J Neurol, Neurosurg Psychiatry 1963; 26: 285–99.

Turner EA. Temporal lobe operations. In: Surgery of the mind. Birmingham, UK: Carver Press, 1982: 126–69.

Vaernat K. Stereotactic amygdalotomy in temporal lobe epilepsy. Confin Neurol 1972; 34: 176–80.

Van Buren JM. Complications of surgical procedures in the diagnosis and treatment of epilepsy. In: Engel J (ed.) Surgical treatment of the epilepsies. New York: Raven Press, 1987: 465–75.

Van Buren JM, Ajmone-Marsan C, Mutsage N, Sadowsky D. Surgery of temporal lobe epilepsy. Adv Neurol 1975; 8: 155–96.

Van Wagenen WP, Herren RY. Surgical division of commissural pathways in the corpus callosum. Arch Neurol Psychiatry 1940; 44: 740–59.

Wada J. A new method for the determination of the side of cerebral speech dominance. A preliminary report on the intra-carotid injection of sodium amytal in man. Med Biol 1949; 14: 221–2.

Wada J. Secondary cerebral functional alteration examined in the kindling model of epilepsy. In: Mayersdorf A, Schmidt RP (eds) Secondary epileptogenesis. New York: Raven Press, 1982; 45–87.

Wieser HG. Selective amygdalo-hippocampectomy: indications, investigative technique and results. In: Symon L (ed.) Advances and technical standards in neurosurgery. vol. 13. Wien: Springer-Verlag, 1986: 39–133.

Wieser HG, Elger CE, Stodieck SRG. The 'foramen ovale electrode'; a new recording method for the preoperative evaluation of patients suffering from mediobasal temporal lobe epilepsy. Electroencephalogr Clin Neurophysiol 1985; 61: 314–22.

Wieser HG, Yasargil MG. Die 'selektiv Amygdalo-Hippokampektomie' als chirurgische Behandlungsmethode der mediobasal-limbischen Epilepsie. Neurochirugia 1982; 25: 39–50.

Wilder BJ, King RL, Schmidt RP. Comparative study of secondary epileptogenesis. Epilepsia 1968; 9: 275–89.

Williamson PD. Corpus callosum section for intractable epilepsy: Criteria for patient selection. In: Reeves AG (ed.) Epilepsy and the corpus callosum. New York: Plenum Press, 1985: 243–57.

Williamson PD, Spencer DD, Spencer SS, Novelly RA, Mattson RH. Complex partial seizures of frontal origin. Ann Neurol 1985; 18: 497–504.

Wilson DH, Reeves AG, Gazzaniga M. 'Central' commissurotomy for intractable generalised epilepsy: Series two. Neurology 1982; 32: 687–97.

Wilson PJE. Cerebral hemispherectomy for infantile hemiplegia: A report of 50 cases. Brain 1970; 93: 147–80.
Wright GDS, McLellan DL, Brice JG. A double-blind trial of chronic cerebellar stimulation in twelve patients with severe epilepsy. J Neurol, Neurosurg Psychiatry 1985; 47: 769–74.
Wyler AR, Bolender NF. Preoperative CT diagnosis of mesial temporal sclerosis for the surgical treatment of epilepsy. Ann Neurol 1983; 13: 59–64.
Yasargil MG, Teddy PG, Roth P. Selective amygdalo-hippocampectomy. Operative anatomy and surgical technique. In: Symon L (ed.) Advances and technical standards in neurosurgery. vol. 12. Wien: Springer-Verlag, 1985: 93–123.

17
Epilepsy in Developing Countries: A Review of Epidemiological, Sociocultural, and Treatment Aspects*

S. D. Shorvon and P. J. Farmer
Institute of Neurology and National Society for Epilepsy Research Group, London, UK

Epilepsy respects no national or racial boundaries; it is found in all populations that have been surveyed around the world, and whilst many of its characteristics are universal, there are specific features of epilepsy in developing countries that are worthy of separate consideration. Most of what is accepted dogma about clinical aspects of epilepsy derives from studies in the developed world, and extrapolation to Third World practice may be often inappropriate—and yet is the general rule. This is all the more likely to occur since hard data from the developing world are sparse and what do exist may be sometimes of doubtful authenticity or originality. Sophisticated cross-cultural clinical research in epilepsy or neurology is in its infancy (far behind that in psychiatry, for instance), and this is an important deficiency. In this chapter, we will discuss four broad areas in which differences do occur and in which findings from investigations in developing countries may be surprising to those whose perspective is wholly oriented to the First World. Such an account is inevitably incomplete and impressionistic: first, because of the lack of comprehensive data from countries in which research does not have a high medical priority, and second, because of the inaccuracy inherent in making generalizations about the enormously diverse countries that constitute the great majority of the world population. The areas to be covered are the epidemiological studies of

---

* This chapter was previously published in Epilepsia 1988; 29, suppl I: S36–S53, and is reproduced by permission of Raven Press, New York.

Chronic Epilepsy, Its Prognosis and Management
Edited by M.R. Trimble. 1989 Published by John Wiley & Sons Ltd

incidence and prevalence, studies of the characteristics of epilepsy in general populations, social or anthropological aspects, and finally the treatment of epilepsy.

This account will be illustrated by some preliminary observations from studies currently in progress in Ecuador, Kenya and Pakistan, with which the authors are associated (see Ellison et al., 1989). There are two particular features of these studies that should be emphasized. First, efforts have been made to identify as random a sample of the population as possible (in two studies by a house-to-house survey), since the problems of extrapolation from clinic-based to population-based studies, so evident in studies in the First World, are even greater in developing countries. Second, in these projects, the social, cultural and psychological aspects of epilepsy are being considered in relation to the epidemiological and treatment features. It is strongly our view that it is only with this perspective that the practical issues important for the control of epilepsy in Third World countries can be fully understood. In these ways, these studies differ from many of the epidemiological and clinical studies reported previously.

Incidence and Prevalence Rates of Epilepsy

Methodological Difficulties in Studies in Developing Countries

Incidence is the number of *new cases* of a given disease occurring in a unit time within a specified population, and prevalence is the proportion of the population *with a given disease* at a specified time. With all chronic diseases, the number of patients accumulates with time and so prevalence rates tend to be high in spite of low incidence rates; thus, meaningful studies of prevalence can be made on smaller populations than are necessary for incidence studies. Moreover, studies of incidence are usually only satisfactorily performed in prospective longitudinal investigations, whereas prevalence can be studied in a cross-sectional survey. For both these reasons, there are many more studies of prevalence of epilepsy than of incidence in developing countries. Another useful measure is the cumulative incidence rate, which is the cumulation of age-specific incidence rates adjusted to fit the age range of a population, and is a measure of the numbers in a population who have *ever developed* the condition at any point in their lives. In a truly chronic condition that never recovers, and assuming that incidence rates are constant over years, cumulative incidence rates should approximate to prevalence rates—the difference being largely explained by differential death rates between the cases and the general population. There have been a small number of studies of cumulative incidence in epilepsy but none in developing countries. Incidence and prevalence studies in epilepsy in developing countries have particular methodological difficulties (Sander and Shorvon, 1987). We will discuss these in some detail herein, as their recognition is important in assessing the findings and conclusions of the published literature.

Table 1. Screening questions for epilepsy used in the WHO screening questionnaire for neurological diseases

a. For subjects of 7 years of age and older:
   1. Have you ever lost consciousness?
   2. Have you ever had episodes where you lost contact with your surroundings?
   3. Have you ever had any shaking of your arms and legs which you could not control?
b. For children under 7 years of age:
   1. Has this child ever lost consciousness?
   2. Does this child have episodes characterized by vagueness and unawareness of surroundings?
   3. Have you ever seen this child shaking and unable to control the arms and legs?

Questionnaire of 15 or 16 questions, screening for neurological diseases in epidemiological surveys.

Case ascertainment poses important problems in all comprehensive epidemiological studies in developing countries. In developed countries, the most common published method of case ascertainment is a review of medical records. These have covered total populations or selected groups, and are usually supplemented by an interview of positively identified cases. There are a number of sources of inaccuracy (see Sander and Shorvon, 1987) and under-reporting is common. In developing countries, however, where medical records are much less complete, this approach will usually grossly underestimate the numbers of epileptics (Stanhope, Brody and Brink, 1972), and should not normally be used in a comprehensive survey. A more useful method is to apply a screening questionnaire in a community or selected population, and then to examine persons giving a positive response to the screen (Lessell, Torres and Kurland, 1962; Mathai et al., 1968; Dada, 1970a; Gomez, Arciniegas and Torres, 1978; Chiofalo et al., 1979; Osuntokun et al., 1982, 1987; Proano, 1984; Li et al., 1985; Marino, Cukiert and Pinho, 1987). An accurate definition of the population at risk (the sample frame) is mandatory, and where census data are not available this may be difficult. Such surveys depend on both the *sensitivity* and *specificity* of the screening questionnaires. These need careful design and should be piloted in known populations; in epilepsy studies, these points are frequently neglected, and some published questionnaires show great naïveté. The screening questionnaires are invariably administered by non-medical personnel, sometimes with inadequate training, which can also compound these difficulties. In Table 1 are shown the three questions relevant to epilepsy in the questionnaire used by the WHO for neurological diseases, and whether this is really a satisfactory screen for epilepsy is surely debatable.

A more detailed screening questionnaire, involving 20 questions, is in use in current studies in Ecuador, with greater accuracy and precision. It is inevitably the case, however, that the more sensitive a questionnaire is, the generally less specific it is, and in order to achieve high sensitivity (i.e. to pick up all cases), a large number of false-positive possible cases will be identified which have to be examined and subsequently rejected. This requires considerable resources and logistic expertise, and may need governmental or commercial support. In any large field study, the use of an existing infrastructure (e.g. personnel, transport, communications) may greatly alleviate logistical difficulties, and the best example of this is the Ecuadorian study, with the collaboration of the governmental (Ministry of Health), professional (Society of Ecuadorian Neurologists and Institute of Neurology, London), and commercial (Ciba-Geigy) organizations (see Ellison et al., 1989).

A major problem in studies using inadequate screening instruments is that cases with partial seizures or mild or inactive epilepsy are often overlooked. Patients may have ignored or misinterpreted the symptoms or indeed have been unaware of them, and this is particularly likely with absence seizures or brief partial seizures (Zielinski, 1974). Sometimes, the condition may be denied or concealed. That concealment is a common problem is shown from a field study in Warsaw (Zielinski, 1974), in which patients known from medical files to have had seizures refused to answer a questionnaire more often than the rest of the population (8% versus 1.4%), and by the finding of Beran et al. (1985) that approximately 1 in 4 people proven to have epilepsy denied this fact when sampled by a postal questionnaire.

In studies of rural populations, it is important to have some understanding of the patient's concepts of and beliefs about epilepsy. In Indonesia, for instance, the question 'Do you suffer from convulsions?' is almost always answered in the negative, but if the question is phrased 'Do you suffer attacks of twitching and cramps in your arms and legs followed by unconsciousness or urinary incontinence?' a person with epilepsy will answer 'Yes' (Chandra, 1988). The reason for this is that in most villages the term 'convulsion' implies an hereditary incurable disease, which is a disgrace for the family. Concealment or denial is probably widespread, and has been reported anecdotally in several African and South American countries (see below). In a recent study from China (Li et al., 1985), compliance rates of 100% were said to apply, which is a unique situation indeed!

That the local attitudes and beliefs of patients should be taken into account in the design and administration of screening questionnaires is very clear, but there is little evidence from the literature that this problem has in fact been acknowledged. The traditional views of illness, symptoms and aetiology in rural areas of developing countries are often very different from the Western medical model, and questions framed in a medical format may well be meaningless to peoples from these cultures.

A further problem in field studies in developing countries concerns the criteria for the diagnosis of epileptic seizures. Syncope is often misdiagnosed as epilepsy, and in one review from Europe, syncope was initially diagnosed as epilepsy in about one-third of cases (Gastaut, 1974). Furthermore, psycho-

Table 2. Criteria for the definition of tonic–clonic seizures used in epilepsy studies in rural areas of Africa, Asia and South America. From Sander and Shorvon (1987)

i. Loss of consciousness from 1 to 30 min
ii. Tonic phase
iii. Clonic phase
iv. Sphincter disturbance
v. Tongue biting
vi. Fall
vii. Injury due to fall
viii. Postictal muscle soreness
ix. Postictal drowsiness, sleep or confusion
x. Transient postictal focal paralysis

A tonic–clonic convulsion is considered to have definitely occurred if criteria i–iii are present with any two of criteria iv–x.

genic attacks may mimic epilepsy, and in specialized epilepsy clinics this may be a problem in up to 20% of cases referred (Jeavons, 1983). Epilepsy is essentially a clinical diagnosis, and in epidemiological studies it is necessary to specify the clinical criteria used for the diagnosis. In Table 2 is an example of the clinical criteria used in the definition of tonic–clonic seizures in current studies in rural areas in three diverse Third World countries, and criteria for complex partial and other seizure types have also been devised on similar lines. In no other published epidemiological study from developing countries have detailed diagnostic criteria been specified. Commonly an operational definition of 'a specialist confirmed diagnosis' is used, but there is enormous variability in subjective specialist opinion, and such a method has been rejected in epidemiological studies of other diseases (e.g. angina and schizophrenia).

It is also necessary to consider what constitutes 'epilepsy'. The inclusion of single seizures, neonatal seizures, febrile seizures, seizures with an obvious precipitant (e.g. alcohol), or seizures in acute illness, may vary from study to study and this may heavily influence incidence and prevalence figures. Many published reports from developed and developing countries have failed to specify whether such seizures have been included, and the evaluation of their results is therefore problematic. A particular source of difficulty concerns patients with inactive epilepsy. It is clear that in most treated patients with epilepsy the seizures cease, but there is no general agreement as to what length of remission should occur before a patient is no longer designated 'epileptic'. Some have defined epilepsy as a condition in which a seizure has occurred in the preceding year, 2 years, 3 years, or 5 years, and some investigators have taken treatment status into account. Many reports, however, appear not to have considered this problem, and it is probably this simple failure to define epilepsy that is particularly responsible for the observed major differences in prevalence data. The importance of this factor is shown by the fact that cumulative incidence figures are more than four times the prevalence figures of active epilepsy (Annegers, Hauser and Elveback, 1979; Goodridge and Shorvon, 1983a, b; Shorvon, 1984).

Incidence Rates

In the developed world, published incidence rates have varied from between 11 cases per 100 000 to 134 cases per 100 000, although most fall between about 20 and 70 cases per 100 000 (see Sander and Shorvon, 1987). Higher rates are found in studies of children than of adults, and age is the most important factor in determining incidence rates. There have been few, if any, satisfactory studies of incidence rates in developing countries. Although it is often claimed that the incidence of epilepsy is higher in developing than in developed countries, there are few data to support this contention (Cruz, Barberis and Schoenberg, 1986).

Prevalence Rates

As mentioned above, prevalence data are more easily obtained than are incidence data, largely because smaller numbers are needed and cross-sectional survey designs may be used. As with incidence rates, reported prevalence rates are very variable; rates as low as 1.5 per 1000 (Sato, 1964) and as high as 31 per 1000 (Chiofalo et al., 1979) have been reported.

In most studies the prevalence of chronic epilepsy has been found to lie between 4 and 10 per 1000 (see Sander and Shorvon, 1987). It is generally claimed that epilepsy is more prevalent (up to twice as prevalent) in developing than in developed countries. What data there are, however, present a much more variable picture (see Table 3).

Marino, Cukiert and Pinho (1987) in Sao Paulo found a prevalence rate of 13.3 per 1000 of the population, excluding febrile or single seizures, and a further 3 per 1000 had a single attack. Chiofalo et al. (1979) found a prevalence rate amongst children of 31 per 1000, and this was higher than two American studies using the same study methodology and the same screening questionnaires. In China, a much lower prevalence rate of 4.4 per 1000 was found by Li et al. (1985) in a screening survey of 63 195 persons in six Chinese cities. It is noticeable in this study that a high proportion of generalized seizures, a very low proportion of complex partial seizures, and a low proportion of inactive cases were found. It seems possible that partial seizures were overlooked using this study methodology.

A similarly low prevalence rate was found in a study from Igbo-Ora, a Nigerian town, using the same screening methods (Osuntokun et al., 1987). In another study from Nigeria, Dada (1970a) estimated a prevalence rate of 13 per 1000. A low prevalence (2.3 per 1000 in adults) was also found in a study from

Table 3. Selected community-based prevalence studies of epilepsy from developing countries

Author	Site	Prevalence rate per 1000	Comment
Gomez, Arciniegas and Torres (1978)	Colombia, Bogota	19.5	Single seizures and febrile seizures not included
Chiofalo et al. (1979)	Chile, Melipilla	28	Children up to age of 9 years. Febrile seizures and single seizures included
Garcia-Pedroza et al. (1983)	Mexico, Mexico City	42	Excluding febrile seizures
Li et al. (1985)	China, six cities	4.4	Excluding single seizures, febrile seizures and symptomatic seizures
Marino, Cukiert and Pinho (1987)	Brazil, Sao Paulo	13.3	Excluding febrile and single seizures
Osuntokun et al. (1987)	Nigeria, Igbo-Ora	5.3	Excluding single seizures, febrile seizures, and symptomatic seizures

Libya (Shridharan et al., 1986), in a prospective hospital rather than community-based study. Thus, although it is likely that prevalence rates are higher in developing than in developed countries, actual figures have varied widely and provide rather shaky support for this view. Study methodology has been generally poor, and it is likely that this is responsible for some conflicting findings. If prevalence rates are higher in developing countries, this probably relates to the younger age of the populations, the different aetiological profiles in different countries (see below), and the effects of socio-economic factors. In practice, though, it is easier to postulate such effects than to demonstrate them. There have been several community-orientated studies of epilepsy in the US that consider race and socio-economic class (Shamansky and Glaser, 1979; Haerer, Anderson and Schoenberg, 1986). The epidemiological rates for epilepsy were found to be higher in blacks than in whites, and in both groups lower in females than in males. Socio-economic class alone, however, was not clearly shown to be an important risk factor. Lower standards of perinatal care may also be relevant, and, as an indication of this, infant mortality rates amongst blacks in America are twice those of whites (Wise et al., 1985).

The Characteristics of Epilepsy in General Populations

Epilepsy is a heterogeneous condition, and simple prevalence and incidence data reveal only a limited amount about the characteristics of the condition in a general population. It is equally important to know the range of seizure types, aetiology, and severity of epilepsy in a population, and the treatment status.

Seizure Type

Many contradictory data have been published about seizure type. The International League Against Epilepsy has proposed a standard classification which is widely accepted and which is based on clinical features and the electroencephalogram (EEG) (Dreifuss et al., 1981). Although an important reason for using a standardized classification is that it allows international comparison, the requirement for EEG means that almost no epidemiological studies in developing countries can truly report seizure type—since the EEG is usually unavailable. This simple fact is often ignored, and a number of recent studies that purport to use the International League Classification report seizure type without the EEG (e.g. Li et al., 1985; Osuntokun et al., 1987). This may be a major source of confusion. Absence seizures, for instance, are subdivided in the International Classification into generalized absence (petit mal) and partial absence (e.g. a form of complex partial seizure). Generalized absence seizures are rare, and in clinical and EEG surveys have a prevalence of under 1% and a cumulative incidence ten times smaller than complex partial seizures (e.g. Juul-Jensen, 1986). In some studies from developing countries, in which the EEG has not been used, the rate of petit mal may be reported to be considerably higher, possibly reflecting the classification of partial absence as generalized absence seizures. A more common misclassification concerns tonic–clonic seizures. Many so-called generalized seizures are in fact secondarily generalized, and should therefore be categorized as partial. The detection of a partial onset may depend on the EEG or the skill of the investigator in uncovering partial features, and, as a general rule, the more sophisticated the study, the higher proportion of partial epilepsy is found. A final point is the almost complete absence of 'unclassified seizures' in published epidemiological reports using the international classifications. In hospital practice—albeit reflecting a highly selected group—about one-third of cases are strictly speaking 'unclassifiable', and in epidemiological surveys this figure might be expected to be higher. Indeed, in one well-conducted survey of epilepsy from Sri Lanka, using international criteria, 49 of 177 patients were deemed unclassifiable (Peiris et al., 1986).

A further problem concerns case ascertainment methods. As mentioned above, partial seizures may be under-reported in studies that use inadequate screening questionnaires, and this is another cause of the under-reporting of partial seizures. In the most detailed studies from Western populations (e.g. Juul-Jensen, 1986), about two-thirds of cases are reported to have partial seizures, and complex partial seizures are more commonly found than simple partial seizures. At the other extreme, in a survey of epilepsy in six cities in China, complex partial seizures accounted for only 2.8% of the cases found, simple partial seizures 4.8%, and 81% showed generalized convulsive seizures (Li et al., 1985). It is likely that this reflects the methodology used rather than any real geographical difference. In developing countries in which more symptomatic epilepsy is found, one might expect a higher rate of partial seizures than in developed countries, and it might indeed be argued that the adequacy of prevalence and incidence data could be assessed by an analysis of the seizure types reported.

Aetiology

In studies from developed countries, an aetiology for the epilepsy can be established in about one-third of cases only (see Sander and Shorvon, 1987). Of course, the proportion of cases with identifiable aetiology depends to some extent on the use of investigations, particularly radiological investigations. In most developing countries, sophisticated radiology will not be available for community-based studies, and aetiology is derived largely on historical grounds. In large-scale epidemiological studies, criteria for aetiological diagnosis and the extent of investigation within the population should therefore be carefully stated. In one study from Benghazi, Libya (Shridharan et al., 1986), where computed tomography (CT) was available, the profile of CT abnormalities found was similar to that in studies from developed countries (in 568 cases there were 5 meningiomas, 5 gliomas, 3 metastatic tumours, 22 focal atrophies, 3 porencephalies, 4 haemorrhages, and 8 infarctions). In a study from an experienced neurological unit in India, however, where CT was not available, tumours were identified in only 0.3% of the epileptic population (Mani, 1987).

The aetiological profile of epilepsy in different parts of the world, however, does show true variation. A number of chronic infectious diseases result in epilepsy, such as schistosomiasis, cysticercosis, paragonimiasis and hydatid diseases. The most important of these is cysticercosis. This condition is endemic in areas of Africa, Asia and South America. In Mexico City, for instance, 1.9% of all general autopsies showed evidence of cysticercosis infection (Miller et al., 1983), and cysticercosis accounts for 28% of all neurological admissions (Davis, 1983). Epilepsy is the commonest clinical manifestation of cerebal cysticercosis (Alarcon and Olivares, 1975). Gadjusek (1978) identified it as the cause of 'an epidemic of burns' due to epilepsy in New Guinea. In Ecuador, it is said to account for nearly one-quarter of all new cases of epilepsy (Placencia, personal communication). Sakamoto (1985) showed it as the aetiology in 13% of cases of epilepsy in his survey from Brazil, and this was the single most important identifiable cause. Paragonimiasis is endemic in the Far East, particularly in Korea, Japan, the Philippines and China. Epilepsy again is a common manifestation (Chang et al., 1958). Epilepsy is a frequent symptom of infection with *Schistosoma japonicum*, and a much less common symptom in central nervous system (CNS) involvement in *Schistosoma mansoni* and *Schistosoma haematobium* infection (Chang, Chu and Fan, 1957; Scrimgeour and Gajdusek, 1985). Epileptic seizures occurred in 35% of 62 cases of cerebral hydatidosis reported from Rumania (Arseni and Marinescu, 1974). Epilepsy may also be seen in other cerebral parasitic diseases (e.g. sparganosis) (Fan and Pezeshkpour, 1986), toxocariasis (Elliot et al., 1985) and ascariasis (Dada, 1970b).

The importance of these conditions varies with geographical location. It is commonly claimed that poor perinatal care will result in a high frequency of epilepsy in developing countries. Perinatal mortality rates may be very high in some developing countries (see Table 4), and there may be considerable perinatal morbidity. In a recent survey from Saudi Arabia, for instance, 13% of all children referred to the King Khalid University Hospital with neurological disorders showed a perinatal cause (Alfrayh and Al Naquib, 1987). The extent to which poor perinatal care results in epilepsy, however, is uncertain, and it is worth noting that birth trauma was said to account for only 2% of cases of epilepsy in a rural inner study from India (Mani, 1987) and 3% from a recent study in Nigeria (Osunkotun et al., 1987). In Table 5 are shown the aetiological findings from eight series of epilepsy from developing countries. The causes vary, but comparisons are difficult because of different methods of case

Table 4. Population, population per physician, and infant mortality rates in the US, UK and eighteen developing countries. From South (Sept. 1985)

Country	Population ($\times 10^6$)[a]	Population per physician	Infant mortality[b] (%)
Afghanistan	17	16 700	21
Angola	8	15 000	17
Bangladesh	96	11 000	13
Brazil	130	1 700	7
China	1021	1 800	7
Colombia	27	1 700	5
Ecuador	8	800	8
India	733	3 700	9
Iran	43	6 000	10
Iraq	14	1 800	7
Kenya	19	7 900	8
Libya	3	700	10
Liberia	2	9 600	9
Malaysia	14	7 900	3
Nigeria	94	12 600	11
Pakistan	89	3 500	12
Peru	18	1 400	8
Sri Lanka	16	7 100	3
United States	255	600	<1
United Kingdom	55	800	<1

[a] Mid-1985 population figures to nearest million.
[b] Percentage of children who die before reaching the age of 1 year.
All figures are based on government statistics that in some instances may be unreliable.

selection and the differing extent of investigation. In isolated communities, specific diseases may have an important impact on aetiology, and an example of this has been found in the Grand Bassa county in Liberia, where a possible degenerative cerebral disease (known locally as See-ee) has resulted in a high prevalence of epilepsy (28 per 1000) (Goudsmit, van der Waals and Gadjusek, 1983; van der Waals, Goudsmit and Gadjusek, 1983). Similarly, Jilek-Aall (1965) found a prevalence rate in Tanzania of 20 per 1000, and considered that a specific degenerative disease accounted for many of these cases (Jilek-Aall, Jilek and Miller, 1979; Jilek and Jilek-Aall, 1977).

Frequency of Seizures

Seizure frequency is an important characteristic of epilepsy in a population, but data concerning this are extremely sparse. In developed countries (see Shorvon, 1988), it has been estimated that of those with active generalized tonic–clonic seizures on treatment, about 15% have seizures less than once a year,

Table 5. Aetiology of epilepsy in eight case series from developing countries

Author	Country	Number	No cause found (%)	Perinatal damage (%)	Head injury (%)	Familial (%)	Cysticercosis (%)	Infective (%)	Tumour (%)	Cerebrovascular disease (%)	Other (%)
de Pasquet, Pietra and Gaudin (1976)	Uruguay	155	52		12	7			11	13	3
Hamdi, Al-Husaini and Al-Hadithi (1977)	Iraq	100	52	1	5			16	4	4	18
Sakamoto (1985)	Brazil	455	63	14	3		13	5	1	3	2
Li et al. (1985)	China	289	79		10			5	1	3	2
Mani (1987)	India	631	88	2	2		2	1	1	2	4
Osuntokun et al. (1987)	Nigeria	101	85	2	6	5			1	2	
Shridharan et al. (1986)	Libya	568	83		5				4	5	4
Bittencourt (1988)	Brazil	147	68	11	13		4			3	2

60% have seizures at a frequency of between one per month and one per year, and 25% have seizures occurring at a frequency of more than one per month. Over one-half of patients with active partial seizures will have seizures occurring more than once per month. Of course, many patients on treatment will have seizures suppressed altogether, and those patients will not appear in these figures. In Mani's study from Bangalore (Mani, 1987), of 627 patients, 308 had seizures occurring less than once per year, 156 occurring between once per year and once every 3 months, and 163 at a frequency of more than once every 3 months. Ninety-four of these patients were untreated. In view of the high proportion of untreated patients in developing countries (see below), it might be expected that higher seizure frequencies occur, but exact data on this point are lacking. It would be possible to use such data to evaluate the effectiveness of treatment programmes in the Third World.

Sociocultural Aspects

Introduction

Any discussion relating to the Third World, on the social effects of epilepsy, attitudes of epileptic patients in particular and communities in general towards the disease and its victims, beliefs about its cause, and treatment strategies by patients, is limited by the relative lack of accessible material in this field. Much of what there is relates to Africa, Nigeria being particularly active. There is useful information from other areas, such as India and Iraq, in some collections of more specifically medical papers. Two ongoing studies in Kenya and Ecuador in which the authors are collaborating provide raw data not yet fully analysed but already interesting, particularly since these are the only studies we can find using an unbiased population, recruited door to door in Ecuador, and by local word of mouth in Kenya. Finally, there are the anecdotal—but not to be discounted—observations of those who have treated epilepsy in the field. We are grateful for access to information from Malawi made available by Dr Anne Watts (Watts, 1985) and to the as yet undocumented work of anthropologist Dr Alison Redmayne among the He He tribe in Tanzania.

Among other things, the literature reveals the problems in gathering information of this kind. Arawatife, Longe and Arawatife (1985), for instance, point out that previous research in Nigeria had concentrated on obtaining evidence from the patients themselves on the social disadvantages of their disease, which may well not be forthcoming since sufferers are likely to be reluctant to admit to such sensitive problems. This paper redressed the balance by questioning non-epileptic patients as well about their attitudes and beliefs. For the same reason, the Ecuador and Kenya studies are questioning both non-epileptic controls and community figures about their and their communities' beliefs and attitudes. Orley (1970) has also suggested, usefully, that some sensitive information can be obtained by asking more indirect questions—e.g. where patients sleep in the house, where they are buried, and so forth.

The evidence of Dr Redmayne is particularly interesting. Although not a physician, in an area short of medical facilities she was drawn into treating her neighbours, but was 16 years in the field before hearing of a single epileptic patient. After the successful treatment of one, other patients appeared in droves. Dr Watts had a similar experience in Malawi. This reluctance of patients to come forward has been borne out by experience in Kenya also, and illustrates very well both the problems of getting evidence from sufferers so unwilling to reveal themselves in the first place and the fact, borne out almost everywhere, that epileptic patients prefer if possible to keep their disease secret from their nearest neighbours, let alone anyone else.

Social Effects of Epilepsy

The hypothesis generally is that epilepsy is a disease incurring considerable social disadvantage, not to say stigma, a hypothesis borne out in the experience of most researchers. The picture revealed by Arawatife, Longe and Arawatife (1985) was, as expected, negative. The paper made the point, however, that research may show a reality different in certain respects from that previously assumed—the experience of other Nigerian observers, for instance, led them to believe that fear of infection was the most significant reason for the shunning of epileptic patients. That, for Arawatife's respondents, this did not turn out to be the case suggests that if the main hypothesis remains valid, the fine details of disadvantage revealed by research may not always be as expected.

Uncontrolled epilepsy must by definition cause considerable disruption of sufferers' lives on a practical level at least. They are subject to accidents when falling, cannot or should not be left alone for this reason, and their work—whether at school if they are children or in the labour market if adult—is inevitably disrupted, both by the seizures themselves and the debility often persisting thereafter. In the Third World, given the lack of treatment programmes, the relative invisibility of patients in the local community, let alone in the wider one where medical programmes are devised, and, lastly, the high proportion of patients involved in more or less subsistence agriculture, it might have been assumed by careless observers that the problems were less severe than they are known to be in developed communities.

This of course is not the case. In some respects the practical disadvantages for epileptic patients are even worse. Very poor people need all hands available to plant and harvest the crops. They cannot easily afford to carry their unfortunates, let alone, as Redmayne has observed in the He He community, spare someone to keep full-time watch on sufferers, even though uncontrolled falls may involve hazards not encountered elsewhere. In Africa, for instance, as in many parts of the Third World, all cooking is done on open fires. Epilepsy is sometimes actually known as 'the burn disease'. Watts (1985) found that the first patients she encountered all presented with bad burns rather than epilepsy. The scarred and mutilated state of some patients taking part in the Kenya study is also apparent. In Tanzania (Jilek-Aall, Jilek and Miller, 1979), the problem is exacerbated by the fear that those pulling the sufferer out may be contaminated by his saliva. In Ecuador, a further hazard is that up in the high Andes, horseback is a common form of transport. In all countries where industry is less strenuously controlled, there are extra hazards from unfenced machinery and so forth.

Any further doubts as to the disadvantages are dispelled by the evidence given by the patients themselves. In India (Virmani, Kaul and Juneja, 1977), only 25% of patients felt that epilepsy had not affected their daily activities. Though in both the Kenya and Ecuador studies many patients claimed their work was not affected by their disease, others recognized considerable disability. Although some of this perceived disability may differ, as in the case of epileptic patients elsewhere, from actual disability in less severely affected patients, there is no doubt that it is felt by all as a considerable burden. Not one patient did not long to be cured. In Kenya a striking number claimed they would go anywhere, do anything, pay anything for cure. A phrase, constantly reiterated, is 'life is more precious than money . . .'—a claim backed by the amount many of these impecunious people had spent seeking treatment from healers of one kind or another. If they did not present themselves to the orthodox medical services, it was not because they were happy to live with their disease, but because either belief that no medical treatment exists or past negative experience with doctors led them to believe it was a waste of time.

Social disadvantage for the person with epilepsy is not of course merely practical. There is also the matter of how he sees himself and is seen by his peers. As already stated, this image is assumed, and, where researched, has often been found to be negative. In Ethiopia, patients were treated as lepers and banished from the community (Giel, 1968). In Arizona (Levy, Neutra and Parker, 1979), in a study not strictly Third World but of interest as revealing the attitudes—mostly extremely negative—of a non-white, tribal and rural community isolated from the mainstream of US life, Navaho patients were thought to have committed incest. In Madagascar, epileptic patients were buried separately (Osuntokun, 1977). In Nigeria, non-epileptic respondents, asked to compare patients cured of psychosis with epileptic ones, discriminated on the whole in favour of the ex-psychotics (Arawatife, Longe and Arawatife, 1985).

Questionnaires administered in Kenya and Ecuador to non-epileptic controls and community leaders revealed some realistic assessment of epilepsy both as a disease and a social condition, but also much prejudice. Informants claimed they would not let their children play with known epileptics, would not marry them, or let their children do so. (This is a common problem—Indian psychiatrists have observed, for instance, that a woman known to have epilepsy has virtually no chance of an arranged marriage.) Epileptic patients are thought to be uneducable, unemployable, and a danger to the community. All of these prejudices may or may not manifest themselves in practice for particular patients. Inability to get married, breakups of marriages and problems with employment seem factors in the lives of epileptic sufferers almost everywhere, but by no means invariably.

Many prejudices, of course, relate to the assumed (in some cases observed) brain damage resulting from uncontrolled seizures. In India (Arjundas, 1977), after a fit children are assumed to be unfit to study further, and about one-third of epileptic patients suffer delays in their education. In Kenya and Ecuador, problems with education appear to arise from the fairly common reluctance and sometimes outright refusal of teachers to have epileptic children in their classes; they are seen as being uneducable and/or a nuisance. Such attitudes may be summed up in the words of one leader in Ecuador—'Oh these people, they're just mad, aren't they.'

Of course, as already stated, there are plenty of examples of patients leading relatively normal marital and working lives, and neither they nor their families seem to suffer significant or at least overt problems, despite their disease. These tend, however, to be less severely affected patients. Families where the mother is the sufferer appear to be less severely disadvantaged than those with an epileptic breadwinner. Patients also believe it advantageous where seizures come at night, unknown to the community. One man in Ecuador, a black from the tropical Chota Valley, set in the high Andes, laid great emphasis on the fact that only his wife saw his seizures, and did certainly seem to have fewer problems than many patients. A man of 58 years, with three wives and 30 children, had, as his chief complaint against his seizures, loss of his 'potencia para mujeres' (potency) for a fortnight after each. Although this might appear frivolous, comparatively speaking, it is a salutary reminder that in the final analysis, no matter how many questionnaires are applied, how many statistics gathered on the attitudes and experience of patients generally the 'dis-ease' as perceived by each patient is his, individually, and may bear little relation to that perceived by similarly afflicted neighbours, let alone sociologists.

Perceived Causes of Epilepsy

Again, accurate understanding is limited by a lack of documentary evidence, as also by a reluctance by some informants, patients, and non-patients to admit their true beliefs (Table 6). In underdeveloped communities, for instance, a strong belief in the supernatural as a cause of epilepsy might be expected, a hypothesis borne out by some of the evidence. The Shona (Gelfland, 1973) can see it as the revenge of aggrieved ancestors, the Yoruba in Nigeria (Osuntokun, 1977) as the sign of visitation by the devil, and many patients in a study in Iraq (Hamdi, Al-Hasaini and Al-Hadithi, 1977) regarded their illness as due

Table 6. Perceived causes of epilepsy (as reported in sociocultural studies in developing countries)

Supernatural
   Witchcraft
   Breaking of taboo
   Seeing ghosts
   Visiting 'dangerous places' (e.g. cemeteries)
   Possession by devils/dissatisfied ancestors
   Will of God/s

Environmental
   Climate (e.g. wind/hot/cold/rain)
   Phases of the moon
   Poverty
   Family problems
   Contagion by others

Physical
   Malaria/other illness
   Heredity
   Bang on the head or other accidents
   Sexual misbehaviour (e.g. incest)
   Other wrongdoing or bad behaviour
   Brain damage
   Drug/alcohol abuse
   Mental/physical weakness

Psychological
   Worry and/or grief either of patient; or close family member = emotional stress
   Guilt
   Anger
   Craving for things the patient can't have
   A tendency to brood/think too much

to 'powers, the ghost, or the evil eye'. In India (Virmani, Kaul and Junejagh, 1977), 6% of the poorer patients and no less than 35% of their families saw it as due to supernatural causes (undefined). The discrepancy between the patients and their families is significant here. It may not be that patients' beliefs are so different but simply that as those affected they are less willing to acknowledge supernatural influences. A further complication is that in a rapidly changing world, people may be reluctant to admit that what they have been taught are socially backward opinions. This is a particularly significant factor in Kenya, for instance, where strong missionary activity in the past 50 years, both Catholic and Protestant, has attempted to outlaw belief in witchcraft. 'We are Christians, we don't believe in such things' was stated repeatedly. The ambivalence remaining, however, was demonstrated very effectively in the evidence of one community leader, a pastor who, evincing witchcraft and so forth as possible causes of epilepsy, claimed that being who he was he ought not to acknowledge such things, but, having been brought up in a tribal village, he could not wholly dismiss them.

Patients too, as they became more at ease with the study team, could begin to acknowledge beliefs previously denied. In Kenya, comparison of 10 matched sets of closed questionnaires given at the beginning of the study with 10 open questionnaires given later found 9 of the patients admitting supernatural causes in the open questionnaires, as against 4 in the closed. During an informal interview with the author, one woman who had been previously reticent claimed witchcraft as the cause of her epilepsy, she had her first fit the day after a quarrel with a discarded lover.

In Ecuador, similarly, the man who feared for his potency claimed to have been bewitched by a former lover. Here, however, in a country where Catholicism has long come to terms with pre-Christian belief, people are more willing to acknowledge the existence of diseases supernatural in origin, such as 'mal hechizo' (witchcraft), and to describe the treatment given them by local 'brujos' (witches) and healers. On the other hand, epilepsy appears to be seen by many traditional healers as a natural disease (Estrella, 1977), and though in the questionnaires reviewed so far in the Ecuador study a few patients, like the man above, may understand the disease in some instances as having supernatural causes, e.g. 'mal hechizo', far more appear to believe its origin is natural (Estrella, 1977). In the long-suffering Andean communities, 'pena y sufrimiento' (trouble and woe, more or less) is seen as a significant cause of many illnesses, if not as an illness (Estrella, 1977) amongst which epilepsy can be included, judging by the answers given to our questions in both the questionnaires and informal interviews with patients. Another cause commonly suggested is 'debilad' (weakness), a view hardly surprising in a chronically undernourished people, and one reflected elsewhere—in both the Kenya and Ecuador studies, poverty is thought to be a factor in many cases, as are extremes of heat and cold. Indeed, natural aetiologies are accepted in all communities studied, either alongside or in place of supernatural ones. In Kenya, for instance, some patients who have had accidents recognize that the 'bang on the head' may be one reason for their disease, and also that heredity may be a factor, where other family members have been known to suffer.

One natural (if not medically accurate) cause suggested can be, of course, contagion. Traces of this belief surface in many places, e.g. Madagascar, Tanzania (Jilek-Aall, Jilek and Miller, 1979), and Nigeria (Arawatife, Longe and Arawatife, 1985). People's attempts to keep away and keep their children away from patients may also often reflect a fear that many observers too have reported. On the other hand, as Arawatife, Longe and Arawatife (1985) discovered, this fear when researched may turn out to be less extensive than at first sight.

Treatment

The one common factor everywhere is the general lack of medical treatment available for people with epilepsy and the lack of programmes to help sufferers, even in a country such as India where medicine is relatively well developed and where there is a move at the moment to improve services for epilepsy. Though this may partly reflect the fact that epilepsy is not a fashionable disease whose control would bring political kudos, as important are the difficulties of treating a condition that is almost always chronic, needing, first, a reliable supply of drugs and, second, long-term compliance on the part of patients whose view of illness tends to lead to expectations of instant cure. It may also relate to the fact, documented above, of epilepsy being a relatively hidden disease so that the scale of the problem is by no means apparent at either the community or national level.

In many countries, Malawi, for instance (Watts, 1985), scientific medicine is thought to have no remedies against epilepsy. In any case, patients traditionally prefer to visit healers for this disease, although they were not always willing to admit this initially. In Ecuador, patients widely use traditional healers as well as local home remedies, such as pulling the sufferer's middle finger, or rubbing them with cologne.

Treatments used both in Africa and Ecuador, reflecting beliefs about the illness that may or may not in different cases tally with the beliefs of patients, defined epilepsy as a foreign body that had to be expelled from the body. For instance, in Malawi (Watts, 1985), potions causing diarrhoea and vomiting were used to expel something moving around in the abdomen; among the Shona (Gelfland, 1973), medicine was given to get rid of the poison imposed by the offended spirit. In Ecuador, in a healing session observed by one of the authors, the 'brujo' lightly whipped his patient with a bunch of herbs smelling like mint and raising bumps on the skin like nettles—this, he claimed, was a sign of the 'germs' coming out. This same healer also claimed to have cured an unmarried woman (i.e. a virgin) by extracting excessive 'hormones' from her with needle and syringe. If he is describing hysteria, it is possible this somewhat dubious remedy may, for psychological reasons, have effected the cure as stated.

In general, however, healers, even if seen to be the best sources of treatment, as in Malawi, do not affect cures. Some healers indeed recognize that their resources are limited in relation to this disease. One patient in Kenya was brought into the study by a healer who had been treating her unsuccessfully for a year. In Ecuador, many healers admitted they could do little (Estrella, 1977) and prescribed mostly cold baths, a quiet life, and valerian, a sedative herb used in Europe against epilepsy from the sixteenth century onwards (Temkin, 1971). Valerian was indeed one element in a prescription given to the patient by the 'brujo' described above.

Redmayne has suggested that one reason patients may be more willing to go to medicine men, apart from the fact these are seen as the appropriate—or only—practitioners, as in Malawi (Watts, 1985), is that, since healers are expected to diagnose the ailment, patients themselves are not expected to divulge their shameful secret. In Nigeria, 32.5% of patients questioned (Danesi, 1984), though recognizing the effectiveness of medical treatment, nevertheless would like to combine this with 'native' or 'church' healing, suggesting that informal medicine still has some part to play in these communities in alleviating the non-medical aspects of the disease. In general, however, it is clear that the availability of formal medicine is the only hope.

The problem, of course, is to use it effectively. Apart from the matter of reliable drug supply, the idea of ongoing treatment has to be sold to patients. Experience in Kenya, which has fair medical services, and where many patients in the study had sought previous help and then failed to persist with treatment, highlights the problem. Some doctors questioned stated that it was a waste of time treating such patients, and patients themselves complained that the disease wasn't taken seriously; that they were just given pills 'as if all they had was malaria'—a much more commonplace disease. The education of not only patients but doctors in this area is obviously crucial. From her successful practice in Malawi, Watts (1985) has described some useful principles (e.g. proper follow-up, proper explanations), and the same priorities are coming to light in both Ecuador and Kenya. The essential facts emerging in both studies, however, are that patients, when they dare to announce themselves, long to be cured, and that successful treatment of the few—as the experience of both Watts and Redmayne has shown—encourages many more to come forward and, as importantly, persist with treatment given.

Medical Management and Treatment

Only orthodox Western medical treatment will be considered here, and not traditional medicine, the sociocultural aspects of which are discussed above. This is not to underestimate the importance of traditional medicine in many developing countries. No epilepsy treatment programme should ignore the force of traditional medicine, and the most successful programmes are those that work in tandem with traditional medicine.

Medical Manpower

Table 4 lists the number of patients per physician in developing countries (based on official government sources, which in some cases may be an overestimate of the true figures; in 1977, for instance, Osuntokun stated that the doctor:population ratio in most African countries has been less than 1:20000). It is clear from even these raw data that the time a physician is able to devote to epileptic patients must be severely restricted. These figures, furthermore, may be misleading because of a significant degree of medical unemployment in many developing countries (the overproduction of medical graduates is an economic necessity for some universities) and because, in most developing countries, medical services are concentrated in large cities and the medical coverage of rural areas may be extremely deficient. In recent years, a number of developing countries have introduced regulations to try to improve rural medical care; one solution is to oblige new medical graduates to spend a certain time (e.g. 1 year) after graduation in posts in rural areas. In Ecuador, for instance, a network of health centres, staffed by a single newly qualified doctor with some paramedical support, has been established throughout the country. In other countries, however, large regions will be very poorly served, and this may seriously compromise the successful treatment of epilepsy.

Another assumption implicit in medical teaching from developed countries is that epilepsy will be treated by specialists, e.g. neurologists or paediatricians. In many developing countries, of course, such specialists are few. In Kenya, for instance, there is only one accredited neurologist in the country, and the great majority of specialist resources—and about 75% of all doctors—are concentrated in Nairobi. In Nigeria, with one-quarter of the population of the whole of Africa, there were only seven neurologists in 1977, concentrated in two university teaching hospitals, and in Ghana there was one neurologist covering a population of 8 million (Osuntokun, 1977). Similar considerations apply in other developing countries. Epilepsy, therefore, is much more likely to be treated in primary care settings than by specialists. Any treatment programme for epilepsy needs to be cognizant of this, and there are implications for diagnosis, investigation and treatment. Recent WHO initiatives have been made, looking at the feasibility of managing epilepsy by paramedical personnel rather than doctors, and although it seems unlikely that such personnel could successfully diagnose or initiate treatment, there may be an important role for paramedical personnel in monitoring therapy and ensuring compliance. Other organizations have also initiated projects, such as the epilepsy programme in Sri Lanka (Meinardi, 1988), in which a community training programme in epilepsy has been instituted, and parallel studies of the role of 'health promoters' in assisting and monitoring treatment in epilepsy in Ecuador and Kenya (see Ellison et al., 1989).

It is interesting to compare the medical manpower situation with that in the USA. In a recent analysis (Kurtze et al., 1986), it was estimated that there would be a requirement for 12 600 neurologists in the USA by 1990. This is a ratio of about 4 neurologists per 100 000 of the population. It was estimated that each neurologist will need annually 340 h of outpatient consultations for epilepsy, 72 h for single seizures, and 52 h for febrile seizures (about 20% of their professional time). This is based on the assumption that between 75% and 100% of new cases and 50% of old cases will be seen by the neurologist, that 50

Table 7. Number of cases per 1000 persons, and prevalence ratio of neurological diseases, detected by WHO screening questionnaire in rural Nigeria. From Osuntokun et al. (1982)

	Number (per 1000)	Prevalance ratio
Epilepsy	33	37
Perceptive disorder	8	9
Completed stroke	4	4
Peripheral neuropathy	14	15
Isolated bilateral optic atrophy	3	3
Myelopathy	3	3
Cerebral palsy	2	2
Cerebral neoplasm	2	2
Primary cerebellar degeneration	1	1

min should be spent on the first consultation, and that 120 min of follow-up were needed over the next 12 months for every new case and 40 min of follow-up for every old case. This perception of care in epilepsy, which is reflected in the treatment approaches taught in major textbooks of epilepsy, is clearly wholly inappropriate in the setting of most developing countries.

Nevertheless, in neurological clinics in developing countries, convulsive disorders form a greater proportion of the caseload than in developed countries. Thus, in Saudi Arabia (Alfrayh and Al Naquib, 1987), for instance, 48% of all cases referred to a children's neurological clinic concerned convulsive disorders, and a similar high proportion of epilepsy cases is seen in neurology clinics in India (Mani, 1987), South America (Placencia, unpublished data), and elsewhere. The prevalence ratios of several neurological disorders from a population survey in Nigeria are shown in Table 7, and epilepsy was the commonest condition identified. Epilepsy, therefore, is a major health care problem in developing countries both for specialist and primary care services.

General Principles of Treatment

The Western model of the management of epilepsy might run somewhat as follows: the patient develops seizures and presents this information to his doctor, who diagnoses epilepsy; investigations are carried out to determine the type and aetiology; chronic therapy with anticonvulsant drugs is initiated, and the dose is monitored at follow-up consultations, often with the assistance of serum level estimations. This Western model clearly does not apply in rural settings in any developing country. First, the development of seizures may not be seen as something with which to visit a doctor. As discussed above, the concepts of cause and the nature of the illness may result in ostracism or incarceration, but not necessarily in seeking medical help. Furthermore, traditional healers are much more likely to be consulted initially than orthodox medical personnel. If a patient does visit a doctor, the language he uses to describe seizures may obscure the diagnosis. For instance, in Indonesia (as noted above) the word convulsion has connotations that mitigate strongly against its use (Chandra, 1988); similarly, amongst the He He in Tanzania, epilepsy was said to be unusual largely because the mission doctors dealing with this rural population were unable to obtain a history from the reticent and frightened patients (Redmayne, personal communication). Even when epilepsy is diagnosed, resources or expertise are usually not available for seizure classification and aetiology. Recent evidence from Pakistan and Ecuador, however, suggests that most patients do visit orthodox practitioners at some point, but that this seldom results in long-term treatment or in regular follow-up (Ellison et al., 1989).

A major difficulty regarding treatment relates to the patient's own conception of Western medical therapy. Often treatment is sought on an on–off basis, with medication taken for a short, well-defined period. In this sense, patients seek cure rather than suppression of seizures, and the concept of long-term regular treatment to prevent recurrence is often alien. A common problem is that treatment is taken intermittently after a seizure in response to the crisis, or when a seizure seems imminent, rather than as a prophylactic.

Local custom should not be overlooked, and, for instance, during Ramadan in Muslim countries, strict fasting is observed and daytime drugs will not be taken. This may result in worsening seizure control, as has been observed in Libya (Shridharan et al., 1986). Many of these problems could be resolved by improving the explanations given to patients. This might be best achieved by programmes directed at the local physicians and general practitioners, who are in a unique position to effect improvements. Physician-directed, rather than the fashionable patient-directed, educative efforts should be a high priority for the international and national agencies concerned with improving the treatment of epilepsy.

However, the most formidable problem in the treatment of epilepsy in most developing countries relates to the availability of treatment. In rural areas, the supply of drugs to health centres is frequently interrupted. Furthermore, one drug may be available one month and another drug the next. As discussed below, interrupted therapy may have serious consequences for patients taking drugs such as phenobarbitone, and the sudden interruption of supply may result in a severe exacerbation of seizures. The WHO initiatives regarding drug prescription are discussed below, but it is important to emphasize that in practice the logistical problems of drug availability and supply are just as important as any of these other issues. Other problems concern the different dosage sizes of tablets (the WHO essential drugs list (see below) recommends, for instance, the use of phenytoin 25 mg tablets, as well as 100 mg tablets, which is surely inviting confusion), and the fact that in many health centres the drug instructions, printed in English, are frequently incomprehensible. Thus, although the importance of regular therapy over a prolonged period of time is heavily stressed in developed countries, this is often very difficult to achieve with the current arrangements in the Third World. Finally, the technology required to monitor dose by serum level is not available in most developing countries—even in major centres.

It is notable that, in some developing countries, lay organizations provide a considerable amount of treatment for epileptic patients. The Kenyan Epilepsy Association, for instance, runs its own epilepsy clinics in four locations staffed by volunteers including two doctors, a psychologist and social workers. Seven hundred and fifty patients per month may be seen in these clinics. In other countries, missionary hospitals may also supplement government health care provision.

The Choice of Anticonvulsant Drugs and WHO Initiatives

It is generally assumed that cost is a major determinant of drug choice in epilepsy in the developing world. The cost of individual anticonvulsant drugs varies enormously; in many countries, phenobarbitone is the cheapest drug, and phenytoin may cost five times as much, carbamazepine fifteen times as much, and valproate 20 times as much. Perhaps because of its cheapness, phenobarbitone is still the most commonly prescribed drug throughout the world. Thus, phenobarbitone and phenytoin accounted for the treatment of 93% of subjects prescribed anticonvulsant therapy in a survey from India (Mani, 1987), and 67% in Pakistan (Ellison, personal communication). Phenobarbitone has been shown to have approximately equal efficacy in generalized tonic–clonic and in partial seizures as other first-line anticonvulsant drugs, although its toxicity is greater. Largely because of its low cost and equal efficacy, it has been a drug chosen for community-based studies of the treatment of epilepsy by the WHO. (WHO collaborative initiatives for an extensive programme for the control of epilepsy are being considered in Brazil, Colombia, Egypt, India, Senegal and Sudan, and other countries in which special projects have been undertaken in epilepsy include Tanzania, Rwanda, Nigeria, Sri Lanka, Liberia, Guinea-Bissau, Botswana, Zambia and Pakistan.) There are a number of disadvantages to phenobarbitone, however (Shorvon, 1986). First, if withdrawn suddenly, it may result in severe withdrawal seizures—sometimes in status epilepticus—and other withdrawal symptoms. This withdrawal effect is probably worse than with any other first-choice anticonvulsant drug. As discussed above, in the developing world the availability of anticonvulsant supplies is often erratic, and it is not uncommon for health centres suddenly to run out of drug supplies (this is indeed the rule in many African, Asian and South American countries). This confers on phenobarbitone therapy a considerable hazard. Second, phenobarbitone is a drug of abuse and is issued only with special precautions in many countries. In the large cities in the developing world, its free availability to epileptic patients may encourage illicit dealing and abuse. Third, phenobarbitone interacts with alcohol, and alcohol is a common precipitating factor for epilepsy, and alcoholism a common problem in some developing countries. Fourth, phenobarbitone is relatively commonly used in successful suicide. Fifth, and perhaps most important, phenobarbitone's profile of toxicity has discouraged its use in developed countries, at least as a first-choice anticonvulsant. The most important toxic effects are hyperactivity in children and sedation in adults, and it is cynical to believe that these side-effects are of no importance in the less priviledged developing countries. This is to put a geographical hierarchy on brain function, which is unacceptable. The International League Against Epilepsy has expressed its worries about the WHO recommendations concerning phenobarbitone, and whether the WHO will modify these recommendations remains to be seen.

Ironically, the low cost of phenobarbitone may exacerbate the problems of its supply. In several developing countries, manufacturers show little interest in a compound with such a low cost (and therefore mark-up), and supplies are often limited simply by a failure of local manufacturers to produce sufficient quantities of the drug.

In recent years the WHO has become more active in prescribing policy. A meeting on the rational use of drugs was held in Nairobi in 1985 (Anon, 1985; Richards, 1986). The 100 experts at the meeting—drawn from governments, drug regulatory authorities, the pharmaceutical industry, and other organizations—invited the WHO to take a leadership role to influence government policy (although without becoming 'a supranational manipulator of governments'). The concept of an 'essential drugs list', a comprehensive list of drugs that should have wide availability, is a central plank of the WHO's rational drug use strategy. With it, as the WHO Director General commented, 'we make a very special effort to try to make this penetrate into government national drug policies. We can only be an international supporter of the governments as they put their drug house in order.' The WHO made three major proposals. First, that governments should adopt national drug policies based on the WHO essential drug concept and use the skill of the WHO in drawing up these policies. Second, they should set up effective national regulatory authorities. Third, efforts should be made to ensure that drug promotion is ethical and that the education of health workers is improved (see Anon, 1985; Richards, 1986). The second report of the WHO expert committee (1985) on the use of essential drugs recommended that the anticonvulsant drugs in the essential drugs list should consist of diazepam, ethosuximide, phenobarbitone, and phenytoin, and that carbamazepine and valproate be included 'when the drugs in the main list are known to be ineffective or inappropriate for a given individual, or for use in rare disorders or in exceptional circumstances' (World Health Organization, 1985). This interventionist policy has become highly controversial, and it is important that these arguments do not draw attention away from other important health issues in the Third World, e.g. the need to establish a better health care superstructure and more effective primary and secondary health care services. In epilepsy, for instance, more reliable drug supply and patient and doctor education would have a much greater impact on health care than the imposition of a rigid drugs policy. It is also worrying that, in the opinion of many, the WHO has made the wrong recommendations regarding anticonvulsant drugs.

In several countries, in response to the WHO initiatives, the concept of 'an essential drugs kit' has been initiated. This is a kit of 40 drugs, based on the essential drugs list, which are supplied to health centres, for distribution largely by paramedical personnel. A typical example is that from Kenya (Anon, 1986). The kits are supplied from central sources, and the supply is notoriously unreliable, due—on the government's own admission—to 'poor planning, unsuitable procurement policies, shortage of foreign exchange, and pilferage.' It is therefore common for even a large hospital pharmacy to run out of an anticonvulsant drug. Phenobarbitone is the only oral anticonvulsant drug in the kit. The emphasis of this programme is surely misplaced, and because of intermittent drug availability, and reliance on prescribing by paramedical personnel, with little training in the principles of epilepsy treatment, there is little evidence that this policy has actually improved the day-to-day treatment of epilepsy at all. Finally, even if drugs are made available to local health clinics, there is no guarantee that these drugs will be distributed to patients. In Tanzania, for instance, phenobarbitone is often requisitioned as rat poison!

One method of assessing the success of drug treatment programmes is to use anticonvulsant drug supply figures to determine the proportion of patients with epilepsy receiving and not receiving treatment. A useful measure is the *treatment gap* (Ellison et al., 1989), which is defined as the percentage of patients in a defined population on any one day, with active epilepsy, not receiving anticonvulsant medication (see Ellison et al. (1989), and Table 8). Treatment gap figures for three developing countries are shown in Table 8, based on an assumed prevalence of non-febrile seizures of 0.5%, almost certainly a low estimate, monotherapy, standard anticonvulsant drug dosage, and drug consumption figures based on IMS (segment N3A) figures, institutional consumption (Ciba-Geigy), and adjusted by local factors (Ellison et al., 1989). These figures are an approximation only and are influenced by many factors, and may be open to various interpretations. Nevertheless, these figures do appear to show that in these three developing countries, between 80% and 94% of patients with active epilepsy are not receiving anticonvulsant medication at any point in time, and there is thus enormous potential for improving medical care. One explanation for this treatment failure, frequently proposed, is that the cost of the drugs prohibits their general utilization. We suspect,

Table 8. Treatment gap figures in three developing countries

Country	Estimated prevalence of epilepsy (1)[a]	Number of patients receiving drug treatment (2)[b]	Treatment gap (%)[c]
Pakistan	450 000	22 000	94
Philippines	270 000	14 000	94
Ecuador	55 000	11 000	80

[a] The estimated prevalence is assuming 0.5% of the population has active non-febrile seizures requiring treatment.
[b] The total number of patients receiving drug treatment derived from drug supply figures based on IMS figures, institutional consumption (Ciba–Geigy), and local data. It is an approximation assuming minimum standard dosage regimens, monotherapy, regular therapy, etc.
[c] The treatment gap is calculated as: $[(1)-(2) \times 100]/(1)$.
See Ellison et al. (1989).

however, that this is an oversimplification, and cost is only one of many factors determining the success of treatment.

It is interesting to note that many patients spend considerable amounts of money on obtaining traditional cures. It is not uncommon, for instance, for a patient to travel hundreds of miles or to donate cattle or treasured items to a healer in Africa or in South America in return for anticonvulsant treatment. Preliminary figures from a survey in Pakistan suggest that up to 20% of a family's income may be spent on health care, and this is borne out by anecdotal findings in several other countries. The treatment gap calculations can be computed for individual anticonvulsant drugs and the results for inexpensive and expensive anticonvulsant drugs compared. In Table 9 are shown treatment gap figures for inexpensive and expensive drugs (with relative costs varying by 20-fold), assuming health care spending of 10% of family income, and similar derivations may be made for other percentage estimates. It is striking to note that the treatment gap is just as great for inexpensive as for more expensive drugs, and the inference from this is that the failure to take anticonvulsant drugs in these communities cannot be explained simply in terms of affordability. Indeed, there is enormous underutilization of very inexpensive drugs (e.g. phenobarbitone, the cost of a course of which in some countries may be only $3 a year) as well as the more expensive anticonvulsants. Nor is this because of governmental control on health spending; for it is a remarkable fact that—whatever statements of intent are made by governments—in the developing world only about 20% of total health care spending is provided by government compared with 80% in developed countries (World Bank figures). Although governments may hesitate to devote resources to health care, it is clear that patients do not. Cost is therefore not the only (or even the major) reason for the large treatment gap in epilepsy, and other causes must include

Table 9. Treatment gap figures for inexpensive and expensive drugs

Country	Relative costs of inexpensive and expensive drugs (1)[a]	Number of patients Receiving treatment (2)[b]	With annual family income >10% cost of 1 year's drug treatment (3)[c]	Treatment gap (%)[d]
Philippines				
Inexpensive	1	7500	220 000	97
Expensive	17	2400	25 000	90
Pakistan				
Inexpensive	1	4700	450 000	99
Expensive	20	1000	111 000	90

[a] Relative costs of an inexpensive and expensive drug in these countries.
[b] Total number of patients receiving treatment with the inexpensive and expensive drugs (based on drug supply figures as in Table 8).
[c] Total number of patients whose family annual income is in excess of 10 × of the cost of a year's treatment with the inexpensive and expensive drugs.
[d] Treatment gap figures estimated for inexpensive and expensive drugs calculated as: [(1)−(2) × 100]/3.
See Ellison et al. (1989).

the irregularities of supply or availability, and the patient/doctor's failure to appreciate the potential for or the principles of drug treatment.

Racial and Geographical Differences in Drug Handling

A small amount of work has been carried out looking at the genetic and racial differences in the metabolism of anticonvulsant drugs. Dam, Larsen and Christiansen (1977) found small but significant differences in the plasma level and clearance of phenytoin in different ethnic populations. Peiris et al. (1986), studying the relationship between dose and serum concentration of carbamazepine, phenytoin, phenobarbitone, and primidone in a Dutch and Sri Lankan population, found no systematic pharmacokinetic difference. Anecdotal evidence from India (Mani, 1987) suggests that effective anticonvulsant dosages in India may be lower than those needed in Europe, although no formal study has been carried out. In many developing countries, liver diseases are frequent, and the influence of abnormal liver function on pharmacokinetics in this setting has not been investigated. Clearly, more work is needed to detect the possible influence of diet, genetic factors, and concomitant local diseases on both pharmacokinetics and pharmacodynamics of the anticonvulsant drugs—before the treatment policies accepted in the developed world can be extrapolated uncritically to developing countries.

Conclusion

We consider that the three most important practical steps that could be taken to improve the medical care of epilepsy in the Third World are: first, to ensure the regular availability of drug supplies; second, to devote resources to the education of general practitioners and other primary care doctors about the simple effective management of epilepsy; and, third, to base this educative effort on an understanding of local cultural attitudes. Other issues, such as the use of an essential drugs list, the training of paramedical personnel, the relative costs of individual anticonvulsants, and the provision of specialist facilities, are secondary to these. The WHO emphasis on the implementation of a rigid drug policy (and particularly the provision of phenobarbitone) and on the training of paramedical personnel may be therefore partly misdirected, and it would be a pity if the prestige and status of the WHO unduly influenced governments away from what may be more important practical initiatives.

Summary

In this chapter, aspects of epilepsy that differ in developing and in developed countries are reviewed. This is inevitably an incomplete and impressionistic survey, because data on many aspects in developing countries are scarce, and because it is difficult to generalize meaningfully about the enormous diversity of countries and populations that make up the developing world. Epidemiological studies of prevalence and incidence are reviewed with an emphasis on the problems inherent in work in this area in developing countries. Data concerning seizure type, aetiology, and severity of seizures in the Third World are contrasted with those from developed countries. Sociocultural aspects of epilepsy have been poorly studied, and yet are fundamental to effective medical management. The social effects of epilepsy and the local perceptions of cause and of treatment are discussed from work in Africa, Asia and South America. The principles and success of treatment in the Third World may differ considerably in developing and developed countries. In the Third World, medical manpower is scarce, and epilepsy is managed essentially by primary care resources, without specialized investigations or personnel. The principles of drug therapy may not be understood by patients, and the supply of drugs is often erratic; and these are major reasons for poor compliance with treatment. World Health Organization (WHO) initiatives have stressed the extensive use of paramedical personnel and of an essential drugs list, but this emphasis may be misdirected, and in practice neither proposal has achieved much success. The recommendation that phenobarbitone be extensively used in the Third World, because of its cheapness and efficacy, is also of doubtful merit, as there are well-known and major drawbacks to the widespread use of this drug. Computations of treatment gap figures in three developing countries suggest that between 80 and 94% of patients with active epilepsy are not receiving anticonvulsant therapy, and cost is only one of a number of reasons for this. The key to improvements in medical treatment lies with a better understanding of the patients' cultural concepts of epilepsy and its treatment, improved drug supply and availability, and efforts to improve education amongst general practitioners and other primary care medical personnel.

Acknowledgement

We acknowledge the help and advice of many persons in the preparation of this report. In particular, we are grateful to Dr Russell Ellison for his consistently stimulating suggestions; Dr J. W. A. Sander, Dr Marcelo Placencia, and other members of the Projecto de Manejo Comunitario de la Epilepsia in Ecuador and the Sociedad Ecuatoriana de Neurologia; Drs Adolf Feksi and Graham Cooper and other members of the epilepsy control project in Kenya; and the sociologists, Mr Gatiti in Kenya, and Miss Jumbo in Ecuador. Also, we acknowledge the financial grant support of Ciba–Geigy (Basel) in these studies.

References

Alarcon G, Olivares L, Cysticercosis cerebral. Manifestaciones en un medio de alta prevelancia. Rev Invest Clin 1975; 27: 209–15.

Alfrayh A, Al Naquib H. The pattern of central nervous disease in children in King Khalid University Hospital in Riyadh, Saudi Arabia. J Trop Paediatr 1987; 33: 124.

Annegers JF, Hauser WA, Elveback L. Remission of seizures and relapse in patients with epilepsy. Epilepsia 1979; 20: 729–37.

Anon. WHO meeting agrees on rational drug strategy. Lancet 1985; ii: 1350–1.

Anon. New drug supplies management system for rural health facilities in Kenya (presentation of Kenya's drug kit to the WHO conference of Experts on the Rational Use of Drugs, Nairobi 1985). Medicus 1986: 13–8.

Arawatife A, Longe AC, Arawatife M. Epilepsy and psychosis: a comparison of societal attitudes. Epilepsia 1985; 26: 1–9.

Arjundas G. Epilepsy in India. In: Penry JK (ed.) Epilepsy: The Eighth International Symposium. New York: Raven Press, 1977: 359–64.

Arseni C, Marinescu V. Epilepsy in cerebral hydatidosis. Epilepsia 1974; 15: 45–54.

Beran RG, Michelazzi J, Hall L, Tsimnadis P, Loh S. False-negative response rate in epidemiologic studies to define prevalence ratios of epilepsy. Neuroepidemiology 1985; 4: 82–5.

Bittencourt PRM. Epilepsy in developing countries. Part two: epilepsy in Latin America. In: Richens AL, Laidlaw J, Oxley J (eds) A textbook of epilepsy. Edinburgh: Churchill Livingstone, 1988: 518–28.

Chandra B. Epilepsy in developing countries. Part one: epilepsy in Indonesia. In: Richens AL, Laidlaw J, Oxley J (eds). A textbook of epilepsy. Edinburgh: Churchill Livingstone, 1988: 511–8.

Chang H-T, Wang C-W, Yu C-F, Hsu C-F, Fang J-C. Paragonimiasis. A clinical study of 200 adult cases. Chin Med J 1958; 77: 3–9.

Chang YC, Chu CC, Fan WK. Cerebral schistosomiasis. Chin Med J 1957; 75: 892–907.

Chiofalo N, Kirschbaum A, Fuentes A, Cordero M, Madsen J. Prevalence of epilepsy in Melipilla, Chile. Epilepsia 1979; 20: 261–6.
Cruz ME, Barberis P, Schoenberg BS. Epidemiology of epilepsy. In: Poeck K, Freund HJ, Ganshirt H (eds) Neurology. Berlin: Springer-Verlag, 1986: 229–39.
Dada T. Epilepsy in Lagos, Nigeria. Afr J Med Sci 1970a; 1: 161–84.
Dada TC. Parasites and epilepsy in Nigeria. Trop Geogr Med 1970b; 22: 313–22.
Dam M, Larsen L, Christiansen J. Phenytoin: ethnic differences in plasma level and clearance. In: Gardner Thorpe C, Janz D, Meinardi H, Pippenger CE (eds) Antiepileptic drug monitoring. Tunbridge Wells: Pitman Press, 1977: 73–9.
Danesi MA. Patient perspectives on epilepsy in a developing country. Epilepsia 1984; 24(2): 184–90.
Davis A. A epidemiologia da teniase e da cisticercose. J Brasil Med 1983; 45(suppl.): 9–14.
Dreifuss F et al. Proposal for revised clinical and electrocephalographic classification of epileptic seizures. Epilepsia 1981; 22: 489–501.
Elliot DL, Tolle SW, Goldberg L, Miller JB. Pet-associated illness. N Engl J Med 1985; 313: 985–95.
Ellison RE, Guvener A, Feksi G, Placencia M, Shorvon S. A study of approaches to antiepileptic drug treatment in four countries in the developing world. In: Dreifuss F. et al. (eds). Advances in epileptology—XVIIth Epilepsy International Symposium. New York: Raven Press, 1989 (in press).
Estrella E. Medicina aborigena. Quito, Ecuador: Editorial Epoca, 1977.
Fan K-J, Pezeshkpour GH. Cerebral sparganosis. Neurology 1986; 36: 1249–51.
Gadjusek DC. Introduction of *Taenia solium* into West New Guinea with a note on an epidemic of burns from cysticercus epilepsy in the Ekari people of the Wissel Lakes area. Papua New Guinea Med J 1978; 21: 329–42.
Gastaut H. Syncopes: generalized anoxic cerebral seizures. In: Vinken PJ, Bruyn GW (eds). Handbook of clinical neurology, Vol. 15. Amsterdam: North Holland, 1974: 815–23.
Gelfland M. Epilepsy in the African. Central Afr J Med. 1973; 3: 11–2.
Giel R. The epileptic outcast. East Afr Med J 1968; 45: 27–31.
Gomez JG, Arciniegas E, Torres J. Prevalence of epilepsy in Bogota, Colombia. Neurology 1978; 28: 90–5.
Goodridge DMG, Shorvon SD. Epileptic seizures in a population of 6000. 1: Demography, diagnosis and classification. Br Med J 1983a; 287: 641–4.
Goodridge DMG, Shorvon SD. Epileptic seizures in a population of 6000. 2: Treatment and prognosis. Br Med J 1983b; 287: 645–7.
Goudsmit J, van der Waals FW, Gadjusek DC. Epilepsy in the Gbawein and Wroughbarh Clan of Grand Bassa County, Liberia: The endemic occurrence of 'See-ee' in the native population. Neuroepidemiology 1983; 2: 35–44.
Hamdi HI, Al-Husaini AA, Al-Hadithi F. The epilepsies: clinical and epidemiological aspects/availability and desirability of services. In: Penry JK (ed.) Epilepsy: The Eighth International Symposium. New York: Raven Press, 1977: 393–9.
Haerer AF, Anderson DW, Schoenberg BS. Prevalence and clinical features in a biracial U.S. population. Epilepsia 1968; 27: 66–75.
Jeavons PM. Non-epileptic attacks in childhood. In: Rose FC (ed.) Research progress in epilepsy. London: Pitman Press, 1983; 224–30.
Jilek WG, Jilek-Aall L. The problem of epilepsy in a rural Tanzanian tribe. Afr J Med Sci 1977; 1: 305–7.
Jilek-Aall L. Epilepsy in the Wapogoro tribe in Tanganyika. Acta Psychiatr Scand 1965; 41: 57–86.

Jilek-Aall L, Jilek W, Miller JR. Clinical and genetic aspects of seizure disorders prevalent in an isolated African population. Epilepsia 1979; 20: 613–22.

Juul-Jensen P. Epidemiology of intractable epilepsy. In: Schmidt D, Morselli PL (eds). Intractable epilepsy, LERS Monograph Series, Vol. 5. New York: Raven Press, 1986: 5–12.

Kurtze JF, Bennett DR, Berg BO et al. On national needs for neurologists in the United States. Neurology 1986; 36: 383–8.

Lessell S, Torres JM, Kurland LT. Seizure disorders in a Guamanian village. Arch Neurol 1962; 7: 37–44.

Levy JE, Neutra R, Parker D. Life careers of Navaho epileptics and convulsion hysterics. Soc Sci Med 1979; 13B: 391–8.

Li S, Schoenberg BS, Chung-Cheng W, Xueming-Ming C, Shu-Shun Z, Bolis CL. Epidemiology of epilepsy in urban areas of the People's Republic of China. Epilepsia 1985; 26: 391–4.

Mani KS. Collaborative epidemiological study on epilepsy in India. Final report of the Bangalore Centre. Bangalore: Department of Neurology, National Institute of Mental Health and Neuro Sciences, 1987.

Marino R Jr, Cukiert A, Pinho E. Epidemiological aspects of epilepsy in Sao Paulo, Brazil. In: Wolf P et al. (eds). Advances in epileptology—XVIth Epilepsy International Symposium. New York: Raven Press, 1987: 759–64.

Mathai KV, Dunn DP, Kurland LT, Reeder FA. Convulsive disorders in the Mariana Islands. Epilepsia 1968; 9: 77–85.

Meinardi H. Epilepsy in developing countries. Part three. In: Richens AL, Laidlaw J, Oxley J (eds). A textbook of epilepsy. Edinburgh: Churchill Livingstone, 1988: 528–32.

Miller BJ, Goldberg MA, Heiner D, Myers A. Cerebral cysticercosis: an overview. Bull Clin Neurosci 1983; 48: 2–5.

Orley JH. Culture and mental illness—a study from Uganda. Nairobi: East African Publishing House, 1970.

Osuntokun BO. Epilepsy in the African continent. In: Penry JK (ed.) Epilepsy—The Eighth International Symposium. New York: Raven Press. 1977: 365–78.

Osuntokun BO, Schoenberg BS, Nottidge VA et al. Research protocol for measuring the prevalence of neurologic disorder in developing countries. Results of a pilot study in Nigeria. Neuroepidemiology 1982; 1: 143–53.

Osuntokun BO, Adeuja AOG, Nottidge VA et al. Prevalence of the epilepsies in Nigerian Africans: a community-based study. Epilepsia 1987; 28: 272–9.

de Pasquet EG, Pietra M, Gaudin ES. Eitiologia de la epilepsia tarda. Acta Neurol Latinamer 1976; 18: 256–75 (quoted in Bittencourt, 1988).

Peiris JB, Karunanayake EH, Joice PDTM, Goedhart DM, Meijer JWA, Meinardi H. Relationship between dose and serum concentration of carbamazepine, phenytoin, phenobarbital and primidone in a Sri Lankan population compared with a European population. Heemdstede: Epilepsy International, 1986.

Proano J. Preliminary results of the neuroepidemiological study in Quiroga, Ecuador. Commun Neurol 1984; 1: 11–20.

Richards T. Drugs in developing countries: inching towards rational policies. Br Med J 1986; 292: 1347–8.

Sakamato AC. Estudio clinico e prognostico das crises epilepticas que niciam na infancia numa populacao Brasileira. Tese de doutorado, Universidade de Sao Paulo, Ribeirao Preto, 1985 (quoted in Bittencourt, 1988).

Sander JWAS, Shorvon SD. Incidence and prevalence studies in epilepsy and their methodological problems: a review. J Neurol Neurosurg Psychiatry 1987; 50: 829–39.

Sato S. The epidemiological and clinico-statistical study of epilepsy in Nigata City. Clin Neurol (Tokyo) 1964; 4: 413–24.
Scrimgeour EM, Gajdusek DC. Involvement of the central nervous system in *Schistosoma mansoni* and *S. haematobium* infection. Brain 1985; 108: 1023–38.
Shamansky S, Glaser G. Socioeconomic characteristics of childhood seizure disorders in the New Haven area: an epidemiological study. Epilepsia 1979; 20: 457–74.
Shridharan R, Radhakrishnan K, Ashok PP, Mousa ME. Epidemiological and clinical study of epilepsy in Benghazi, Libya. Epilepsia 1986; 27: 60–5.
Shorvon SD. The temporal aspects of prognosis in epilepsy. J Neurol Neurosurg Psychiatry 1984; 47: 1157–65.
Shorvon SD. Drugs in developing countries. Br Med J 1986; 292: 1666–7.
Shorvon SD. Medical services. In: Richens AL, Laidlaw J, Oxley J (eds) A textbook of epilepsy. Edinburgh: Churchill Livingstone, 1988: 611–30.
Stanhope JM, Brody JA, Brink E. Convulsions among the Chamorro people of Guam, Mariana Island. Am J Epidemiol 1972; 95: 292–8.
Temkin O. The falling sickness (revised edition). Baltimore and London: The Johns Hopkins Press, 1971.
van der Waals FW, Goudsmit J, Gadjusek DC. See-ee: clinical characteristics of highly prevalent seizure disorders in the Gbawein and Wroughbarh Clan region of Grand Bassa County, Liberia. Neuroepidemiology 1983; 2: 35–44.
Virmani V, Kaul V, Juneja J. Sociocultural and economic implications of epilepsy in India. In: Penry JK; (ed.) Epilepsy: The Eighth International Symposium. New York: Raven Press, 1977: 385–92.
Watts A. Primary care of epileptic patients in a rural area of Tanzania. (Unpublished paper, presented at World Federation of Mental Health (Mind) Conference, 1985.)
Wise PH, Kotelchuck M, Wilson ML, Mills M. Racial and Socioeconomic disparities in childhood mortality in Boston. N Engl J Med 1985; 313: 360–6.
World Health Organization. The use of essential drugs. Second report of the WHO expert committee. World Health Organization. Technical report series 722. Geneva: World Health Organization, 1985.
Zielinski JJ. Epidemiological and medicosocial problems of epilepsy in Warsaw. Final report on research program no. 19-P-58325-F-01, Warsaw Psychoneurological Institute, 1974.

18

Advances in Genetics and Their Application to Epilepsy*

H. Meierkord
Institute of Neurology, London, UK

Introduction

Genetics is a young discipline. Its scientific beginning dates back to Mendel's laws of inheritance (Mendel, 1866) and the fast development of molecular genetics most importantly includes the description of the double helical structure of deoxyribonucleic acid by Watson and Crick (1953), the discovery of restriction endonucleases (Smith and Wilcox, 1970) and other important steps eventually leading to the sophisticated technology of recombinant DNA. Rosenberg (1983) announced 'the coming of a new age' in a paper on recombinant DNA and neurological disease. Can the application of modern molecular genetics to the epilepsies lead to a 'new age' in epileptology as well? If so, how can gene technology be applied to epilepsy?

The epilepsies are in fact a particularly interesting group of syndromes to study genetically because they represent common conditions in the general population, and with the EEG a non-invasive tool for identifying subclinically affected carriers is available. The epilepsies can therefore perhaps serve as a model for a group of neurological conditions showing polygenic or multifactorial patterns of inheritance, i.e. caused by a number of different environmental and genetic factors. Multiple sclerosis (Acheson, 1985) and myasthenia gravis (Compston et al., 1980) are other examples of conditions comprising environmental and genetic factors aetiologically.

---

* This essay won second prize in the Sanofi 'Epilepsy Essay Competition 1989'.

Evidence for Hereditary Factors in Epilepsy

The epilepsies constitute a highly heterogeneous group of diseases, which necessitates a clear distinction of different syndromes (phenotypes) in genetic studies. This is done below for six forms of epilepsy which appear to be suitable for molecular genetic studies, extending the group of syndromes suggested by Delgado-Escueta and Greenberg (1984).

There is considerable evidence from pedigree, EEG, twin and animal studies that hereditary factors are involved in the aetiology of some forms of epilepsy (Noebels, 1984; Rich et al., 1986; Seyfried and Glaser, 1985; Tsuboi and Okada, 1985). The question is no longer whether or not genes are involved but rather in which way they are acting in different epileptic syndromes. A small proportion of patients, however, has a straightforward diagnosable Mendelian trait (see below).

For the primary generalized forms a genetic background has been assumed for a long time; there is also evidence, however, that genetic factors are involved in the aetiology of focal epilepsy; this form is usually thought of as being due to exogenous factors (Andermann, 1982).

Generalized Epilepsy

Epilepsy with simple absences The attacks in this syndrome are frequent, show childhood onset and are characterized by a sudden arrest of normal behaviour. The typical EEG trait is the bilaterally synchronous and symmetrical 3 Hz spike–wave complex. The pattern of inheritance is controversial.

Metrakos and Metrakos (1961) stated that the 3-Hz spike and wave pattern was due to an autosomal dominant gene with variable features according to the age of patients, with a low expression at a very young age, a maximal expression at 4–16 years and a gradual decline after that. Doose et al. (1973), however, observed a bimodal age distribution of spike–wave abnormalities in siblings of patients, with peaks occurring at 5–6 years and 11–14 years. They found that 6.7% of siblings of 239 probands with absence seizures also had seizures, and of 242 siblings, 22.3% had EEG abnormalities, including generalized spike and wave patterns. They felt that their results suggested a polygenic pattern of inheritance.

Juvenile myoclonic epilepsy The disorder shows a peak age of onset between 13 and 15 years, consisting of irregular myoclonic jerks of shoulders and arms, grand mal convulsions on awakening, and absence seizures. Photosensitivity is often present. The characteristic EEG pattern is the 4–6 Hz diffuse polyspike–wave complex. A positive family history is common, with 13–50% of relatives being affected. Tsuboi and Christian (1973) found the incidence of affected relatives to be 27% among their JME patients, which was significantly higher than the incidence of 9.9% in 466 non-selected patients with epilepsy. The incidence of epilepsy in first-degree relatives (4.1%) was higher than that among the general population, which, according to Hauser and Kurland (1975), is 0.38%. The EEGs of 390 first-degree relatives (asymptomatic and symptomatic) of 136 probands showed specific epileptiform abnormalities in 15%. This would be against the possibility of autosomal recessive inheritance. Sex-linked inheritance can be excluded because males and females are equally affected. Autosomal dominant inheritance with low penetrance or polygenic inheritance is possible in this condition.

Epilepsy with 'grand mal' seizures   In this syndrome, tonic–clonic seizures occur exclusively and the interictal EEG trait shows generalized 3-Hz spike–wave and polyspike–wave complexes. The attacks tend to occur during diurnal and nocturnal hours. The pattern of inheritance is unclear but probably multifactorial. Eisner, Pauli and Livingston (1959) found a seizure rate of 5.26% for siblings and parents of patients, which is considerably higher than the control rate of 1.75%.

Focal Epilepsy

Rolandic epilepsy (benign epilepsy with centrotemporal sharp waves)   The characteristic seizures seen in patients with this syndrome are focal seizures with involvement of the face. Occasionally, secondary generalization can occur. The typical EEG pattern shows spikes of high amplitude followed by slow waves which are at a maximum in the centrotemporal region. The onset is between 5 and 9 years of age, and the condition is benign and tends to disappear after 15–16 years of age.

There is considerable evidence in the literature that Rolandic epilepsy is a genetic disease. Some evidence stems from the twin study by Kajitani et al. (1980), who investigated three pairs of monozygotic twins who all had benign focal epileptiform discharges of childhood in the EEG between the ages of 5 and 11 years; only three patients had seizures. Bray and Wiser (1965) investigated twelve pedigrees with positive family histories, and concluded that this condition is an autosomal dominant disease with an age-dependent expression. This mode of inheritance was strongly supported by the study of Heijbel, Blom and Rasmuson (1975) and has now been generally accepted.

Other Forms (showing Mendelian Inheritance)

Primary reading epilepsy   Although this is a rare condition, it is worthwhile considering for genetic studies because there is strong evidence that it is inherited as an autosomal dominant trait (Matthews and Wright, 1967). The clinical features are well established: jaw jerking is triggered by reading and accompanied by abnormal EEG discharges, often over the temporal region of the dominant hemisphere.

Benign neonatal familial convulsions This syndrome is characterized by short, generalized clonic convulsions with an age of onset between 2 days and 3 months. According to several reports, the pattern of inheritance is autosomal dominant (Plouin, 1985).

Approaching the Epilepsies by Means of Molecular Genetics

The group of syndromes discussed here is characterized by epileptic seizures in the absence of known structural abnormalities of the brain. A definite primary protein defect has not yet been identified, and the chromosomal localization of the responsible gene(s) is unknown.

The question is, what approach should be chosen, as no primary defect has been identified? Gusella et al. (1984) suggested a strategy which reverses the traditional strategy based upon defining a biochemical abnormality, before direct isolation of the disease gene is possible, as in phenylketonuria. The alternative approach is to identify an altered protein by analysis of the gene that encodes it. If certain genes responsible for special forms of epilepsy could be identified, it should be possible to determine certain protein products which might be involved in the aetiology of epilepsy. This would make possible a meticulous study of the pathophysiology of different epileptic syndromes, leading to a deeper understanding of it.

Linkage Analysis Using Markers and Techniques Used in Molecular Genetics

In order to define the chromosomal map position of an 'epilepsy' gene, linkage analyses using certain markers is suggested.

What is linkage analysis and how can it be applied to the search for the chromosomal site of an epilepsy gene?

In every meiosis, crossing over between pairs of chromosomes occurs with great frequency. As a result, recombination of genes may occur at any point of the chromosome. The further apart two genes are on the same chromosome, the greater the likelihood that a crossing over will occur in the space between them. Two different genes are said to be linked when they are close to each other on the same chromosome. They are not linked in the genetic sense of the word when they are far apart from each other but still on the same chromosome. The relative distance between genes on any particular chromosome is measured by the frequency at which crossing over occurs between homologous chromosomes. Distances are measured in 'map units': one map unit is equal to 1% crossing over. A map unit is frequently referred to as a centiMorgan (cM), which is roughly equal to 1000 kilobases (kb) or 10^6 base pairs (Emery, 1984). The idea of linkage analysis is to find markers whose chromosomal locations are known and which are linked to the disease (epilepsy) gene. If, for example, the marker gene and the epilepsy gene were located 10 cM apart, they would be passed on together from parents to offspring 90% of the time.

The likelihood of linkage between two genetic loci is assessed statistically using so-called lod scores. Lod means 'log of the odds'; linkage between two loci at a given distance is considered to be proven or excluded if the lod score is greater than $+3$ or -2 respectively. A lod score of $+3$, for example, means that the odds in favour of linkage are 1000 to 1.

How should we choose suitable markers?

There are two large groups of markers, phenotypic markers and DNA markers. The first group comprises, among others, red blood cell antigens, red blood cell enzymes and serum proteins that are polymorphic. About 30 of these are currently available. They can be separated electrophoretically or by antigen–antibody reaction. The second group of markers is based on direct analysis of the DNA; they are referred to as restriction fragment length polymorphisms (RFLPs).

RFLPs are detected by the use of type II restriction endonucleases, a group of enzymes found in bacteria which cleave DNA at sequence-specific sites (Malcolm, 1981). They cleave DNA at these sites and do not cut it anywhere else. An alteration in the human genome as small as a single base change, located in the DNA at one of these recognition sequences, will thus eliminate cleavage at that site. By using the method of Southern blotting, DNA from leukocytes is incubated with a given restriction endonuclease and a large number of fragments is produced. The fragments are electrophoresed on an agarose gel; small fragments migrate faster than large ones. The fragments are transferred to nitrocellulose or nylon membrane filters loaded onto filter paper which hangs in a bath of salt solution. The solution is drawn up through the gel by the filter wicks, and the DNA fragments are deposited on the filter. Then they are bound to the filter by baking or ultraviolet irradiation (Harding and Rosenberg, 1988).

DNA fragments can then be hybridized to radioactively labelled sequences of human DNA (probe) mapping to a particular position in the genome. This radioactive probe binds to its complementary sequence and is therefore retained on the filter only at positions marking the fragment sizes generated from that locus. The positions can be detected by autoradiography.

To determine linkage between markers and the disease gene, informative families have to be available. Especially in autosomal dominant disorders (Rolandic epilepsy, primary reading epilepsy, benign neonatal convulsions), large multigeneration families are necessary to track the defective gene by analysing the maximum number of informative meioses (Harding and Rosenberg, 1988).

According to Botstein et al. (1980), it is possible to map the entire human genome with polymorphic DNA markers. About 200 evenly spaced markers will be required to provide complete genotypic information. With such a set, any locus of interest will be less than 10 map units from a marker locus. This would allow chromosomal localization for the majority of Mendelian disorders (White et al., 1985).

Candidate Genes

A further useful approach to identifying epilepsy genes is the use of 'candidate gene markers'. As has been mentioned above, no definite single abnormal gene product has been identified so far in the primary generalized epilepsies. However, from animal studies it is known that certain proteins are involved in the pathophysiology of different epileptic syndromes. The amount of GABA, for example, has been found to be decreased in substantia nigra and periventricular grey matter in the Mongolian gerbil model (Olsen et al., 1984). Its significance in the pathogenesis of the epilepsies is further stressed by the finding that the GABA a receptor is part of a complex on which receptor sites for benzodiazepines, picrotoxin and barbiturates are found (Meldrum, 1985). Valproic acid, the anticonvulsant of choice for the primary generalized epilepsies, acts through the GABA system as well; it probably increases the amount of GABA at its receptor (Loescher, 1981). The $GABA_A$ receptor from bovine brain has recently been cloned and both subunits sequenced (Schofield et al., 1987). The hypothesis could be tested that mutations in the genes encoding the GABA receptor are responsible for the susceptibility to primary generalized epilepsy of the type JME, epilepsy with absences or epilepsy with tonic–clonic seizures. If a strong correlation was found, it would mean that this particular gene would be involved in the disease process.

In a similar fashion, receptors of other transmitters (excitatory) and genes that play a role in neural cell development could be studied, especially with regard to the age-dependent expression of the pathological phenotype in many epileptic syndromes.

Advantages of RFLPs

Why are RFLPs useful as markers in linkage studies for certain epileptic syndromes?

The traditional markers are insufficient in number, so that many chromosomal regions are not available for investigation. They are also insufficiently polymorphic, so that many families are not informative at the locus of interest. In the human DNA sequence, a large number of variations are present. The resulting variation in the primary amino acid sequence is responsible for the phenotypic differences between individuals (colour of hair, for example). With different restriction endonucleases, these different DNA sequence variants can be detected, and by means of recombinant DNA, an increasing number will be available in the future.

From Linkage to Gene Cloning

If linkage is established between a marker and a disease gene, it is still a large step to isolate the mutant gene.

The aim, however, of using methods of molecular genetics in epileptology is to identify the defective gene and its abnormal product. How can responsible genes be identified once linkage has been established? We have to bear in mind that even closely linked markers are usually more than a million base pairs away from the disease gene. One approach is so-called 'chromosome walking', a way of identifying overlapping DNA sequences.

After identification of a gene specific for a certain form of epilepsy, it can be cloned (production of many identical copies of a defined DNA fragment). This is done by inserting DNA fragments into vectors such as phages, cosmids or plasmids. For example, a DNA fragment containing a human gene sequence can be inserted into a plasmid. A vector containing a 'foreign' DNA sequence is called a recombinant. *Escherichia coli* infected with recombinants in culture will then produce multiple copies of the inserted DNA fragment (Emery, 1984). The next step is to sequence the gene and establish what protein it encodes.

Association and Linkage in Some Forms of Epilepsy

Association and linkage are distinct phenomena: association means the occurrence together of two characteristics, e.g. blood group O and peptic ulcers at a frequency greater than would be predicted on the basis of chance; linkage has been described above. It is interesting to note that according to two reports (Fichsel and Kessler, 1980; Rivas, 1983) an association has been found between epilepsy with absences and alleles of the major histocompatibility complex on chromosome 6. An association with the HLA system has also been found for other diseases, mostly showing a polygenic pattern of inheritance with incomplete penetrance, and not following simple Mendelian rules as is characteristic for the majority of the epileptic syndromes. This is especially interesting because in the analysis of 20 large families with JME, positive linkage has been found to the HLA locus (chromosome 6) as well (Durner et al., 1988), the lod score being 1.8. An abnormality on chromosome 6 could therefore turn out to be responsible for certain forms of epilepsy.

In Situ Hybridization and cDNA Libraries

Further progress in the understanding of the pathophysiology of the epilepsies can be expected by the application of in situ hybridization techniques for the analysis of gene expression in heterogeneous cell types of the brain. Their application to epilepsy is currently speculative but theoretically possible.

The technique can be used to study the levels of specific mRNAs in specific cell types of the brain (Griffin, 1988). In situ hybridization is a hybridization with an appropriate probe carried out directly on a chromosome preparation or histological section. The DNA is denatured by, for instance, treating chromosomes in metaphase with basic solutions. Radioactive mRNA is then added and during renaturing binding of the mRNA only to the complementary DNA sequences occurs. By means of autoradiography the binding sites can be shown. They are identical to the gene locus of the given mRNA.

There is some evidence from post mortem stability studies of different human brain constituents that intact mRNA can be isolated from human brain if the premortem hypoxia and the length of the post mortem interval can be minimized (Morrison, 1988). Experiments with frog oocytes injected with RNA from fetal human brain have shown that certain proteins, cholinesterases and a number of functional ion channels can be synthesized. This indicates that intact mRNAs for these proteins are still present in the RNA isolates.

It also has been found that these mRNAs are still polyadenylated. This makes it possible to construct human brain cDNA libraries; by the use of the enzyme reverse transcriptase, a complementary DNA to a given mRNA sequence (cDNA) is synthesized. The mRNAs can be extracted from certain regions of interest within the brain. The cDNA is cloned and used as a hybridization probe to screen a human DNA library.

The practical value of a cDNA library is that only those sequences are represented which are transcribed. The mRNA does not contain intervening sequences. Therefore, the distribution of cDNA clones is the same as the expression of the related genes and thus sequences that encode specific mRNAs can be identified. In epilepsy research this method could be of great value in determining lesions in neurotransmitter-synthesizing enzymes or abnormalities in transmitter-receptor proteins.

In situ hybridization could also be used to extend the pathological examination of brains of patients with epilepsy. The regulation, for example, of mRNAs in specific cell types can be studied, as intact mRNA is available in routine neuropathological tissue sections.

There is some evidence that in brains of patients with certain forms of primary generalized epilepsy, developmental abnormalities can be found (Meencke and Janz, 1984). The authors hypothesized that a genetic cause may be responsible for the maturation disturbances found in the stratum moleculare of the cerebrum and in the cerebellar cortex. Studies of the differential distribution of mRNAs could shed further light on the question of developmental abnormalities in brains of patients with primary generalized epilepsy.

Summary

Advances in genetics can be applied to the epilepsies after identification of well-studied families with defined epileptic syndromes. Epidemiological studies and registers could help in the tracing of such families. Then linkage studies can be carried out in order to determine the site of the abnormal gene. The gene can be cloned and sequenced, and the protein it encodes determined. At that stage gene therapy for the epilepsies could become possible.

The neuropathological approach to the epilepsies can be extended by studying mRNA distributions in specific brain areas. Through cDNA libraries, research into neurotransmitter systems and their abnormalities in specific forms of epilepsy is possible. The results could lead to a better understanding of the pathophysiology of the epilepsies and new methods of treatment, especially for chronic and resistant seizure disorders.

References

Acheson ED. The epidemiology of multiple sclerosis. In: Matthews WB (ed.) McAlpine's multiple sclerosis. Edinburgh: Churchill Livingstone, 1985: 3–46.

Andermann E. Multifactorial inheritance of generalised and focal epilepsy. In: Andersen VE, Hauser WA, Penry JK, Sing CF (eds) Genetic basis of the epilepsies. New York: Raven Press, 1982: 355–74.

Botstein D, White RL, Skolnick M, Davis RW. Construction of a genetic linkage map in man using restriction fragment length polymorphisms. Am J Hum Genet 1980; 32: 314–31.

Bray PF, Wiser WC. Hereditary characteristics of familial temporal-central focal epilepsy. Pediatrics 1965; 36: 207–11.

Compston DAS, Vincent A, Newsom-Davis J, Batchelor JR. Clinical pathological HLA antigen and immunological evidence for disease heterogeneity in myasthenia gravis. Brain 1980; 103: 579–601.

Delgado-Escueta AV, Greenberg D. The search for epilepsies ideal for clinical and molecular genetic studies. Ann Neurol 1984; 16 (suppl.) 2: 1–11.

Doose H, Gerken H, Horstmann T, Voelzke E. Genetic factors in spike–wave absences. Epilepsia 1973; 16: 285–93.

Durner M, Janz D, Scaramelli A, Weissbecker K, Spence A. Kopplungsanalyse bei Epilepsie mit Impulsiv-Petit-Mal (IPM). In: Scheffuer D, Speckmann EJ, Wolt P (eds) Epilepsie-Blaetter (suppl.). Rundbrief und Zeitschrift der Deutschen Sektion der Internationalen Liga gegen Epilepsie. Bielefeld: Bethel-Verlag, 1988: 8.

Eisner V, Pauli LL, Livingston S. Hereditary aspects of epilepsy. Johns Hopkins Hospital Bulletin 1959; 105: 245–71.

Emery AEH. An introduction to recombinant DNA. Chichester: John Wiley, 1984.

Fichsel H, Kessler M. Immunogenetics of 3/s-sw absence epilepsy: frequency of HLA antigens and haplotypes in patients and relatives. In: Canger R, Angeleri F, Penry JK (eds) Advances in epileptology: XI Epilepsy International Symposium. New York: Raven Press, 1980: 475–7.

Griffin S. In situ hybridization: visualizing brain messenger RNA. In: Rosenberg RN, Harding AE (eds) The molecular biology of neurological disease. London: Butterworths, 1988: 35–43.

Gusella JF, Tanzi RE, Anderson MA, Hobbs W, Gibbons K, Raschtchian R, Gilliam TC, Wallace M, Wexler NS, Conneally PM. DNA markers for nervous system disease. Science 1984; 225: 1320–6.

Harding AE, Rosenberg RN. Molecular genetics and neurological disease: basic principles and methods. In: Rosenberg RN, Harding AE (eds) The molecular biology of neurological disease. London: Butterworths, 1988: 1–21.

Hauser WA, Kurland LT. The epidemiology of epilepsy in Rochester, Minnesota, 1935 through 1967. Epilepsia 1975; 16: 1–66.

Heijbel I, Blom S, Rasmuson M. Benign epilepsy of childhood with centrotemporal EEG foci: a genetic study. Epilepsia 1975; 16: 285–93.

Kajitani T, Nakamura M, Ueoka K, Kobuchi S. Three pairs of monozygotic twins with rolandic discharges. In: Wada JA, Penry IK (eds) Advances in epileptology: the Xth Epilepsy International Symposium. New York: Raven Press, 1980: 171–5.

Loescher W. Valproate induced changes in GABA metabolism at the subcellular level. Biochem Pharmacol 1981; 30: 1364–6.

Malcolm ADB. The use of restriction enzymes in genetic engineering. In: Williamson R (ed.) Genetic engineering. vol. 2. London: Academic Press, 1981: 129–173.

Matthews WB, Wright FK. Hereditary primary reading epilepsy. Neurology (Minneap) 1967; 17: 919–21.

Meencke H-J, Janz D. Neuropathological findings in primary generalized epilepsy: a study of eight cases. Epilepsia 1984; 25(1): 8–21.

Meldrum BS. GABA and other amino acids. In: Frey H-H, Janz D (eds) Antiepileptic drugs. vol. 74. Handbook of experimental pharmacology. Berlin, Heidelberg, New York: Springer, 1985: 153–88.

Mendel G. Versuche ueber Pflanzenhybriden, Bruenn (Sonderdruck), 1866. (Faksimile—Nachdruck 1983. Goettingen: Arkana-Verlag.)

Metrakos K, Metrakos JD. Genetics of convulsive disorders II. Genetic and electroencephalographic studies in centrencephalic epilepsy. Neurology (Minneap) 1961; 11: 474–83.

Morrison MR. Messenger RNA levels in neurological disease. In: Rosenberg RN, Harding AE (eds) The molecular biology of neurological disease. London: Butterworths, 1988: 135–52.

Noebels JL. Isolating single genes of the inherited epilepsies. Ann Neurol 1984; 16 (suppl.): 18–21.

Olsen RW, Snowman AM, Lee R et al. Role of γ-aminobutyric acid receptor–ionophore complex in seizure disorders. Ann Neurol 1984; 16 (suppl.): 90–7.

Plouin P. Benign neonatal convulsions (Familial and non-familial). In: Roger J, Dravet C, Bureau M, Dreifuss FE, Wolf P (eds) Epileptic syndromes in infancy, childhood and adolescence. London: John Libbey Eurotext Ltd, 1985: 2–11.

Rich SS, Anneggers JF, Hauser WA, Anderson VE. Complex segregation analysis of febrile convulsions. Am J Hum Genet 1986. Cited in: Anderson VE, Hauser WA Genetics. In: Laidlaw J, Richens A, Oxley J (eds) A textbook of epilepsy. Edinburgh: Churchill Livingstone, 1988: 49–77.

Rivas ML. Genetic analysis of petit mal epilepsy. I. Evaluation of HLA, blood groups, serum proteins and red cell enzymes. Epilepsia 1983; 24: 115.

Rosenberg RN. Recombinant DNA and neurological disease. The coming of a new age. Neurology 1983; 33: 622–5.

Schofield PR, Darlison MG, Fugita N et al. Sequence and functional expression of the GABA a receptor shows a ligand-gated receptor super family. Nature 1987; 328: 221–7.

Seyfried TN, Glaser GH. A review of mouse mutants as genetic models of epilepsy. Epilepsia 1985; 26: 143–50.

Smith HO, Wilcox KW. A restriction enzyme from *Haemophilus influenzae*. I. Purification and general properties. J Mol Biol 1970; 51: 379–91.

Tsuboi T, Christian W. On the genetics of the primary generalized epilepsy with sporadic myoclonias of the impulsive petit mal type: a clinical and electroencephalographic study of 399 probands. Humangenetik 1973; 19: 155–82.

Tsuboi T, Okada S. The genetics of epilepsy. In: Saki T, Tsuboi T (eds) Genetic aspects of human behaviour. Tokyo: Igaku-Shoin, 1985: 113–27.

Watson JD, Crick FHC. Molecular structure of nucleic acids—a structure for deoxyribose nucleic acid. Nature 1953; 171: 737–8.

White R, Skolnick M. DNA sequence polymorphism and the genetics of epilepsy. In: Anderson VE, Hauser WA, Penry JK, Sing CF (eds) Genetic basis of the epilepsies. New York: Raven Press, 1982: 311–16.

White R, Leppert M, Bishop DT et al. Construction of linkage maps with DNA markers for human chromosomes. Nature 1985; 313: 101–5.

Index

Absence seizures
  in children, 76–78
  classification, 45–46, 216–17
  genetic factors in, 244–5
  myoclonic, 80
  prognosis, 31
  therapy, 153
Accident risk assessment, 23
ACTH for infantile spasms, 155
Aetiology of epilepsy
  in children, 156–7
  in developing countries, 217–19
  as perceived by population, 224–6
Aggression, 137
  following temporal lobe resection, 196–7
Amino acid
  antagonists, excitatory, antiepileptic activity of, 8
  systems abnormalities, excitatory, 5–8
Amnesia, post-traumatic, 88
Amygdalo-hippocampectomy, 197–8
  advantages, 48
Amygdalotomy, 201
Anticonvulsants, *see* Antiepileptics
Antiepileptics
  for absence seizures, 153
  adjunctive therapy in resistant epilepsy, 165–76
  for children, 157–9
  choice, monitoring of epilepsy and, 45–46
  cognitive impairment and, 106-7
  compliance in developing countries, 231
  costs, 232, 235
  effect on prognosis, 26–27
  for infantile spasms, 154–5
  lack of energy and, 124
  for Lennox–Gastaut syndrome, 155
  polytherapy, 158–9
  prescribing strategy, 143–6, 233–4

  racial and genetic effects on metabolism, 236
  resistance to, 27–33
  response failure, 16–17
  sexual drive and, 125
  for single seizures, 18
  supply problems, 231–2, 234
  tolerance avoidance strategies, 183–7
  for tonic–clonic seizures, 153
  for traumatic epilepsy, 94–99
  withdrawal, 146–8, 158
  see also specific drugs
Anxiety in epileptics, 122
Aspartate transaminase metabolism abnormalities, 6–7
Attacks, *see* Seizures
Auditory learning deficit following temporal lobe resection, 196

Behaviour problems
  in children, 160–1
  following temporal lobe resection, 196
  with seizures, 133–41
Benzodiazepines
  for infantile spasms, 155
  tolerance avoidance strategies, 183–7
Bimanual–bipedal seizures, 42–43
Biotinidase deficiency, 157
Blitz–Nick–Salaam–Krampfe syndrome, *see* West syndrome
Brain, *see* Cerebral
Bullet injuries to head, epilepsy following, 91–92

Callosotomy, 201
Candidate gene markers, 248
Carbamazepine
  cognitive impairment and, 106
  combination therapy, 166–8, 174
  for traumatic epilepsy, 96–97, 98
  withdrawal, 147
Cardiac dysrhythmias diagnosis, 37–38

Carotid amytal test, 49
Centro-parietal resection, 198–9
Cerebellar changes, 2
  stimulation, 202
Cerebral
  abnormalities, developmental, 156
  blood flow measurement, 66–70
  damage, epilepsy and, 104
  disease, epilepsy and, 219
  lesions, drug resistance in, 28–29
  metabolic rate measurement, 66–70
  stimulation, 202
Ceroid lipofuscinosis
  juvenile, 81
  neuronal, 157
Cherry red spot myoclonus syndrome, 81
Children and chronic epilepsy, 73–85
  diagnosis in, 152–9
  educational achievement in, 118
  management of epilepsy in, 151–64
  neuropsychiatric study in, 107
Chromosomal abnormalities, 3
Classification
  of epilepsy, 216–17
  of seizure type, 45–46
  of seizures in children, 74–76
Clinical evaluation preoperatively, 47–48
Clinics for epileptics in developing
    countries, 232
Clobazam therapy
  cognitive impairment and, 106
  combination, 168–75
  effect on benzodiazepine tolerance,
    183, 186–7
  indications, 153
  interactions 173
  response factors, 177–82
  tolerance, 181
Clonazepam, cognitive impairment and,
    106
Cloning, genetic, 249
Clorazepate withdrawal, 184
Cognitive impairment
  following temporal lobe resection,
    196
  in epilepsy, 103–11
Compliance
  in children, 159
  related to response, 16
Contagion, fear of, 226
Convulsive status epilepticus frequency,
    29

Corpus callosotomy in children, 160
Corpus callosum section, 201
Cortical degeneration, 2
CT scans
  in children, 157
  in developing countries, 218
  in drug-resistant epilepsy, 60–66
    preoperatively, 49
  preoperative, 191

Dementia, epilepsy and, 107–10
Dependence problems, 126–7
Depression, 138
Depth recording in EEG, 50–54
N-Desmethylclobazam serum levels,
    170–1, 174
Developing countries, epilepsy in, 210–
    41
Diagnosis in children, 152–9
Differential diagnosis of epilepsy, 37–45
Disability perception by doctor, 25–26
  by patient, 22
  by society, 22–25
Disconnection procedures, 201–2
DNA markers, 247–9
cDNA libraries, 250
Drugs, see Antiepileptics
Dysplasia, epilepsy and, 2–3

ECG monitoring in epilepsy, 38
Educational standards, epilepsy and, 118
EEG
  in childhood epileptic syndromes, 78–
    82
  for epileptic risk assessment following
    head injury, 92–93
  monitoring of epilepsy, 38–55
  in children, 74
  preoperative, 192
Employment problems, 116–20
Encephalitis, Rasmussen's, 200
Encephalopathy, early myoclonic, 80
Epidemiology of epilepsy
  in children, 73
  in developing countries, 210–16
Epileptic
  character, period of, 134
  deterioration, period of, 133–4
  syndromes in children, 76–78, 154–6
Epilepticus focus resection, 160
Epileptogenesis, secondary, 189–90
Eye movement monitoring, 55

Index

Family life, 124–5
Febrile convulsions prognosis, 32
Fictitious epilepsy, 152
Financial problems, 125
Flumazenil effect on benzodiazepine tolerance, 184
Focal
  cells, secondary firing of, 189–90
  epilepsy, behavioural problems with, 135
  following trauma, 94
  genetic factors in, 245
  prognosis, 29, 31–32
Folate levels following antiepileptics, 109–10
Foramen ovale electrode use, 44–45, 50
Frontal lobe resection, 198

GABA
  levels in epilepsy, 248
  subsensitivity, 183–4
GABAergic neuronal loss, inhibitory, 2, 4–5
Gaucher's disease, juvenile, 81
Generalized epilepsy
  behavioural problems with, 135
  classification, 75–76
  genetic factors, 244
  therapy, 160–70
Genetics, epilepsy and, 243–53
Geschwind syndrome, 136
Glioma, CT scan for, 60–62
Glutamate dehydrogenase metabolism abnormalities, 6–7
Glutamic acid decarboxylase decrease, 4–5
Grand mal seizures
  genetic factors in, 245
  prognosis, 30

Haematomas
  intracranial, epilepsy following, 92
  post-traumatic, epilepsy and, 89
Hamartomas, 3
Healers, epilepsy and, 227–8
Hemispherectomy, 199–200
  in children, 160
Herbs for epilepsy therapy, 227
Hereditary factor evidence, 244–6
Hippocampal
  removal, 194–7
  sclerosis, unilateral, 2

HLA system, epilepsy and, 249
Housing for epileptics, 126–7
Hybridization, in situ, 250
Hydatid disease, epilepsy and, 218
Hypergraphia, 136–7

Incidence of epilepsy in developing countries, 210–14
Infantile spasms, see West's syndrome
Infectious diseases, epilepsy and, 218
Ionic transport defects, 4

Janz's syndrome, see Myoclonic epilepsy, juvenile
Juvenile myoclonic epilepsy, see Myoclonic epilepsy, juvenile

Kainate receptor abnormalities, 7–8
Ketogenic diet for children, 155
Kindling, 190
  model, 5–6, 19
Kluver–Bucy syndrome, 135, 137
Kojewnikow's syndrome, 82

Lafora body disease, 81
Lesiure activities study, 121–4
Lennox–Gastaut syndrome, 79–80
  in children, 79
  PET in, 68
  prognosis, 29, 31
  therapy, 155
Linkage analysis, 246–7
Lobectomy
  frontal, 198
  results, 145
  temporal, 194–8
Lobotomy, temporal, 202
Localization-related syndromes, 76–78

Manpower against epilepsy in developing countries, 228–9
Markers for epilepsy, 247
Medical assessment criteria, 25–26
Membrane function abnormality, 3–14
Metabolic disorders causing epilepsy in children, 157
N-Methyl-D-aspartate receptor system changes, 5–6
Microdysgenesis, 3
Minnesota Multi-Phasic Personality Inventory, 136
Monitoring of chronic epilepsy, 37–57

Mortality following temporal lobe resection, 196
MRI scans, preoperative, 49, 63–64, 191
Munchausen's syndrome by proxy in children, 152
Myoclonic
  encephalopathy, early, 80
  epilepsy
    absence, 80
    astatic, *see* Lennox–Gastaut syndrome
    juvenile, 78
      genetic factors in, 244–5
      prognosis, 31
      severe, 80
      therapy, 155–6
    progressive, 81
    therapy, 153

Neonatal
  familial convulsions, benign, genetic factors in, 246
  seizures, 81
Neurologist availability in developing countries, 229–30
Neuronal dysgenesis, 3
Neurophysiological examination preoperatively, 192
Neuropsychological assessment preoperatively, 49, 191
Normality, period of, 134

Occipital resection, 198–9
Occupational
  hazards in epilepsy, 222–3
  assessment, 22–25
  problems, 116–20, 161

Pallidal lesions, stereotactic, 200
Parental attitudes to epilepsy, 152, 160–1
Paroxysmal episodes in children, 152
Partial epilepsy
  benign, in children, 154
  classification, 75, 217
  monitoring, 38, *39–36, 51–53*
  PET in, 68–70
  therapy, 169–70, *171*
Pathophysiology of chronic epilepsy, 1–11
Patient's perception of disease, 22
Perinatal care, epilepsy and, 218

Personality changes, 136
PET scans
  in drug-resistant epilepsy, 66–70
  preoperatively, 49
Petit mal, impulsive, *see* Myoclonic epilepsy, juvenile
Phenobarbitone
  cognitive impairment and, 109
  costs, 232, 233
  hazards, 232–3
  indications, 153
  for traumatic epilepsy, 94–96, 98
  withdrawal, 232
Phenotypic markers, 247
Phenytoin
  cognitive impairment and, 106, 109
  combination therapy, 174
  costs, 232
  for traumatic epilepsy, 94–96, 98
  withdrawal, 147
Phosphorylation mechanism defects, 4
Photosensitive epilepsy, 54–55
Prejudice against epilepsy, 119–20
  in developing countries, 222–4
Preoperative assessment, 46–54
Prevalence rates of chronic epilepsy, 14–15
  in developing countries, 210–16
Primidone combination therapy, 166–8
Prognosis of chronic epilepsy, 13–20
  in childhood, 83
  determination, 154
  following treatment, 26–27
  in symptomatic epilepsy, 28
  in traumatic epilepsy, 87–94
Prophylaxis in traumatic epilepsy, 94–99
Pseudoseizures
  diagnosis, 37–45
  in children, 152
Psychomotor peculiarity, period of, 134–5
Psychosis, 138–9
  following temporal lobe resection, 197
Psychosocial management in children, 160–1
Pyknolepsy prognosis, 29, 31
Pyridoxine dependency, 157

Quinolinic acid abnormality, 7

Rasmussen's encephalitis, 200

Index

Reading epilepsy, primary, genetic aspects in, 245–6
Reflex seizures detection, 54–55
Remission
  in children, 73–74
  following treatment, 26–27
  spontaneous, 15–16
  in structural lesions, 28–29
  in trauma-induced epilepsy, 28
Resistant epilepsy
  adjunctive therapy in, 165–70
  clobazam therapy for, 177–80
  scans in, 60–70
Restriction fragment length polymorphisms, 247, 248–9
mRNA levels, 250–1
Rolandic epilepsy, genetic factors in, 245

Schistosomiasis, epilepsy and, 218
Schizophrenic symptoms, 138–9
Schneiderian first-rank symptoms, 139
Screening questionnaires, 211–12
See-ee, epilepsy and, 219
Seizures
  classification, 45–46
  in children, 74–76
  control following temporal lobe resection, 195
  following surgery, 198–200
  following trauma
    early, 87–90, 99
    late, 90–94, 99
  frequency, determination of, 46
  in developing countries, 219–21
  timing of, 22
  type characteristics in developing countries, 216–17
    determination in children, 153–4
  drug resistance and, 29–30
  variables, cognitive impairment and, 104–5
  see also specific types of seizures
Self-induced seizure detection, 54–55
Severity assessment, 21–36
Sexual problems, 125
Sheltered employment, 120
  housing, 126–7
Single seizures, prognosis of, 18
Sleep
  epilepsy, traumatic, 93–94
  slow wave, continuous spike waves in, 81

Social
  assessment of epileptics, 114–29
  disability perception, 22–25
Sociocultural aspects of epilepsy in developing countries, 221–6
Sodium valproate
  combination therapy, 166–8
  withdrawal, 147
Sporting activity in epilepsy, 122–3
Stereotactic lesions, 200–1
Stigma attached to epilepsy, 221–4
Sturge–Weber disease, surgery in, 160
Subdural recording in EEG, 50–54
Subjective handicap perception, 22
Subpial transection, multiple, 202
Suicide following temporal lobe resection, 196
Supersensitivity development, 2
Surgery for chronic epilepsy, 189–207
  in children, 159–60
Syncope diagnosis, 37

Temporal
  lesions, stereotactic, 200–1
  lobe abnormalities, 135–6, 139
    resection, 193, 194–8
      deep structure removal, 197–8
      neocortical and deep structure removal, 194–7
      neocortical removal, 194
      scarring detection, 191
    lobectomy results, 145
    lobotomy, 202
    sclerosis, mesial, detection of, 191
Therapy, *see* Antiepileptics; Surgery; Treatment
Tonic seizures therapy, 153
Tonic–clonic seizures
  classification, 217
  criteria for definition, 213
  genetic factors in, 245
  prognosis, 29
  therapy, 153
Traumatic epilepsy
  prognosis, 28, 87–94
  prophylaxis, 94–99
Treatment
  of epilepsy in developing countries, 227–36
  gap, 234–6
Tumours causing epilepsy in childhood, 156–7

Unconsciousness, seizures following, 88

Valproic acid
  indications, 153
  for infantile spasms, 155
  metabolism, 158
  for traumatic epilepsy, 98
Vascular abnormalities, 2–3
Verbal memory deficit prevention, 194

Wada test, 191
West syndrome in children, 78–79
  prognosis, 29, 31
  therapy, 154–5
Witchcraft as cause of epilepsy, 224–6

Xenon-enhanced CT scans, 64–65, 67

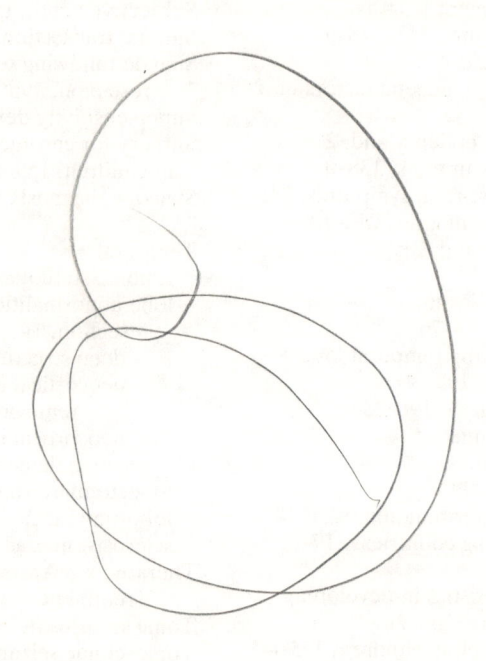